NEUROLOGIC EMERGENCIES

3RD EDITION

NEUROLOGIC EMERGENCIES

GREGORY L. HENRY, MD
Clinical Professor of Emergency Medicine
The University of Michigan Medical School
Ann Arbor, Michigan

NEAL LITTLE, MD
Clinical Professor of Emergency Medicine
The University of Michigan Medical School
Ann Arbor, Michigan

ANDREW JAGODA, MD
Professor of Emergency Medicine
Mount Sinai School of Medicine
New York, New York

THOMAS R. PELLEGRINO, MD
Professor
Department of Neurology
Eastern Virginia Medical School
Norfolk, Virginia

DOUGLAS J. QUINT, MD
Professor of Neuroradiology and MRI
The University of Michigan Medical School
Ann Arbor, Michigan

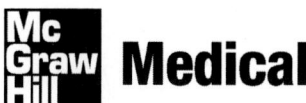

New York   Chicago   San Francisco   Lisbon   London   Madrid
Mexico City   Milan   New Delhi   San Juan   Seoul   Singapore
Sydney   Toronto

The McGraw·Hill Companies

Neurologic Emergencies
Copyright © 2010, 2003, 1985 by The McGraw-Hill Companies, Inc. All rights reserved. Printed in the United States of America. Except as permitted under the United States Copyright Act of 1976, no part of this publication may be reproduced or distributed in any form or by any means, or stored in a database or retrieval system, without the prior written permission of the publisher.

1 2 3 4 5 6 7 8 9 0 WDQ WDQ 14 13 12 11 10

ISBN 978-0-07-163521-9
MHID 0-07-163521-1

This book was set in Times Roman by Aptara, Inc.
The editors were Anne M. Sydor and Karen Davis.
The production supervisor was Sherri Souffrance.
Production management was provided by Indu Jawwad, Aptara, Inc.
The interior text designer was Marsha Cohen/Parallelogram.
The index was prepared by Aptara, Inc.
Worldcolor was printer and binder.

This book is printed on acid-free paper.

Library of Congress Cataloging-in-Publication Data
Neurologic emergencies / Gregory L. Henry . . . [et al.]. — 3rd ed.
    p. ; cm.
    Includes bibliographical references and index.
    Summary: "This book gives a logical approach to rapid investigation and treatment for neurologic emergencies"—Provided by publisher.
    ISBN-13: 978-0-07-163521-9 (hardcover: alk. paper)
    ISBN-10: 0-07-163521-1 (hardcover: alk. paper)   1. Neurologic emergencies.   I. Henry, Gregory L.
    [DNLM: 1. Nervous System Diseases—diagnosis.   2. Diagnosis, Differential.   3. Emergencies.   4. Evidence-Based Medicine. WL 141 N48373 2010]
    RC350.7.H398 2010
    616.8′0425—dc22
                                                            2009047855

McGraw-Hill books are available at special quantity discounts to use as premiums and sales promotions, or for use in corporate training programs. To contact a representative please visit the Contact Us pages at www.mhprofessional.com.

CONTENTS

We are pleased to offer the third edition of our textbook *Neurologic Emergencies.* It has been both an exciting challenge and a privilege to update and improve upon the core concepts presented in the first and second editions. We believe that organizing our book around the ways in which patients present continues to be a useful and productive approach. Patients usually present with complaints and findings, not with diagnoses, and the great challenge in neurologic emergencies, as in all others, is to quickly synthesize those presenting problems utilizing an organized diagnostic approach.

Since the book's first edition in 1985, there have been significant changes in health care. Acute care providers have assumed a leading role in the diagnosis and management of neurologic and neurosurgical emergencies, and time-dependent therapies have made the expedited, systematic evaluation of patients with neurologic complaints a fundamental competency. Coordinated research networks are providing quality evidence to assist clinical decision-making and treatment interventions. Most important, the role of prehospital and emergency care has been recognized as essential to maximizing patient outcomes in many acute neurologic processes.

Although the organization of the nervous system and the most common disorders that affect it have not changed over time, our approach to initial diagnosis and management continues to evolve. In particular, diagnostic imaging continues to become increasingly more sophisticated. Consequently, we have asked Dr. Douglas Quint, a neuroradiologist at the University of Michigan, to provide a primer on neuroimaging technologies and to ensure consistency throughout the book on the appropriate utilization of neuroimaging.

We have tried to strike a balance between readability and completeness. We have systematically reviewed the literature and this edition of the book has been updated applying the best available evidence. The challenge here, as in all of medicine, is what to do when no or little evidence exists. In these cases we have drawn on our more than 100 years of combined clinical experience managing patients with neurologic complaints. In the absence of good evidence, each author recognizes that the strategies discussed simply represent one way of approaching a given problem and should be interpreted in that context; others may favor different approaches. This is one aspect of the text that makes it particularly appealing to have it available as an online version linked to other texts and literature references that may address similar issues from a different perspective, or in different contexts.

This book represents one starting point, while laying the foundation for others. Good neurologic outcomes are dependent on a coordinated continuum of care that promotes effective resource utilization and communication between health care providers; this book is designed to facilitate both. A growing body of evidence supports the benefit of acute interventions in many neurologic emergencies. It is anticipated that the field of neurologic emergencies will continue to evolve with new diagnostic tools and treatment options, placing increasing attention on early recognition and management. Due to the time-dependent nature of many acute interventions in neurologic emergencies, it is almost certain that the role played by the acute care provider will become increasingly more critical. The authors hope that the framework we have provided here will promote the focused evaluations needed in order to assure the best outcomes possible for patients presenting with neurologic emergencies.

1

A REVIEW OF ESSENTIAL CLINICAL NEUROANATOMY

The charm of neurology, above all other branches of practical medicine, lies in the way it forces us into daily contact with principles. A knowledge of the structure and functions of the nervous system is necessary to explain the simplest phenomena of disease; this can be only obtained by thinking scientifically.

—Sir Henry Head

Neuroanatomy is frequently considered by medical students to be one of the least enjoyable and most technically intricate disciplines that they must study. The amount of neuroanatomy necessary to practice good clinical emergency medicine, however, is limited. Basic principles apply to each of the various nervous system modalities that can be tested. Mastery of these simple principles and a fundamental understanding of the overall organization of the nervous system allows for accurate localization of disease entities. This chapter attempts to review the basic anatomic concepts necessary to evaluate the historical and physical findings most often seen with acute neurologic problems. This addition of the text will take a more modern approach. Advances in imaging techniques including, but not limited to, MRI, MRA, CT, CTA, perfusion CT, etc., have brought us to a clearer understanding of structure and function. The chapter on neuroimaging (Chapter 2) will reiterate many concepts from this anatomic discussion.

BASIC ORGANIZATION OF THE NERVOUS SYSTEM

The human nervous system is composed of carefully integrated units that are involved with informing the organism about what is happening within the body and the world around it. The nervous system processes the information and sends out signals to various end organs to adjust to internal and external environmental changes. All changes in

1

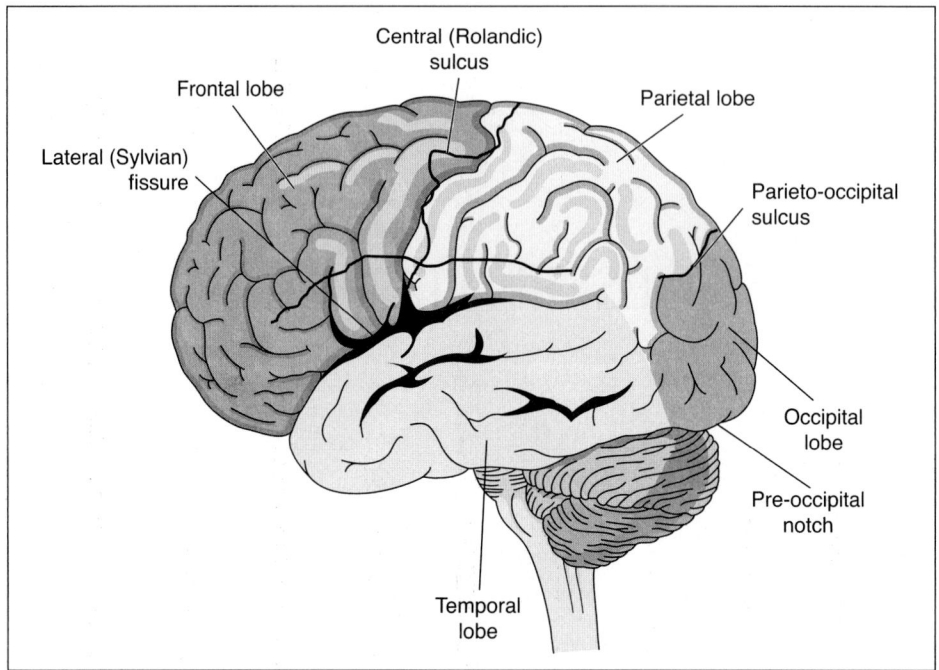

FIGURE 1-1 Lateral view of the brain showing the four lobes (frontal, parietal, temporal, occipital) and the cerebellum.

autonomic function, position, and response to the external world are neurologic events. We test the nervous system in everyone we meet every day.

The central nervous system consists of the brain and the spinal cord. It is completely encased within the skull and spinal column, thereby having osseous protection for its vital structures. The major areas of the brain include the cerebral cortex, subcortical structures, brainstem, and cerebellum (Fig. 1-1).[1–3] The cerebral hemispheres are separated by the medial longitudinal fissure (where the falx cerebri is located) but are connected at their base by the corpus callosum, which provides a pathway that allows the two halves of the cerebrum to communicate with each other. Both the right and left cortex are further subdivided into four lobes. The frontal lobe is the most anterior and largest of the lobes. Although anatomically the right and left frontal lobes appear the same, they have distinctly different functions. In nearly all right-handed individuals and in at least 50% of left-handed individuals, left-hemisphere dominance provides that the areas for initiation of speech and language lie in the frontal lobe on the left side of the brain.[4]

Lying immediately adjacent to and posterior to the frontal lobes are the parietal lobes. Parietal lobes form a principal receiving area for sensory information as well as information from other parts of the body. The parietal lobes are particularly involved in recognition of self with regard to body image and position. Spatial orientation and three-dimensional understanding of objects are parietal lobe functions. The occipital lobes occupy the most posterior portion of the cerebral hemispheres. In the occipital lobes, the visual system terminates and visual impulses come to cognition.[4]

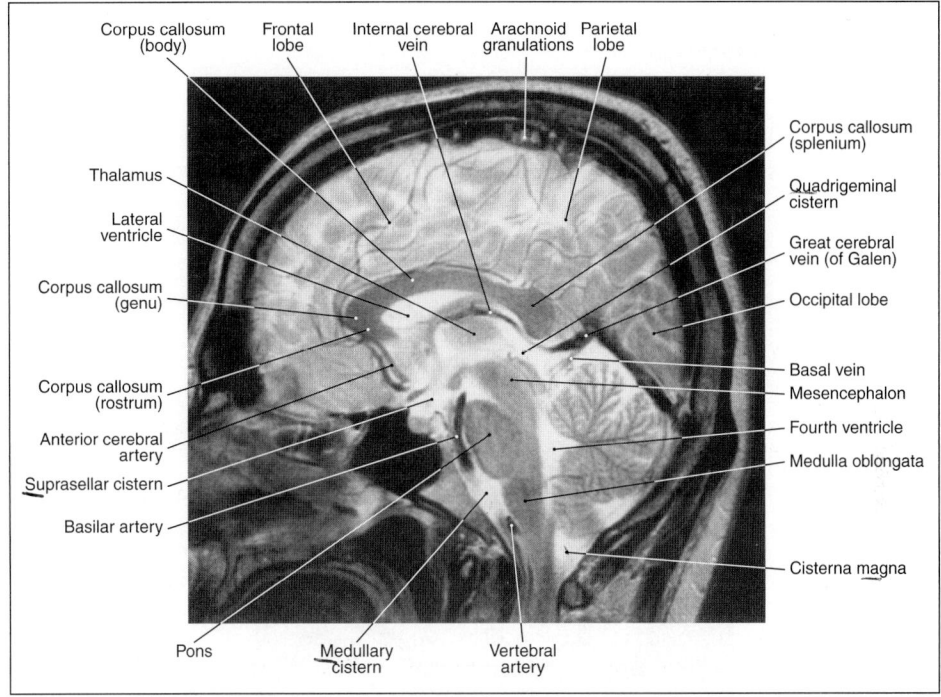

Corpus callosum (body) — Frontal lobe — Internal cerebral vein — Arachnoid granulations — Parietal lobe

Thalamus

Lateral ventricle

Corpus callosum (genu)

Corpus callosum (rostrum)

Anterior cerebral artery

Suprasellar cistern

Basilar artery

Corpus callosum (splenium)

Quadrigeminal cistern

Great cerebral vein (of Galen)

Occipital lobe

Basal vein

Mesencephalon

Fourth ventricle

Medulla oblongata

Cisterna magna

Pons — Medullary cistern — Vertebral artery

FIGURE 1-2 **T2-weighted MRI of the brain in midsagittal cut. In this T2 sequence, cerebrospinal fluid spaces appear white, while brain substance is in shades of gray.** (Reproduced with permission from Afifi A, Bergman R. *Functional Neuroanatomy.* 2nd ed. New York: McGraw-Hill; 2005.)

Moving inwardly from the cortex are deeper structures: the basal ganglia and the thalamus (Figs. 1-2 and 1-3). The basal ganglia are a group of nuclei that lie between the cortex and the internal capsule. The various elements of the basal ganglia constitute the extrapyramidal tracts, which help to control motor movements.

The thalami are located just lateral to the third ventricle bilaterally and form the core of the brain. The nuclei of the thalamus perform a variety of functions, including monitoring homeostasis and relaying information to specific cortical areas.

The hypothalamic nuclei, which are located just inferior to the thalami and form the floor and part of the inferior ventrolateral walls of the third ventricle, also form part of the roof of the suprasellar cistern and are therefore located just above the optic chiasm. They are also connected both structurally (through the pituitary stalk) and, also through the arterial circulation, directly to the pituitary gland.[1,2] Regulation of appetite and body temperature are strongly influenced by the hypothalamic nuclei. The parasympathetic autonomic nervous system receives substantial input from the hypothalamus. Stimulation of the rostral portions of the hypothalamus, on the other hand, causes excitation of the sympathetic system.

The thalami, which make up the dorsal portion of the diencephalon, serve as the principal relay station for impulses of all types sent to the cerebral cortex. Many impulses come to cognition at the level of the thalamus, although precise localization and integration of this material requires cortical interpretation.

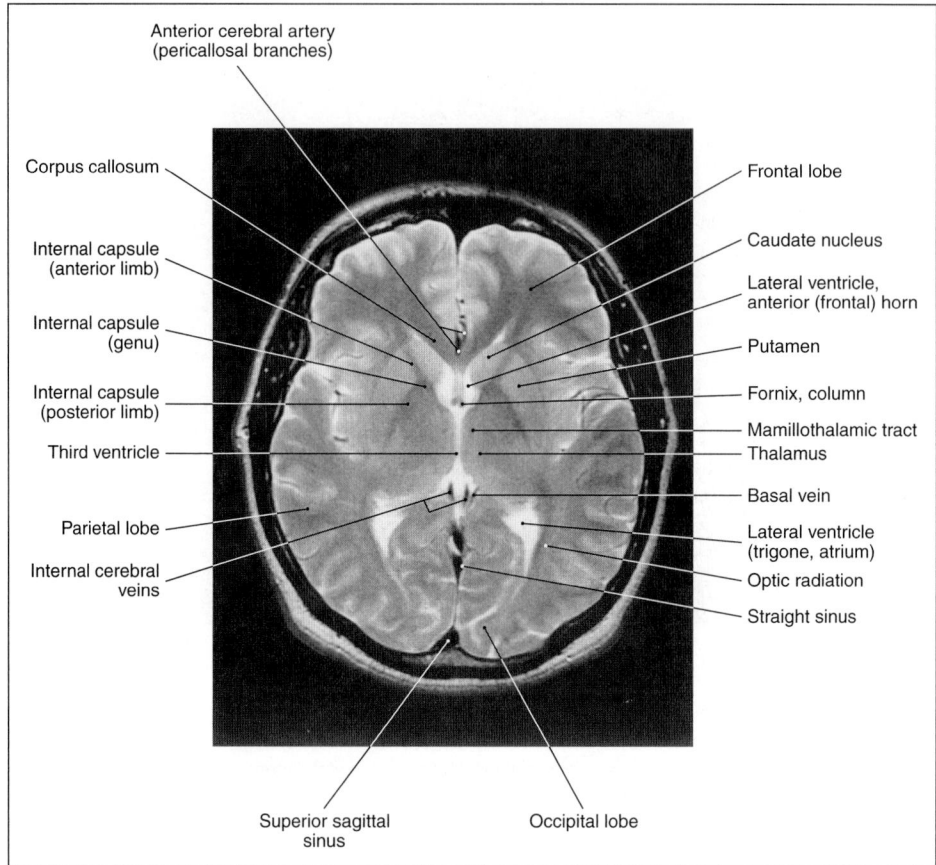

FIGURE 1-3   **T2-weighted axial MRI through the thalamus.**   (Reproduced with permission from Afifi A, Bergman R. *Functional Neuroanatomy.* 2nd ed. New York: McGraw-Hill; 2005.)

The space within the skull is divided into three fossae: the anterior, middle, and posterior cranial fossae. The cerebral cortex, the subcortex, the basal ganglia, and the majority of the thalamic structures are considered to be anterior and middle cranial fossae elements. Lying below the tentorium cerebelli is the posterior fossa, where the cerebellum and most of the brainstem are located. The brainstem is composed of the midbrain, pons, and medulla. These distinct anatomic regions are interconnected with multiple tracts, making their physiologic function an interrelated process (Fig. 1-4). Cranial nerves III through XII are outgrowths of the brainstem, and their nuclei are located within these regions. The brainstem also functions as a conduit for carrying information down to the spinal cord and transmitting information cephalad from the spinal cord to the nuclei in the thalamus.[1,2]

The brainstem proceeds caudally to become the spinal cord at the craniovertebral junction. The spinal cord runs from the medulla (cervicomedullary junction) to its termination as the conus medullaris in the upper lumbar region. Although literally dozens of tracts have been identified in the spinal cord (Fig. 1-5), only three are of major importance for emergency medicine and clinical purposes.[4] These tracts include the dorsal

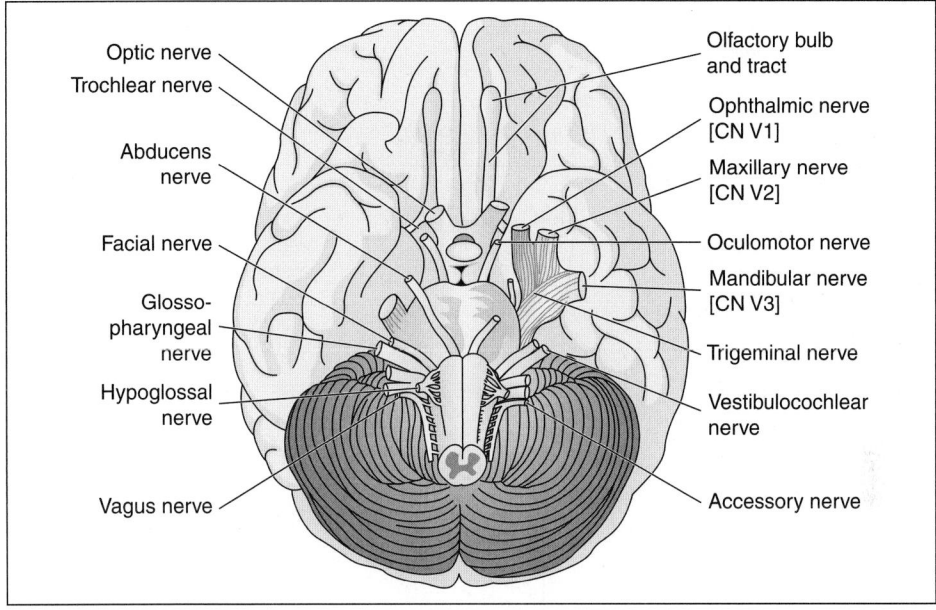

FIGURE 1-4   Ventral view of the brain showing the cranial nerves.

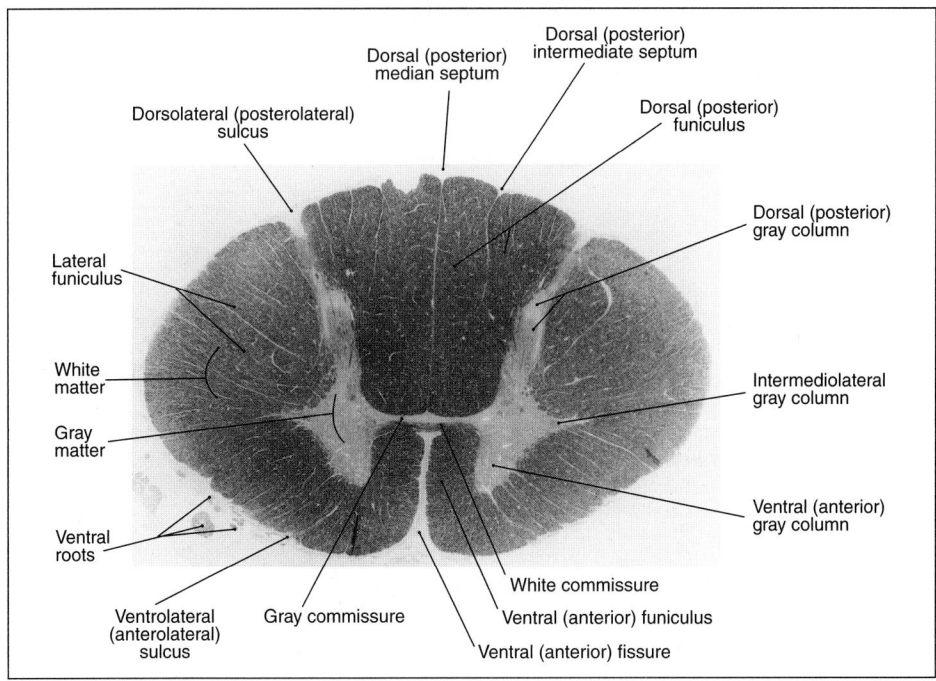

FIGURE 1-5   Photomicrograph of spinal cord showing division into gray and white matter, the sulci and fissures, gray matter columns, and white matter funiculi.   (Reproduced with permission from Afifi A, Bergman R. *Functional Neuroanatomy*. 2nd ed. New York: McGraw-Hill; 2005.)

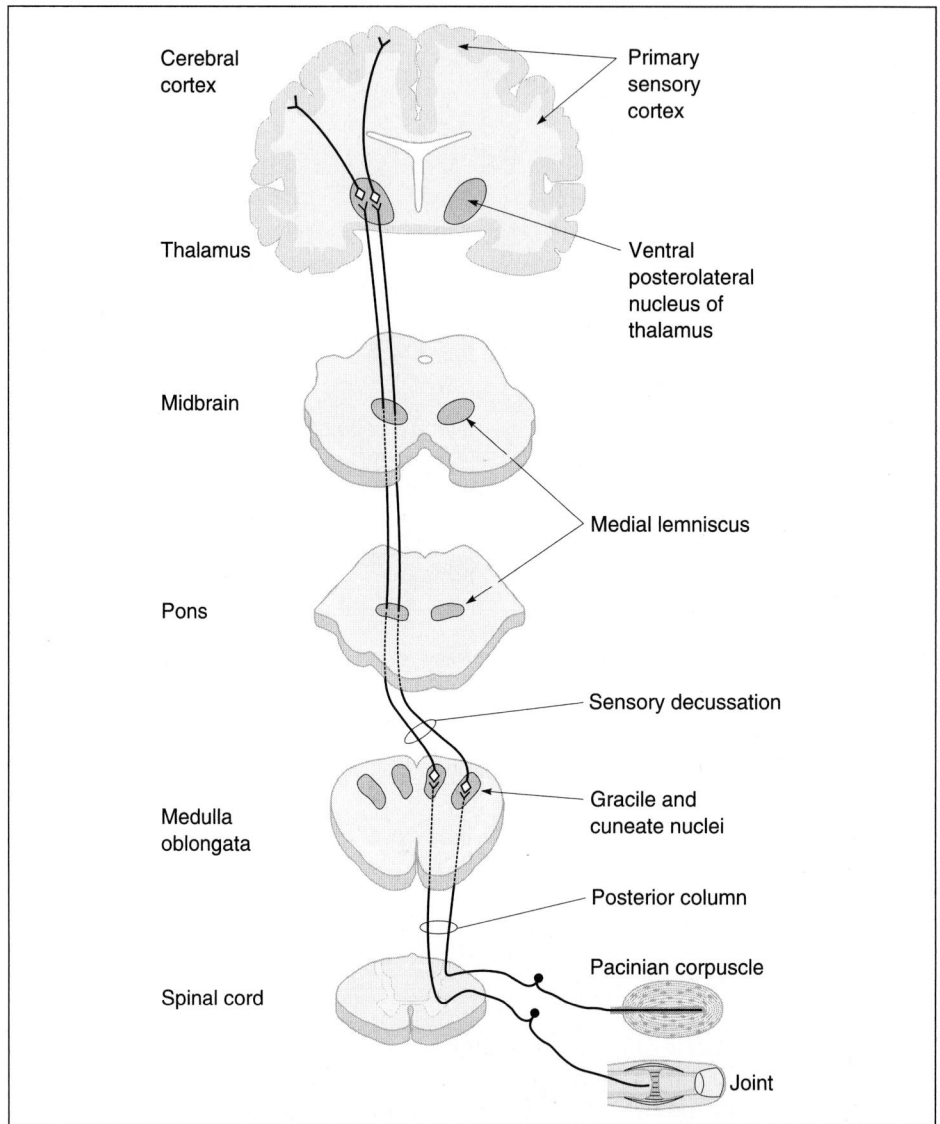

FIGURE 1-6 **Schematic diagram of the posterior column pathway.** (Reproduced with permission from Afifi A, Bergman R. *Functional Neuroanatomy*. 2nd ed. New York: McGraw-Hill; 2005.)

columns, the descending motor pathways, and the ascending lateral spinothalamic tracts. The dorsal columns carry vibration and position sense from the spinal cord to the brainstem, where the tracts cross (in the lower medulla) and ascend to the thalamus and eventually to the sensory cortex (Fig. 1-6).[3,4] The axons of the lateral spinothalamic tracts cross immediately after entering the spinal cord, ascend directly to the contralateral (from side of entrance) thalamus, and are then projected to the cerebral cortex. The lateral spinothalamic tracts carry pain and temperature sensation. The lateral corticospinal tract, or descending motor pathway, arises in the cerebral hemisphere, crosses to the opposite

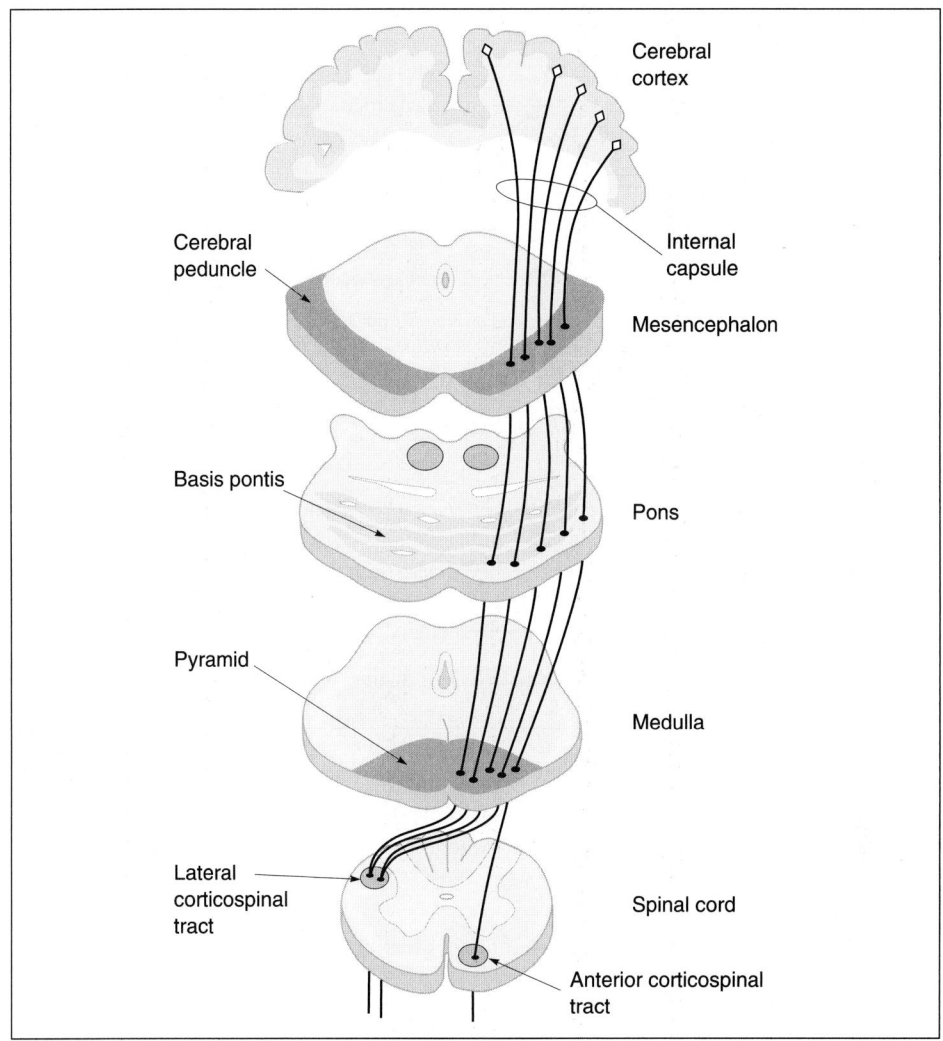

FIGURE 1-7 **Schematic diagram of the corticospinal pathway.**   (Reproduced with permission from Afifi A, Bergman R. *Functional Neuroanatomy*. 2nd ed. New York: McGraw-Hill; 2005.)

side in the medulla, carries motor information caudad in the spinal cord, and then connects to the anterior horn cells whose axons then connect to the muscles through the peripheral nerves (Fig. 1-7).[4] There are moderate variations of the spinal cord at its various levels, but the relationship of the tracts remains fundamentally the same (Fig. 1-8).

Lying in the posterior fossa directly behind the brainstem is the cerebellum. The cerebellum can be thought of as having a central, midline portion (vermis), and larger bilateral hemispheres. Descending cerebellar pathways cross immediately and then recross so that they give their input to the ipsilateral side of the body.[2] The midline cerebellar structures basically control and coordinate musculature involved with axial muscle functioning. The muscles most involved are those controlling the central core of the body with regard to sitting and standing and posturing of the neck and back. The lateral

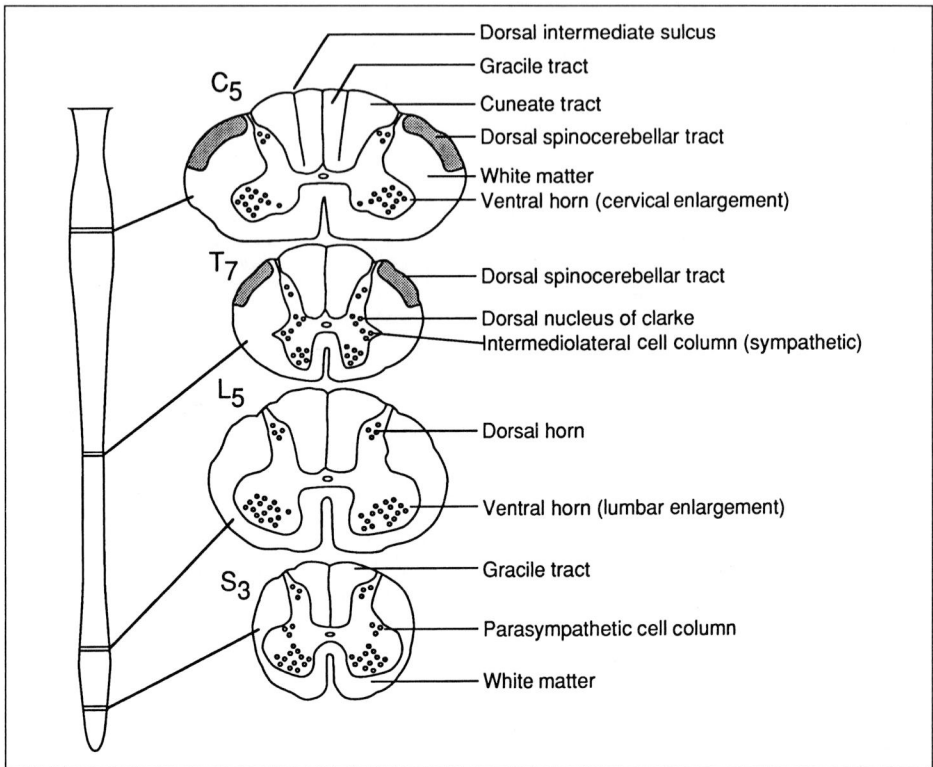

FIGURE 1-8 Schematic diagram showing variations in spinal cord segments at different levels. (Reproduced with permission from Afifi A, Bergman R. *Functional Neuroanatomy*. 2nd ed. New York: McGraw-Hill; 2005.)

flocculonodular cerebellar lobes exert their controlling influences on the finer motor coordination of the extremities (Fig. 1-4).[1,4]

The tissues of the central nervous system are bathed in cerebrospinal fluid (CSF). This fluid, an ultrafiltrate of blood, is produced by the choroid plexus of the lateral ventricles (Fig. 1-9). CSF moves from the lateral ventricles into the third ventricle through the respective foramina of Monro and then through the narrow aqueduct of Sylvius into the fourth ventricle. CSF exits the fourth ventricle through the foramina of Luschka (paired lateral structures that open into the cerebellomedullary cistern) and the midline foramen of Magendie (at the caudal aspect of the fourth ventricle) into the basal cistern and subarachnoid spaces. CSF surrounds the entire brain and spinal cord. CSF absorption is considered to occur at the level of the arachnoid granulations, though that concept is currently being challenged. The normal 70-kg-adult nervous system contains approximately 130 mL of CSF. The normal production of CSF is about 500 mL/d (approximately 1 cm^3 every 3 minutes), or a rate sufficient to replace itself some three to four times over in a 24-hour period.[5,6]

The structures of the nervous system outside the bony protection of the skull and spinal cord constitute the peripheral nervous system. The cranial nerves and spinal nerves with their associated ganglia are the elements of the peripheral nervous system. Cranial nerves vary considerably in the type of fibers they carry. Some fibers are purely motor, such as the ones that innervate the ocular muscles and the IV and VI cranial

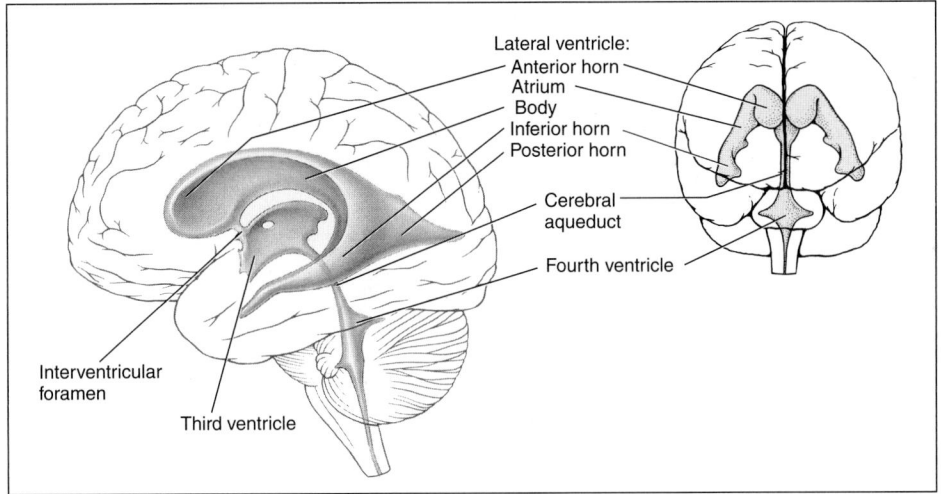

FIGURE 1-9 Ventricular system. The lateral ventricles, third ventricle, cerebral aqueduct, and fourth ventricle are seen from the lateral brain surface (left) and the front (right). The lateral ventricle is divided into four main components: anterior (or frontal) horn, body, inferior (or temporal) horn, and the posterior (or occipital) horn. The interventricular foramen (of Monro) connects each lateral ventricle with the third ventricle. The cerebral aqueduct connects the third and fourth ventricles.   (Reproduced with permission from Martin J. *Neuroanatomy: A Text and Atlas.* 3th ed. New York: McGraw-Hill; 2003.)

nerves. Many, however, have mixed functions, carrying both sensory and motor, and autonomic fibers.

The motor fibers of the peripheral nerves are divided into somatic fibers that terminate in skeletal muscle, and autonomic motor fibers that innervate smooth muscle, cardiac muscle, and various glands. All spinal nerve roots are mixed nerves carrying both motor and sensory elements (Fig. 1-10).

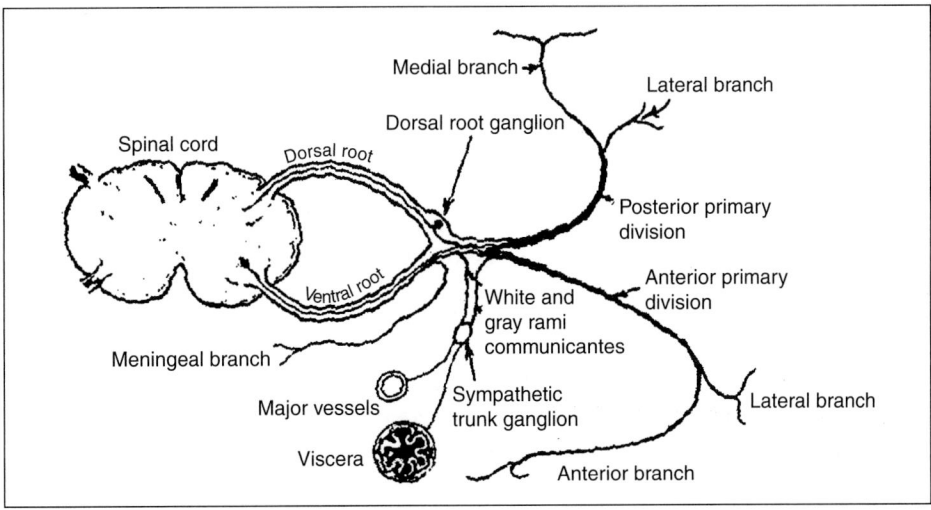

FIGURE 1-10 **Peripheral nerve organization.**   (From Chusid J. *Correlative Neuroanatomy and Functional Neurology.* 14th ed. Los Altos, CA: Lange; 1970:113.)

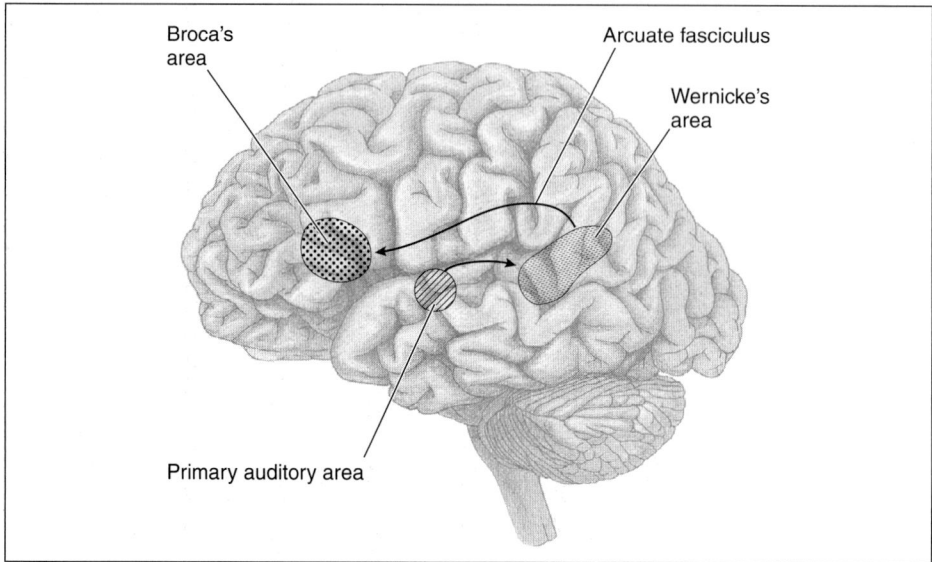

FIGURE 1-11 **Schematic diagram showing transmission of auditory symbols from the primary auditory cortex to Wernicke's area for comprehension, and via the arcuate fasciculus to Broca's area of speech.** (Reproduced with permission from Afifi A, Bergman R. *Functional Neuroanatomy*. 2nd ed. New York: McGraw-Hill; 2005.)

The roots of the peripheral nerves combine in the cervical and lumbosacral regions to form intricate plexi (the brachial and lumbosacral plexi, respectively). These combined nerve bundles then subdivide to form specific peripheral nerves.

Speech

Human verbal output requires careful integration of multiple areas of the nervous system (Fig. 1-11). Language is formulated in the frontal lobes. Specific motor direction proceeds from Broca's area in the frontal lobe. This information is then conveyed through the corticobulbar tracts to the various brainstem nuclei, which innervate the muscles involved in moving the jaw, lips, tongue, and palate to form speech. Careful integration of these movements is provided via input from cerebellar tracts.

The principal areas for receiving, interpreting, and initiating speech are all located around the Sylvian and Rolandic fissure regions. The vascular supply to these areas is principally from branches of the middle cerebral artery. Wernicke's area, which lies in the primary auditory cortex in the posterior temporal lobe, receives speech and performs a monitoring function. It has connections to the angular gyrus of the parietal lobe, which interprets and integrates auditory input and connects it to other areas of the brain for interpretation.

The arcuate fasciculus then connects these posterior speech areas to Broca's area in the motor strip. Although the total integration of speech is complex, there are some useful general concepts.

One has difficulty in testing speech if there is a hearing abnormality. If this is suspected, hearing should be tested to make sure that deafness is not part of the difficulty

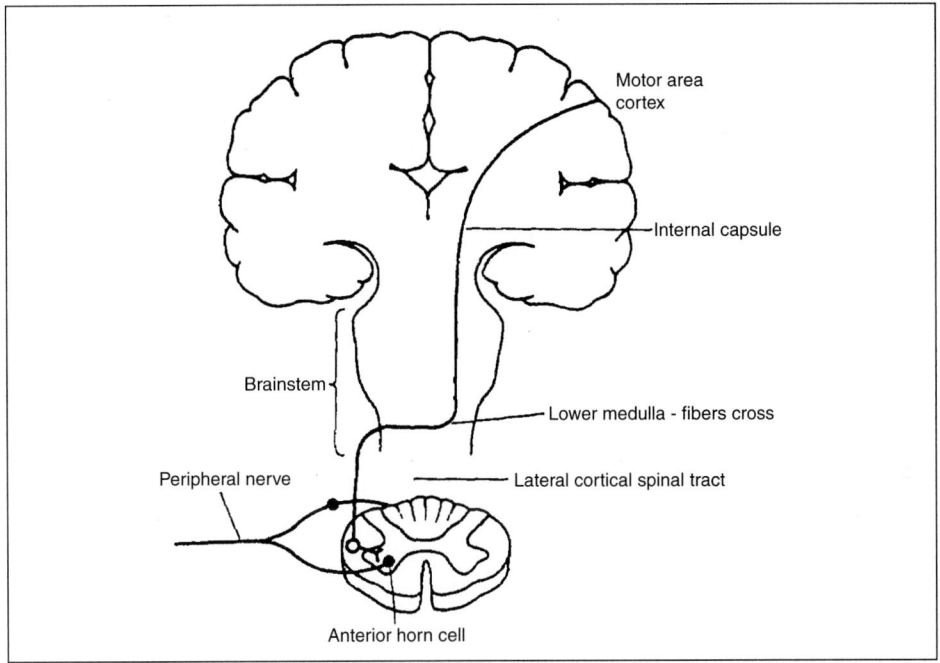

FIGURE 1-12   **Motor system.**

with speech. Basic understanding of speech and the production of speech are dominant hemisphere functions. Problems in understanding speech, translating that understanding into actions, or word finding are all generally lumped under the aphasic/dysphasic syndromes.[7,8]

Motor Pathways

Voluntary motor activity is initiated from the frontal lobes of the cerebral cortex and proceeds through the ipsilateral internal capsule to enter the brainstem (Fig. 1-12). Motor impulses that pass to the various brainstem nuclei travel in the corticobulbar tracts. Motor impulses that arise here, and are to proceed farther down the spinal cord to the rest of the body, travel in the lateral corticospinal tract. Motor impulses for brainstem nuclei basically cross at the level of those nuclei. All other motor impulses for the rest of the body cross at the lower end of the medulla in the area of the motor decussation (Table 1-1).

In the spinal cord, the descending lateral corticospinal tract fibers synapse with anterior horn cell nuclei at appropriate levels.

Motor impulses from these anterior horn cells then exit the spinal cord through the anterior spinal roots to enter the peripheral nerves.[3,4] Finally, motor activity is activated when the peripheral nerve forms a junction with the muscle. The peripheral nerve stimulates this nerve–muscle junction causing skeletal muscle contraction. The cerebellum exerts its influence on the ipsilateral motor tract.[4] The function of the cerebellum is to continuously adjust, coordinate, and refine motor movements in a smooth and integrated pattern (Tables 1-2 and 1-3).[2,9–11]

TABLE 1-1

CROSSINGS IN THE NERVOUS SYSTEM

Pathway	Function	Crosses	Interpretation
Pyramidal tract	Motor	Lower medulla	Lesion below crossing gives ipsilateral signs
Spinothalamic tract	Pain and temperature (body)	On entry to spinal cord	Lesion is always contralateral to pain and temperature loss (except face)
Spinal tract of fifth nerve	Pain and temperature (face)	Midpons (runs throughout medulla)	If lesion is in medulla or lower pons, ipsilateral loss; above midpons, contralateral loss
Dorsal spinal columns	Position and vibration	Lower medulla	Lesion below crossing gives ipsilateral signs
Cerebellar tracts	Coordination of movement	Crosses twice (on entry to cerebellum and in midbrain)	Because of "double crossing" lesions of cerebellum or cerebellar tracts usually produce signs and symptoms ipsilateral to lesion
Gaze fibers	Coordinates lateral gaze	Midpons	
Cranial nerves	Cranial nerves	Just above cranial nerve nuclei	Lesion is ipsilateral when cranial nerve nuclei are involved

Sensory System

Sensory modalities are usually divided into dorsal column functions and lateral spinothalamic tract functions. The dorsal columns receive sensory information (position and vibration) from the dorsal root ganglia of the peripheral nerves (Fig. 1-13). This information then ascends the spinal cord ipsilaterally until it reaches the medulla and the level of the sensory decussation. At the level of the lower medulla, this sensory information crosses and ascends through the medial lemniscus to the thalamus and from the thalamus to the ipsilateral cortex.

Lateral spinothalamic tract modalities, which include pain and temperature, enter the spinal cord through the dorsal root ganglion and immediately cross to the contralateral side of the cord and ascend in the contralateral spinothalamic tract. These fibers then proceed up through the brainstem without further crossing to terminate in the thalamus.[1,3-5]

Facial sensation, which is slightly more complex, is handled through the trigeminal nerve (fifth cranial nerve). Pain and temperature sensation from the face enter the brainstem in the midbrain and form the sensory root of the trigeminal nerve. The fibers then descend through the pons and medulla in the spinal tract of the nerve, cross to the opposite side, and

TABLE 1-2
INNERVATION OF SELECTED MUSCLES OF THE UPPER LIMBS

Muscle	Main Root	Peripheral Nerve	Main Action
Supraspinatus	C5	Suprascapular	Abduction of arm
Infraspinatus	C5	Suprascapular	External rotation of arm at shoulder
Deltoid	C5	Axillary	Abduction of arm
Biceps	C5, C6	Musculocutaneous	Elbow flexion
Brachioradialis	C5, C6	Radial	Elbow flexion
Extensor carpi radialis longus	C6, C7	Radial	Wrist extension
Flexor carpi radialis	C6, C7	Median	Wrist flexion
Extensor carpi ulnaris	C7	Radial	Wrist extension
Extensor digitorum	C7	Radial	Finger extension
Triceps	C8	Radial	Extension of elbow
Flexor carpi ulnaris	C8	Ulnar	Wrist extension
Abductor pollicis brevis	T1	Median	Abduction of thumb
Opponens pollicis	T1	Median	Opposition of thumb
First dorsal interosseous	T1	Ulnar	Abduction of index finger
Abductor digiti minimi	T1	Ulnar	Abduction of little finger

Source: From Simon R, Greenberg D, Aminoff M. *Clinical Neurology.* 7th ed. New York: McGraw-Hill; 2009.

ascend with other pain and temperature fibers of the body.[1,2,12] Lesions in the upper pons will thus affect both facial and body fibers from the same side of the body. Lesions in the lateral part of the medulla or lower pons that damage the spinal tract of the trigeminal nerve and the lateral spinothalamic tract will cause alternating analgesia, that is, loss of pain and temperature on the same side of the face and the opposite side of the body. This alternating analgesia is the hallmark for a brainstem lesion.

Awareness of touch and pain takes place at the level of the thalamus. Precise localization and integration of sensory information requires cortical localization. It is with the aid of cortical centers that precise localization of a stimulus can be made. Intricate sensory tasks such as graphesthesia (recognition of numbers written in the hands) and stereognosis (identification of objects placed in the hands) require extensive cortical evaluation.

Dermatomes are the topographical sensory representation of the various nerve root distributions.

If pathology is at the level of the nerve root before it has a chance to recombine to form a plexus or a specific peripheral nerve, the area of abnormality will reflect the specific nerve root distribution. Cutaneous or peripheral nerve form patterns are based on combinations of multiple nerve roots with various alignments (Fig. 1-14).

TABLE 1-3

INNERVATION OF SELECTED MUSCLES OF THE LOWER LIMBS

Muscle	Main Root	Peripheral Nerve	Main Action
Iliopsoas	L2, L3	Femoral	Hip flexion
Quadriceps femoris	L3, L4	Femoral	Knee extension
Adductors	L2, L3, L4	Obturator	Adduction of thigh
Gluteus maximus	L5, S1, S2	Inferior gluteal	Hip extension
Gluteus medius and minimus, tensor fasciae latae	L4, L5, S1	Superior gluteal	Hip abduction
Hamstrings	L5, S1	Sciatic	Knee flexion
Tibialis anterior	L4, L5	Peroneal	Dorsiflexion of ankle
Extensor digitorum longus	L5, S1	Peroneal	Dorsiflexion of toes
Extensor digitorum brevis	S1	Peroneal	Dorsiflexion of toes
Peronei	L5, S1	Peroneal	Eversion of foot
Tibialis posterior	L4	Tibial	Inversion of foot
Gastrocnemius	S1, S2	Tibial	Plantar flexion of ankle
Soleus	S1, S2	Tibial	Plantar flexion of ankle

Source: From Simon et al. *Clinical Neurology*. 7th ed. New York: McGraw-Hill; 2009.

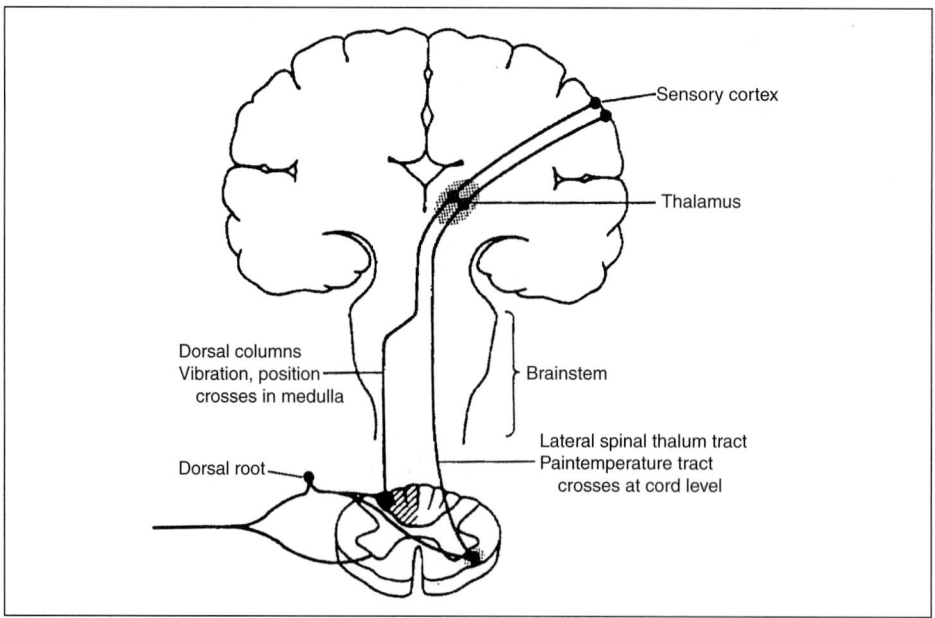

FIGURE 1-13   **Sensory system.**

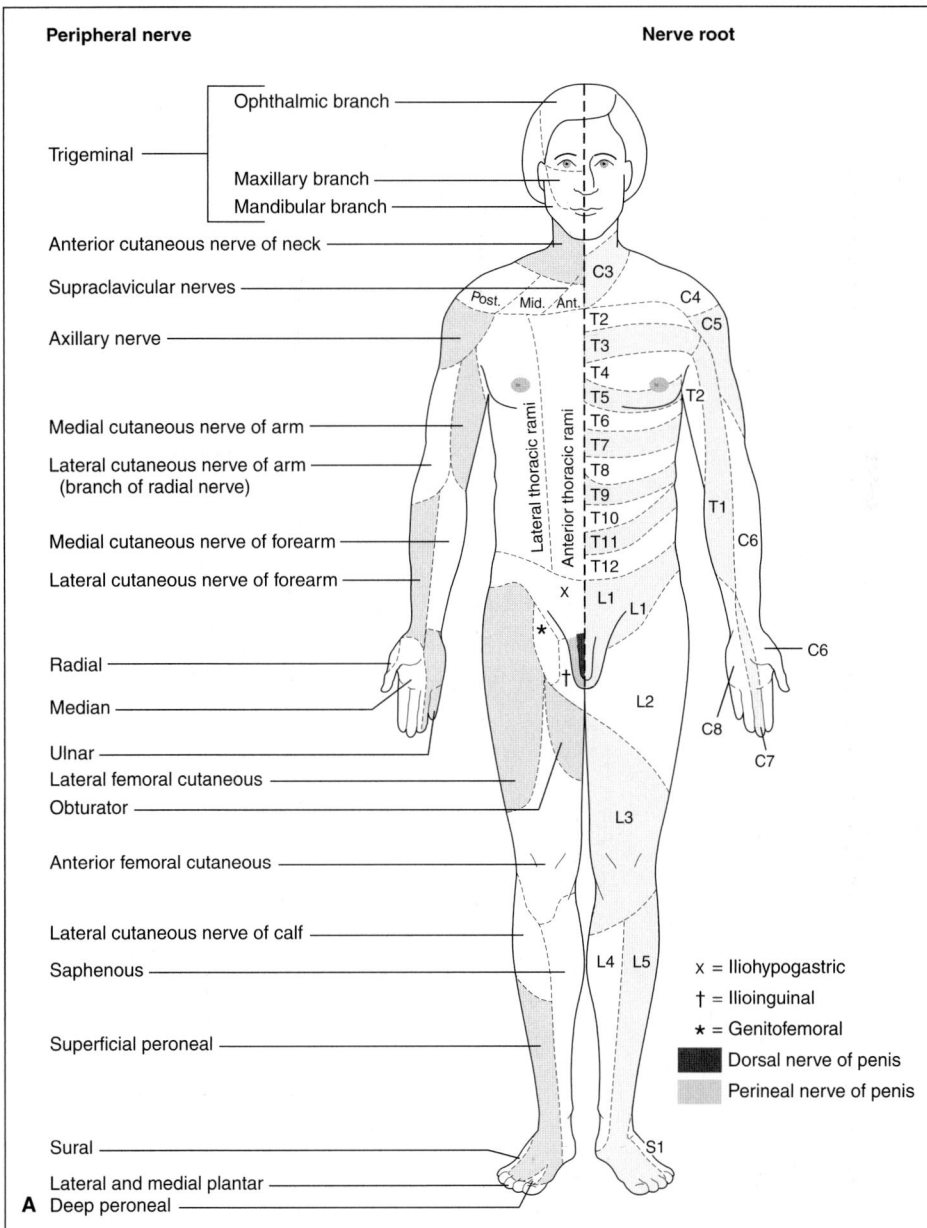

FIGURE 1-14 (A) Cutaneous innervation (anterior view). The segmental or radicular (nerve root) distribution is shown on the left side of the body, and the peripheral nerve distribution on the right side of the body. (*continued*)

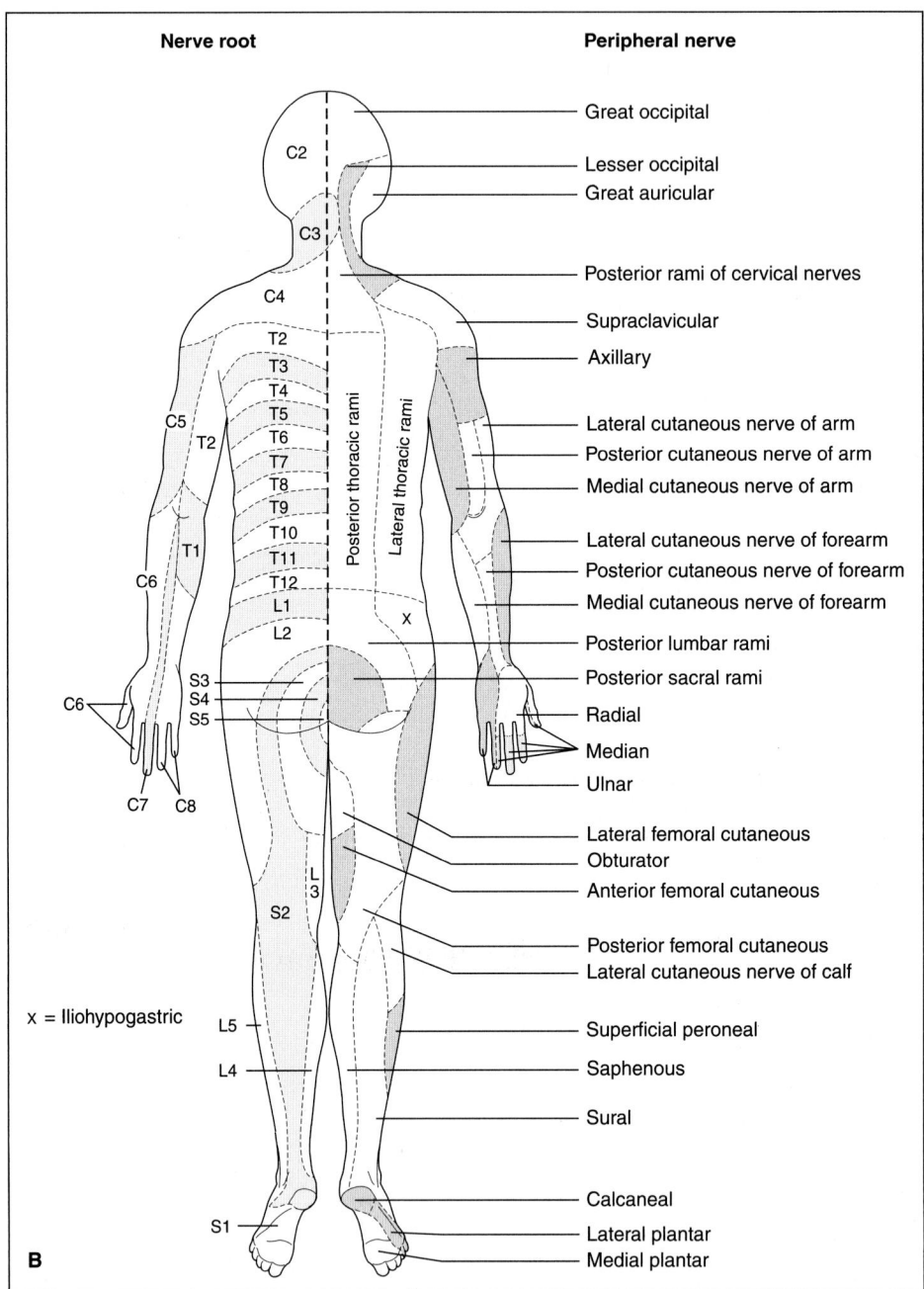

FIGURE 1-14 (*Continued*) (B) Cutaneous innervation (posterior view). The segmental or radicular (nerve root) distribution is shown on the left side of the body, and the peripheral nerve distribution on the right side of the body. (Reproduced with permission from Simon R, Greenberg D, Aminoff M. *Clinical Neurology.* 7th ed. New York: McGraw-Hill; 2009:208-209. 0-07-154644-8.)

Vision

The visual pathways are divided into three distinct regions (Fig. 1-15). Vision from the retina to the level of the optic chiasm is carried in a single optic nerve. At the level of the optic chiasm, optic nerve projections from both eyes redistribute to form the optic tracts. Specifically, it is in this region (i.e., the optic chiasm) that the left visual world as perceived in each eye and the right visual world as perceived in each eye are selectively recombined to form the optic tracts. Visual input then passes through the optic tracts to the respective lateral geniculate bodies, where separate bilateral superior and inferior optic radiations then proceed posteriorly to terminate in the occipital cortex.[1,11,13]

Blindness in one eye represents disease anywhere along the visual axis from the front of the cornea posteriorly to the level of the optic chiasm.

Common optic chiasm lesions include pituitary tumors and intrinsic chiasmal ischemic changes. Such processes classically involve the temporal visual field optic nerve fibers (i.e., medial retina visual receptor projections) from each eye, which cross in the more central portion of the optic chiasm (Fig. 1-15). Such intrinsic and extrinsic chiasmal lesions can produce the classic bitemporal hemianopsia. An asymmetric bitemporal hemianopsia usually implies that the chiasmal lesion is not perfectly symmetric but still denotes a lesion at the level of the chiasm.

If an optic tract is involved in a pathologic process, a homonymous hemianopsia often results. After an optic tract synapses in the lateral geniculate nucleus, optic radiations project through the parietal (superior branch) and temporal (inferior branch) lobes to the occipital region. Lesions of a specific optic radiation branch can result in a quadrantanopia.

The pupils are complex neurologic structures that receive input from both the autonomic nervous system and the visual reflex arcs. Light stimulus is received through the second cranial nerve and is passed to the midbrain nuclei that control pupillary dilation. The pupillary response is affected by visual fibers proximal to the lateral geniculate bodies or by lesions involving the parasympathetic fibers of the third cranial nerve (Fig. 1-16).

The anatomy of extraocular movements is important to understand because it serves as the basis for clinical examination of the functioning of the brainstem. In awake patients, voluntary eye movements are under the control of the frontal eye fields. There are centers in each frontal lobe that initiate voluntary eye movement. Information is passed through the subcortical structures and descending motor pathways to pontine gaze centers (Fig. 1-17).

Coordination of the eye movements themselves is then carried out through the medial longitudinal fasciculus, which lies in the center of the brainstem. This tract connects the third, fourth, and sixth cranial nerve nuclei, and therefore can coordinate and conjugate eye movements.[3,4,14] There is a constant input to the pontine gaze centers from each frontal eye pole. Ocular tracking and pursuit movements are coordinated by the posterior visual centers located in the occipital lobes. Once the frontal eye poles have locked onto an object, smooth pursuit is ensured by the posterior cortical centers that send information to the brainstem.

The Autonomic Nervous System

The autonomic nervous system is made up of the sympathetic and the parasympathetic nervous systems. Sympathetic fibers arise from the thoracic and lumbar regions and

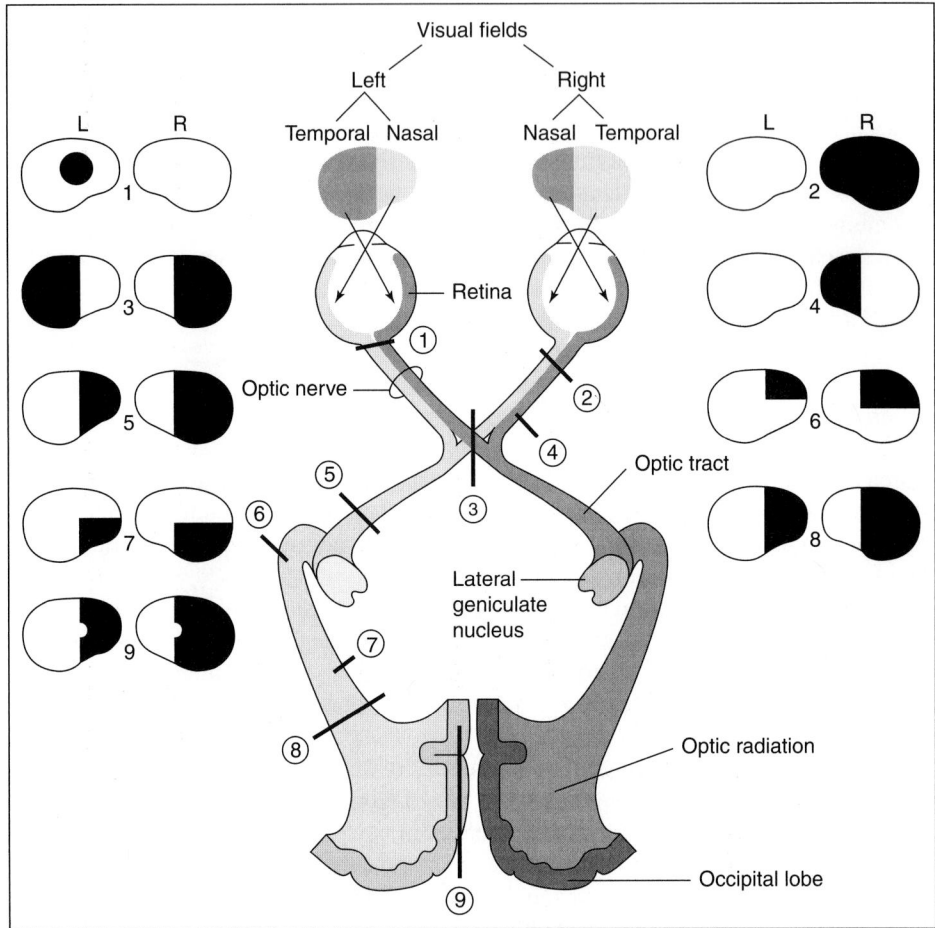

FIGURE 1-15 Common visual field defects and their anatomic bases. (1) Central scotoma caused by inflammation of the optic disk (optic neuritis) or optic nerve (retrobulbar neuritis). (2) Total blindness of the right eye caused by a complete lesion of the right optic nerve. (3) Bitemporal hemianopia caused by pressure exerted on the optic chiasm by a pituitary tumor. (4) Right nasal hemianopia caused by a perichiasmal lesion (e.g., calcified internal carotid artery). (5) Right homonymous hemianopia caused by a lesion of the left optic tract. (6) Right homonymous superior quadrantanopia caused by partial involvement of the optic radiation by a lesion in the left temporal lobe (Meyer loop). (7) Right homonymous inferior quadrantanopia caused by partial involvement of the optic radiation by a lesion in the left parietal lobe. (8) Right homonymous hemianopia caused by a complete lesion of the left optic radiation. (A similar defect may also result from lesion 9.) (9) Right homonymous hemianopia (with macular sparing) resulting from posterior cerebral artery occlusion.   (Reproduced with permission from Simon R, Greenberg D, Aminoff M. *Clinical Neurology.* 7th ed. New York: McGraw-Hill; 2009.)

synapse in the autonomic chain ganglia. Fibers of the parasympathetic system are from the brainstem nuclei and the sacral cord levels. They synapse directly on nuclei of the organ systems involved (Fig. 1-18).[13,15]

The sympathetic system is the alarm system of the body. Its stimulation produces tachycardia, dilation of the bronchi, release of adrenaline, decrease in bowel activity, and inhibition of micturition, as well as increased sweating and dilation of the pupils.

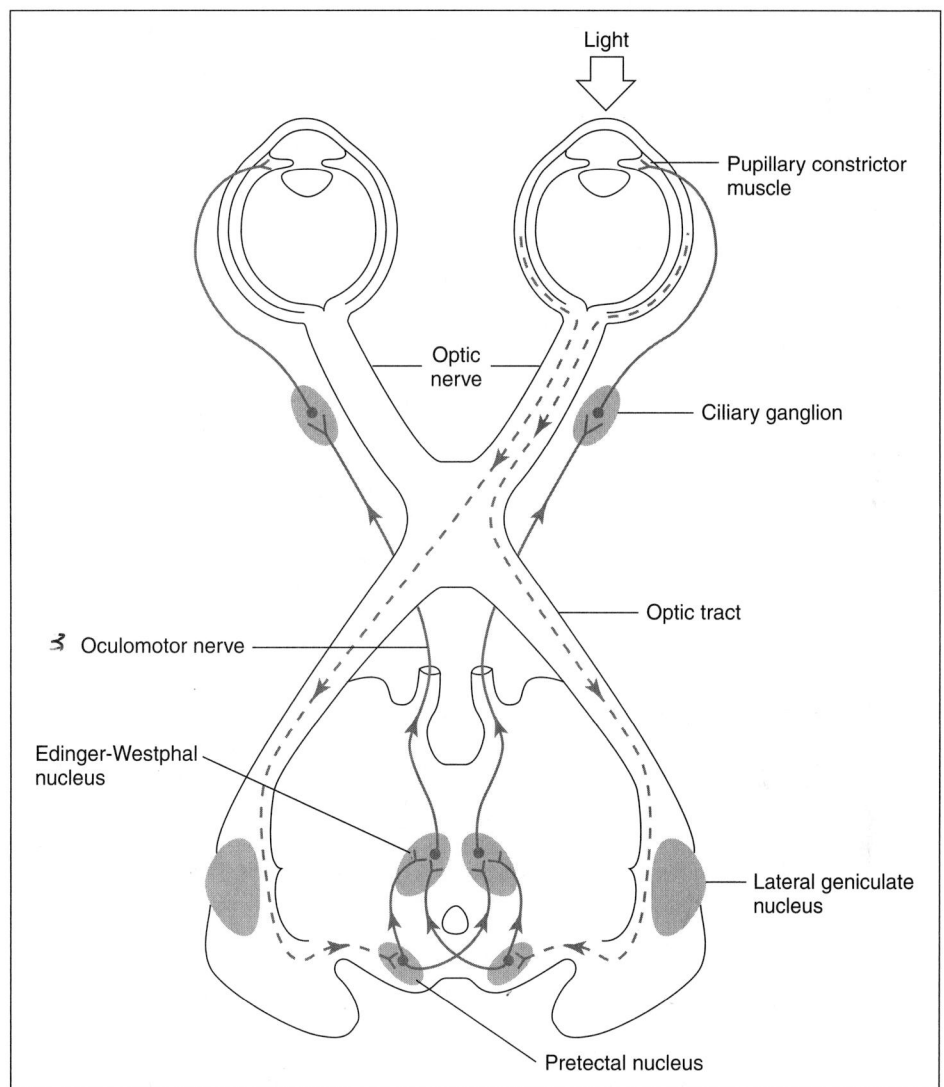

FIGURE 1-16 **Anatomic basis of the papillary light reflex. The afferent visual pathways from the retina to the pretectal nuclei of the midbrain are represented by dashed lines and the efferent pupilloconstrictor pathways from the midbrain to the retinas by solid lines. Note that illumination of one eye results in bilateral papillary constriction.** (Reproduced with permission from Simon R, Greenberg D, Aminoff M. *Clinical Neurology.* 7th ed. New York: McGraw-Hill; 2009.)

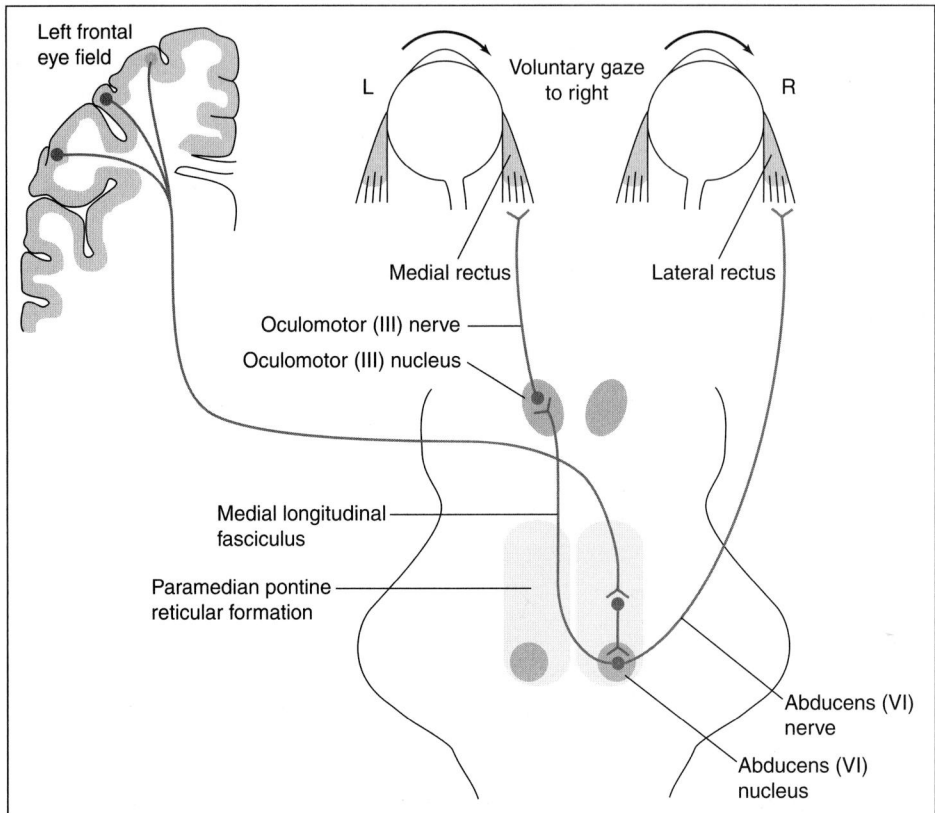

FIGURE 1-17 Neuronal pathways involved in horizontal gaze. (Reproduced with permission from Simon R, Greenberg D, Aminoff M. *Clinical Neurology.* 7th ed. New York: McGraw-Hill; 2009.)

Stimulation of the parasympathetic system causes quite the opposite effects, including bradycardia, constriction of the bronchi, and increased salivation and lacrimation, as well as increased bowel motility and constriction of the pupils.[13,15]

The effects of the autonomic nervous system are vast and complex and are frequently blended with other systems of the body. On a purely neurologic basis, with the exception of some very isolated lesions, the autonomic nervous system findings are often difficult to distinguish from other systems of the body. Except for their effects on vital signs, these systems are not usually tested in the acute care setting.

Innervation of the Bladder

Motor control of the process of urination is divided into three parts. Control of the external sphincters is under voluntary control and is mediated through the pudendal nerve supplied by the S2, S3, and S4 nerve roots (Fig. 1-19). The internal sphincter control and contraction of the detrusor muscle of the bladder is primarily regulated by the parasympathetic nervous system, originating in the sacral roots S2, S3, and S4. These

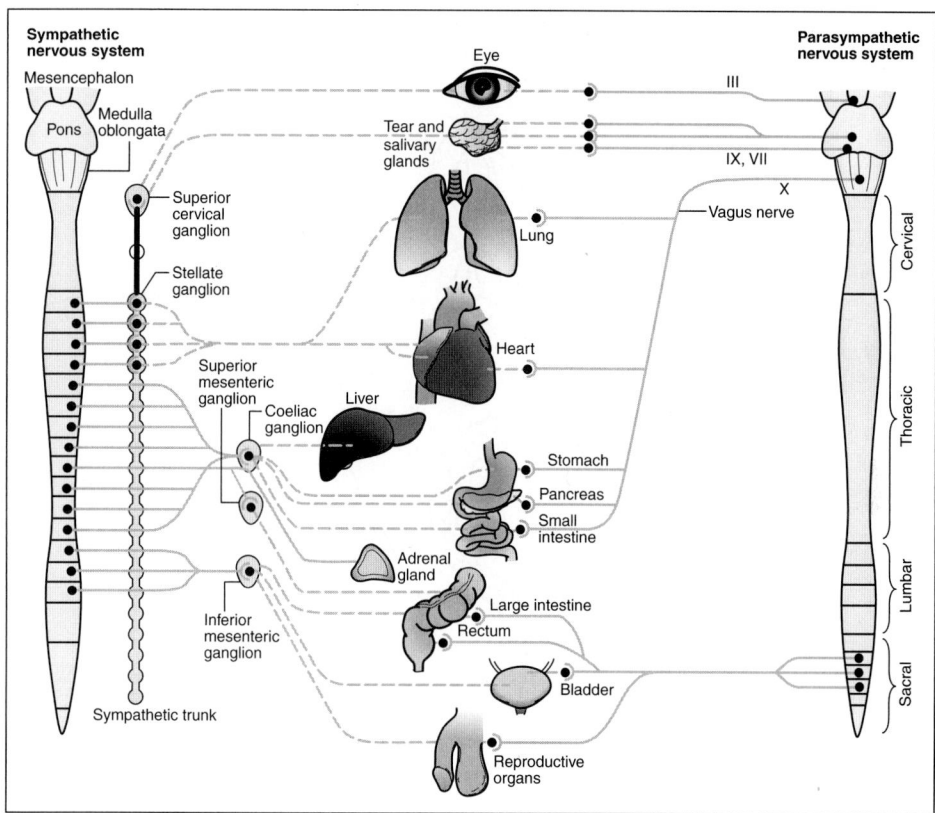

FIGURE 1-18   Organization of the autonomic nervous system. The sympathetic nervous system is shown on the left, and the parasympathetic nervous system is shown on the right. Note that the postganglionic neurons for the sympathetic nervous system are located in the sympathetic trunk ganglia and the prevertebral ganglia (e.g., celiac ganglion). The postganglionic neurons for the parasympathetic nervous system are located in terminal ganglia close to the target organ.   (Reproduced with permission from Nestler E. *Molecular Neuropharmacology.* 2nd ed. New York: McGraw-Hill; 2008.)

parasympathetic fibers terminate on ganglia located in the wall of the bladder itself. Stimulation of parasympathetic fibers causes emptying of the bladder by contraction of the detrusor muscle and relaxation of the internal sphincter muscle.[4,9]

The sympathetic nervous system plays a minor role in bladder function. Sympathetic supply to the bladder comes through the sympathetic chain ganglia supplied by the upper lumbar and lower thoracic segments. Postganglionic fibers then proceed to enter the wall of the bladder and the internal sphincter. The precise actions of the sympathetic nerves with regards to the detrusor muscle are less well understood. A loss of sympathetic supply to the bladder does not measurably affect its function.[9] In the absence of central inhibition and control of the external sphincter muscles, reflex emptying of the bladder occurs either with increased pressure in the wall of the bladder or by stimulation of skin over the thighs.

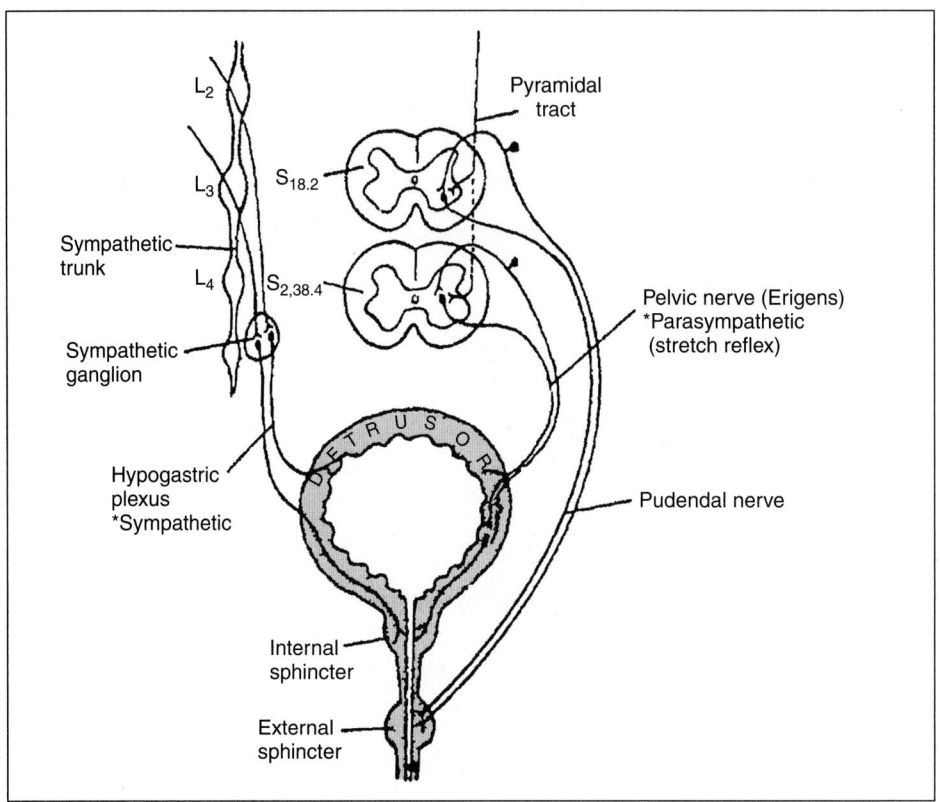

FIGURE 1-19   **Innervation of the bladder.**   (From Clark RG. *Clinical Neuroanatomy and Neurophysiology.* 5th ed. Philadelphia: Davis, 1975:125.)

Vascular Anatomy

Arterial Supply

The arterial supply to the brain and spinal cord can be divided into an anterior and posterior circulation (Figs. 1-20 and 1-21).[16] The anterior intracranial circulation is the portion of the vascular network supplied by the carotid arteries. The left common carotid artery arises directly from the aortic arch and the right common carotid artery arises from the innominate branch of the aortic arch. Both common carotid arteries ascend in their respective lateral neck regions and bifurcate into internal and external carotid arteries at about the C4 level. The internal carotid arteries continue cephalad through the skull base and terminate at the base of their respective cerebral hemispheres dividing into anterior and middle cerebral arteries. The proximal anterior cerebral arteries (A1 segments) extend medially where a small communication between the two, the anterior communicating artery, is usually present. The A1 segments and the anterior communicating artery make up the anterior most portion of the circle of Willis, a potential route of collateral flow between cerebral hemispheres bilaterally and also between the anterior and posterior circulations of the brain (explained later in the chapter). The more distal anterior cerebral arteries (A2 segments and

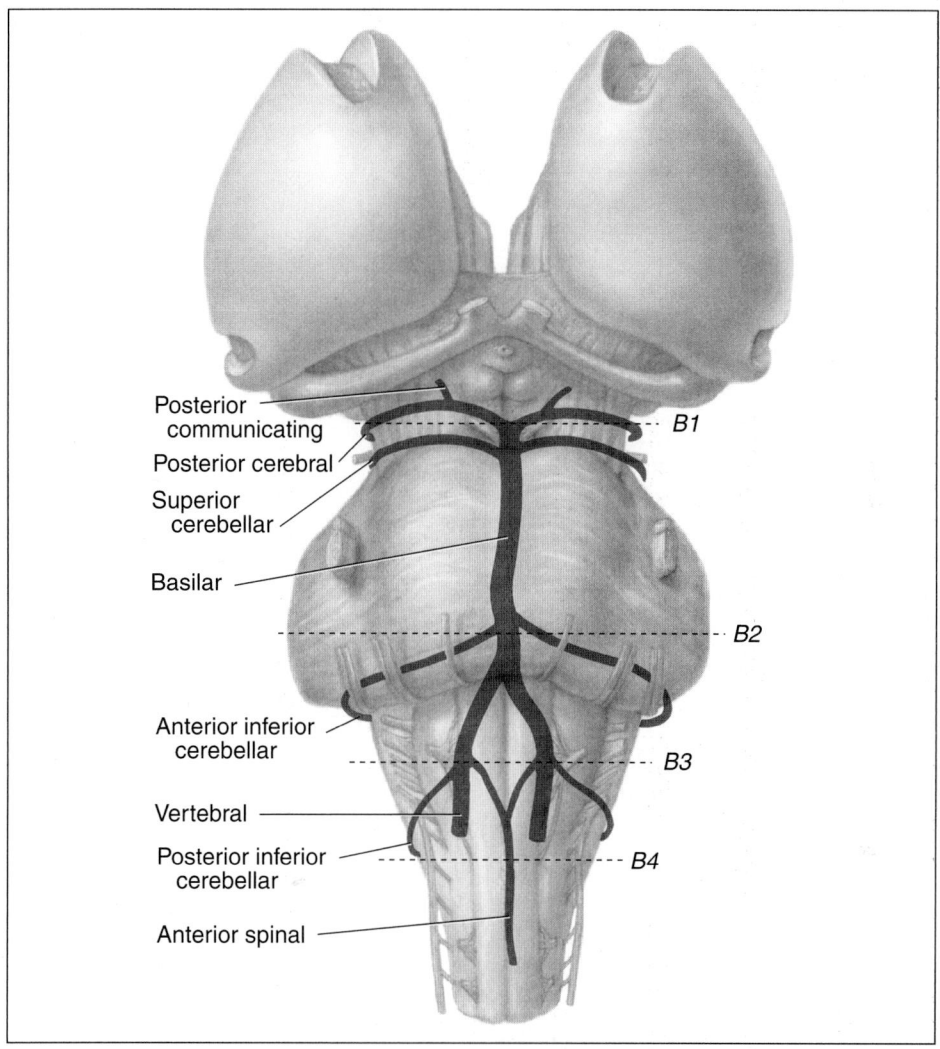

Posterior
communicating
Posterior cerebral
Superior
cerebellar

Basilar

Anterior inferior
cerebellar

Vertebral

Posterior inferior
cerebellar

Anterior spinal

B1

B2

B3

B4

FIGURE 1-20   Arterial circulation of the brainstem is schematically illustrated on a view of the ventral surface of the brainstem.   (Reproduced with permission from Martin J. *Neuroanatomy: A Text and Atlas.* 3th ed. New York: McGraw-Hill; 2003.)

beyond) then extend superiorly and posteriorly along the medial surface of the respective cerebral hemispheres, just superficial to the corpus callosum, supplying blood to the medial aspects of the frontal and anterior/midparietal lobes, including the region of the motor cortex. The motor and sensory portions of the brain particularly concerned with the lower extremities are located on the medial aspects of the cerebral hemispheres and therefore usually supplied by these branches of the anterior cerebral artery.[16]

The middle cerebral artery is the other major terminal branch of the internal carotid artery; it initially extends laterally (M1 segment) and then turns posterosuperiorly within the Sylvian fissure region (M2 and distal branches). It supplies the majority of the frontal,

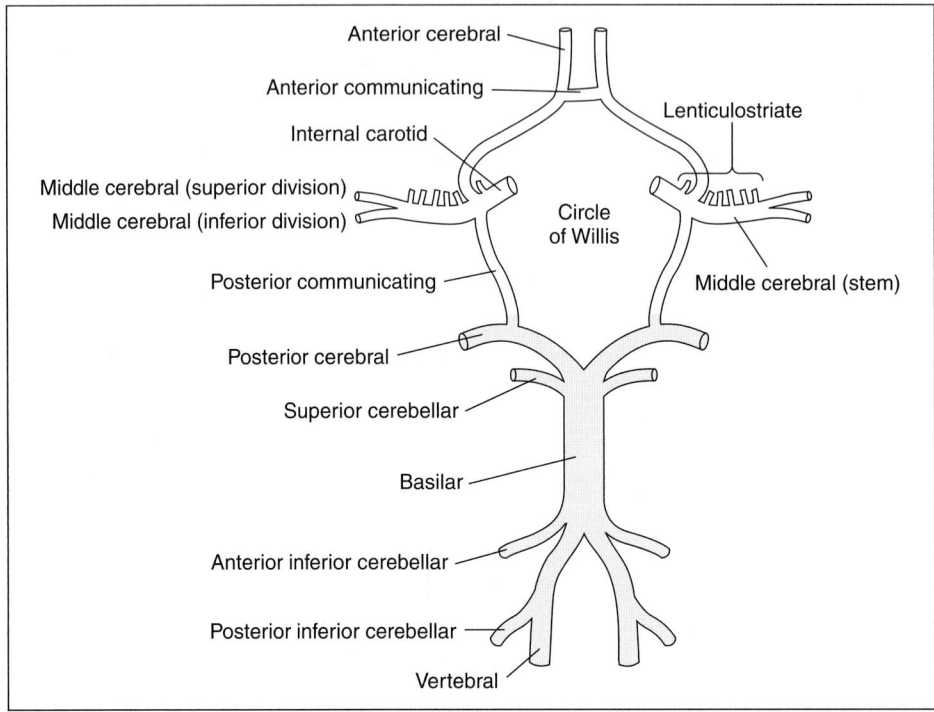

FIGURE 1-21 **Arteries of the anterior (white) and posterior (blue) cerebral circulation in relation to the circle of Willis.** (Reproduced with permission from Simon R, Greenberg D, Aminoff M. *Clinical Neurology.* 7th ed. New York: McGraw-Hill; 2009.)

parietal, and temporal lobes and portions of the upper occipital regions. Lenticulostriate branches from the M1 segment supply blood to the internal capsule and basal ganglion structures. The anterior circulation is connected to the posterior circulation through the posterior communicating arteries (which make up the lateral portion of the circle of Willis).

The posterior communicating arteries are variably patent in any given patient and may or may not be a viable route of collateral flow between the anterior and posterior circulations.

The more inferior (posterior) portions of the central nervous system (the cerebellum, the brainstem, and the cervical spinal cord) are supplied by posterior circulation (Figs. 1-22 and 1-23). Vascular supply to these regions in the neck and head is predominantly from the two vertebral arteries, which extend from their respective subclavian arteries at the thoracic inlet, cephalad through the foramina transversaria in the lateral aspects of the cervical vertebra and enter the posterior fossa through the foramen magnum before joining to form the basilar artery, anterior to the pontomedullary junction of the brainstem. The basilar artery then continues cephalad along the anterior aspect of the mid and upper brainstem. It has small branches that supply the brainstem and the cerebellum. It terminates at the basilar artery "tip" just anterior to the midbrain as the paired posterior cerebral arteries and superior cerebellar arteries, which pass around the upper brainstem and supply the parieto-occipital and superior cerebellar regions bilaterally, respectively. The posterior communicating arteries, when patent, anastomose with the proximal portions of the posterior cerebral arteries (P1 segments), which are considered to make up the posterior aspect of the circle of Willis. As mentioned above, the posterior communicating arteries are variably patent in any given

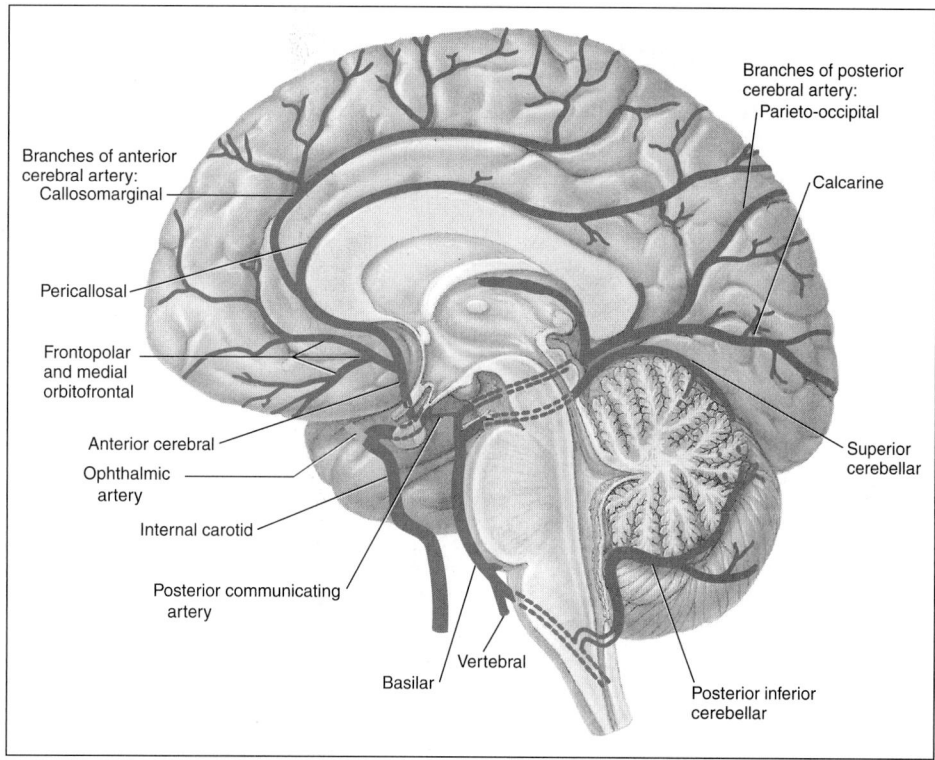

FIGURE 1-22   The courses of the three cerebral arteries are illustrated in the view of midsagittal surfaces of the cerebral hemisphere. Note that the anterior cerebral artery courses around the genu of the corpus callosum.   (Reproduced with permission from Martin J. *Neuroanatomy: A Text and Atlas.* 3th ed. New York: McGraw-Hill; 2003.)

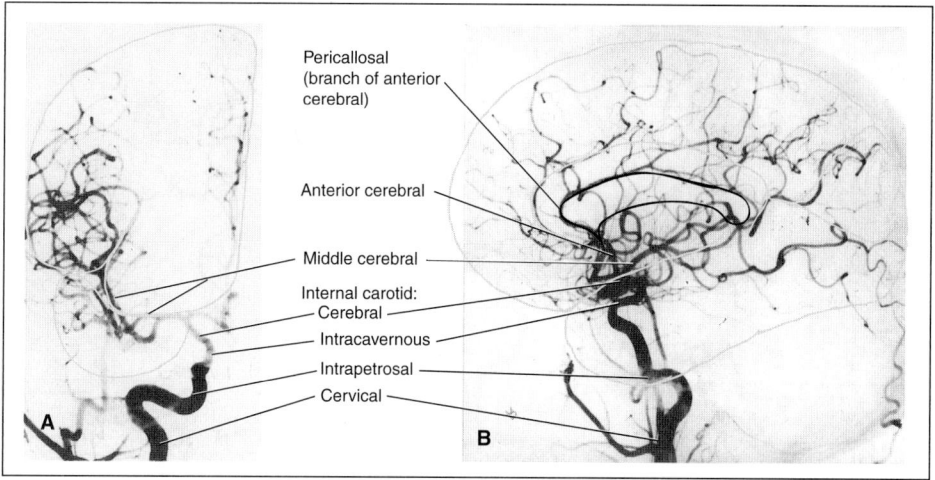

FIGURE 1-23   Cerebral angiograms of the anterior circulation are shown in frontal (A) and lateral (B) projections. Overlaying each angiogram is a schematic drawing of the cerebral hemispheres, showing the approximate location of the surface landmarks in relation to the arteries.   (*Angiograms courtesy of Dr. Neal Rutledge, University of Texas at Austin.*) (Reproduced with permission from Martin J. *Neuroanatomy: A Text and Atlas.* 3th ed. New York: McGraw-Hill; 2003.)

patient and may or may not be a viable route of collateral flow between the anterior and posterior circulations. In fact, the entire circle of Willis (the A1 segments bilaterally, anterior communicating artery, the distal internal carotid arteries, the posterior communicating arteries bilaterally, and the P1 segments bilaterally) is patent in about only 50% of patients.

Because of the range of structures supplied, the posterior circulation pathologic processes are much more likely to result in bilateral symptomatology. They are also more likely to affect consciousness, equilibrium, balance, and the coordination of muscle movements.

The blood supply to the spinal cord[17,18] is predominantly through the several feeding vessels arising from the vertebral, thyrocervical, and the costocervical trunk arterial branches of the subclavian arteries in the cervical region; from the intercostal arterial branches of the aorta in the thoracic region; and from the lumbosacral arterial branches of the aorta (and sometimes the iliac system) in the lumbosacral region. The exact level of the blood vessels, which ultimately supply the spinal cord, is variable in each portion of the spine and varies from person to person. These vessels are not symmetric and are not found at every spinal level. These radiculomedullary arterial branches enter the spinal canal through the neural foramina and separate into anterior and posterior branches that supply the dura, nerves, and the spinal cord. The larger anterior radiculomedullary branch supplies the midline anterior spinal artery along the ventral aspect of the spinal cord; the smaller posterior radiculomedullary branches supply the paired posterolateral posterior spinal arteries. The anterior spinal artery supplies the anterior two-thirds of the spinal

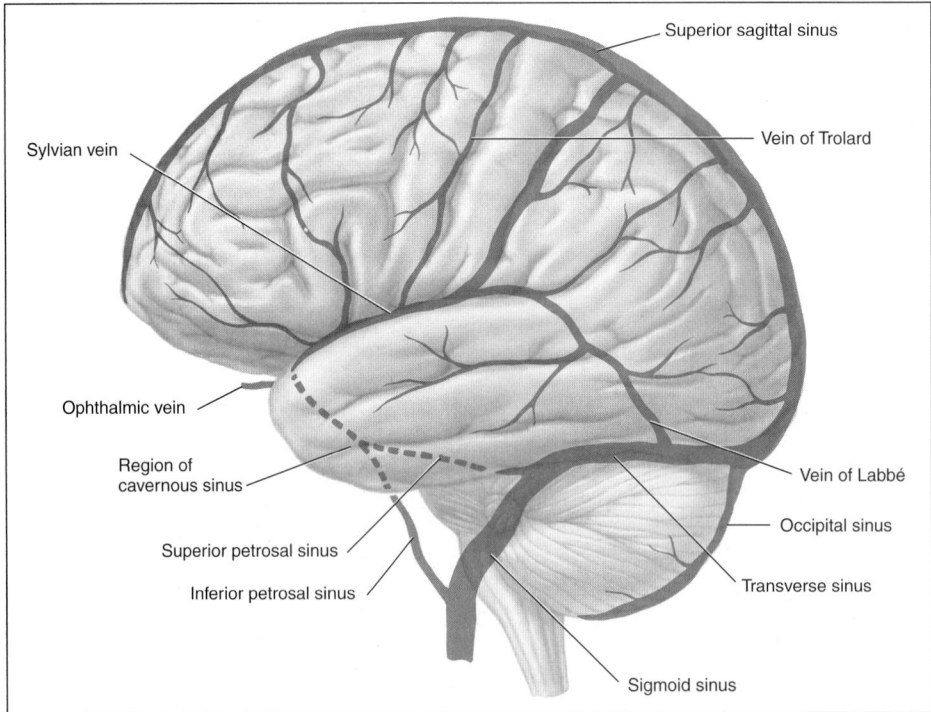

FIGURE 1-24 **Lateral view of the brain, showing major superficial veins and the dural sinuses.** (Reproduced with permission from Martin J. *Neuroanatomy: A Text and Atlas.* 3th ed. New York: McGraw-Hill; 2003.)

cord (including the corticospinal tracts) while the posterior spinal arteries supply the posterior one-third of the spinal cord (including the dorsal columns), though these vascular distributions are somewhat variable. The anterior and posterior spinal arteries then supply a meshwork of collateral vessels, which surround the length of the spinal cord. Watershed regions of vascular perfusion exist within the spinal cord depending on the exact levels that the above-described radiculomedullary branches enter the spinal canal; the most common spinal cord watershed region involves the midthoracic cord. The lack of redundancy (i.e., collateral vascular perfusion) of the vascular supply to the spinal cord results in the cord being vulnerable to vascular insults in the setting of trauma (including surgery particularly that which involves the aorta), aortic dissection, atherosclerosis, or hypotensive events.

Venous Drainage

The venous drainage of the brain involves both the supratentorial and infratentorial external and internal systems which eventually join to form the major dural venous sinuses, superior sagittal sinus, inferior sagittal sinus, straight sinus, torcular herophili, transverse sinuses, and sigmoid sinuses to drain out the head at the skull base through the internal jugular veins.[1,5,19] Dysfunction of the venous system (e.g., dural venous sinus thrombosis or cortical venous thrombosis), because of its somewhat variable regional anatomy and relatively low pressures, can be subtle in onset and initially difficult to diagnose. While a range of systemic and local processes can affect any portion of the superficial or deep venous system drainage from the face posteriorly through a cavernous sinus, they can also lead to intracranial venous problems (Figs. 1-24 and 1-25).

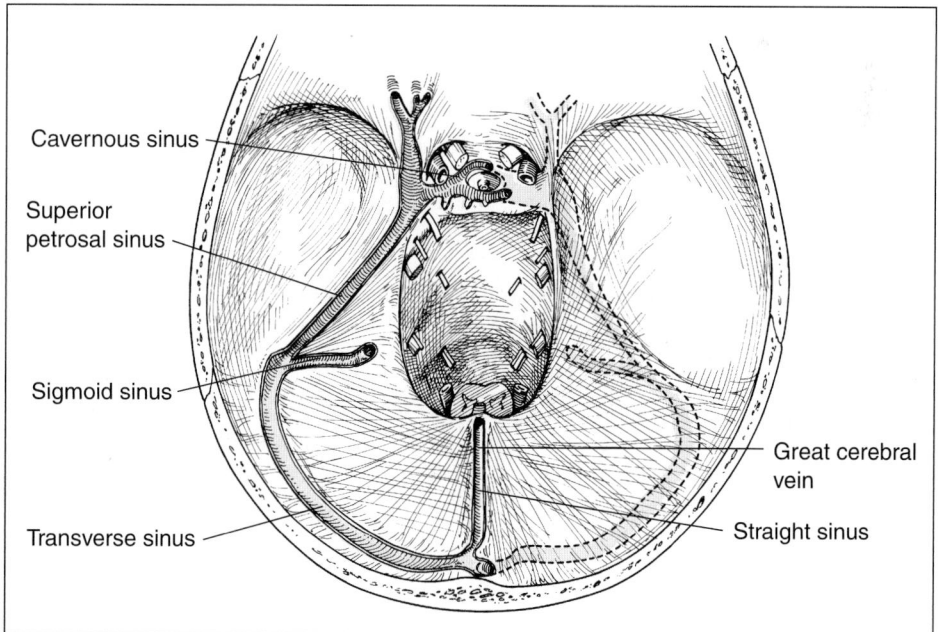

Cavernous sinus

Superior
petrosal sinus

Sigmoid sinus

Great cerebral
vein

Transverse sinus

Straight sinus

FIGURE 1-25 View of the ventral surface of the anterior and middle cranial fossae, and the sinuses on the dorsal surface of the tentorium cerebelli and the ventral cranium.   (Reproduced with permission from Martin J. *Neuroanatomy: A Text and Atlas.* 3th ed. New York: McGraw-Hill; 2003.)

SUMMARY

Functional neuroanatomy should be the basis on which evaluation of all neurologic symptomatology rests. Careful integration of the patient's complaints and proper neurologic examination may help pinpoint the anatomic location of the majority of neurologic problems.

REFERENCES

1. Afifi A, Bergman R. *Functional Neuroanatomy Text and Atlas*. 2nd ed. New York: Lange Medical Books/McGraw-Hill; 2005.
2. Aminoff M, Greenberg D, Simon R. *Clinical Neurology*. 6th ed. New York, NY: Lange Medical Books/ McGraw-Hill; 2005.
3. Bender M, Randolph S, Stacy C. Neurology of the visual and oculomotor systems. In: Joint R, Griggs R, eds. *Baker's Clinical Neurology*. Philadelphia: Lippincott Williams & Wilkins; 2000.
4. Campbell W. *Pocket Guide and Tool Kit to DeJong's Neurologic Examination*. Philadelphia: McGraw-Hill/Williams & Wilkins; 2008.
5. Chusid J. *Correlative Neuroanatomy and Functional Anatomy*. Los Altos, CA: Lange; 1970.
6. Roos KL. Cerebral spinal fluid. In: Joint R, Griggs R, eds. *Baker's Clinical Neurology*. Philadelphia: Lippincott Williams & Wilkins; 2000.
7. Geschwind N. Language and the brain. *Sci Am*. 1972;226:76-83.
8. Geschwind N. The organization of language and the brain. *Science*. 1970;170:940.
9. Haerer A. *DeJong's The Neurologic Examination*. 5th ed. New York: Lippincott-Raven; 1992.
10. House E, Pansky B. *Functional Approach to Neuroanatomy*. 2nd ed. New York: McGraw-Hill; 1967.
11. Kandel E, Schwartz J, Jessell T. *Principles of Neural Science*. 4th ed. New York: McGraw-Hill; 2000.
12. Duus P. *Topical Diagnosis in Neurology*. 3rd ed. New York: Thieme; 1998.
13. Martin J. *Neuroanatomy: A Text and Atlas*. 3rd ed. New York: McGraw Hill; 2003.
14. Simpson J, Magee K. *Clinical Evaluation of the Nervous System*. Ann Arbor, MI: Overbeck; 1970.
15. Low P et al. Clinical autonomic disorders. In: Joint R, Griggs R, eds. *Baker's Clinical Neurology*. Philadelphia: Lippincott Williams & Wilkins; 1998.
16. Toole J, Cole M. Ischemic cerebrovascular disease. In: Joint R, Griggs R, eds. *Baker's Clinical Neurology*. Philadelphia: Lippincott Williams & Wilkins; 1998.
17. Doppman JL, Di Chiro G, Ommaya AK. *Selective Arteriography of the Spinal Cord*. St Louis, MO: Warren H. Green, Inc; 1969:3-17.
18. Harnsberger HR, Osborn AG, MacDonald AJ, et al. *Diagnostic and Surgical Imaging Anatomy: Brain, Head & Neck, Spine*. Salt Lake City, UT: Amirsys, Inc; 2007:III-152-III-161.
19. Crosby E, Humphrey T, Lauer E. *Correlative Anatomy of the Nervous System*. New York: MacMillan; 1962.

2

EMERGENT NEUROIMAGING

There are many different imaging modalities that can be used to evaluate new or progressive neurologic symptoms, each with their own advantages, disadvantages, and cost. It is important to appreciate these differences and use imaging only when warranted and also in a timely, cost-efficient manner.

This chapter is divided into two sections. The first section reviews the most common imaging modalities that are used for the evaluation of patients who present for work-up of acute neurologic changes. The second section reviews respective imaging approaches to several of the more common clinical presentations of acute neurologic symptoms.

Finally, it should be realized that not all imaging modalities are available in every setting where patients are emergently evaluated and treated. Thus, depending on available resources, the imaging modality of choice for a given clinical setting may vary. For example, plain radiographic or ultrasound imaging may suffice when CT and/or MRI are either not available or of limited access.

IMAGING MODALITIES

Plain Radiographs

Plain radiographs (also called "X-rays") are obtained by passing an X-ray beam through a patient with the photons that pass through the patient striking a film or detector and generating an image.

While in the pre-CT/MRI era there were many clinical indications for plain X-rays to evaluate acute neurologic changes, there are currently only a few indications for plain radiographs when CT and/or MRI are readily available (Table 2-1). Searching for a foreign body, such as in a patient with symptoms following a traumatic injury (including being shot, impaled with some other foreign material, etc.), can be performed with plain radiographs, which are excellent for identifying bullet fragments, knife tips, etc. However,

TABLE 2-1

INDICATIONS FOR PLAIN RADIOGRAPHS WHEN EVALUATING
ACUTE NEUROLOGIC CHANGES

- Evaluation of spinal trauma (or suspected spinal trauma) looking for posttraumatic/pathologic fractures or spinal misalignment that might benefit from emergent realignment even before CT or MR evaluation
- Screening search for retained foreign bodies (bullet fragments, knife tips, etc.)
- Screening search for foreign material that might contraindicate advanced imaging (e.g., pre-MRI)
- Suspected child abuse
- Shunt dysfunction (evaluation of the extracranial shunt tubing; the ventricular system is evaluated with CT/MRI)

it should be remembered that some foreign bodies such as wood or plastic may be difficult to identify on plain X-rays and may ultimately require CT (or, as in the case of suspected foreign material within the orbit, sometimes ultrasound is the better test) for their detection. Also, because of the lack of tomographic capability, even if well seen on plain radiographs, the exact location of a foreign body may still be difficult to determine and might require CT again for exact localization.

Linear, nondisplaced skull fractures may be better detected on plain radiographs than on CT because of the higher *spatial* resolution of plain X-rays,[1] but their detection is rarely of clinical importance (i.e., no intervention is needed to treat most nondisplaced skull fractures) with the important exception of suspected child abuse where the detection of a "benign-appearing" nondisplaced skull fracture can dramatically affect patient management. Therefore, in suspected child abuse patients, even if a CT of the head has already been performed, plain radiographs (in two planes) may also need to be performed.[2]

Plain X-rays to search for radiopaque intracorporeal material that might represent a contraindication to emergent MRI are occasionally necessary. Suspected ventriculoperitoneal shunt dysfunction as a potential etiology of acute decline of neurologic function often includes a CT scan to assess the appearance of the intracranial ventricular system, but can also require plain radiographs to assess the extracranial course of a shunt catheter system for discontinuities.

Assuming that CT scanning is readily available, plain radiographs are no longer indicated for the initial evaluation of acute head trauma (as one cannot visualize intracranial compartment structures on plain radiographs), facial trauma (poor characterization of the extent of osseous and soft tissue injuries on plain X-rays), potentially aggressive sinus inflammatory change (poor sensitivity/specificity to the presence and extent of inflammatory changes), and, in many instances, for the evaluation for possible spinal fractures. CT is also better for the characterization of some osseous lesions, localization of foreign material, and delineation of displaced calvarial or spinal fracture fragments.

However, in many clinical settings, plain radiographs are appropriate for evaluation. For example, for evaluation of the spine, in the absence of the availability of CT, plain radiographs are the imaging modality of choice. Also, even if CT is available, plain radiographic evaluation (or no imaging evaluation at all) may be appropriate, particularly in the clinical setting where the probability of significant injury is low.[3,4] Sometimes, in the setting of acute symptoms, a rapidly acquired spinal radiograph may be all that is necessary to initiate aggressive therapeutic intervention.

Finally, opacification of a significant portion of a paranasal sinus or frank expansion of a paranasal sinus can often be detected on dedicated plain radiographic evaluation of the maxillofacial region and may be enough to begin therapy.

Computed Tomography

CT uses a highly collimated X-ray beam generated by an X-ray tube, which is mounted on a "ring" through which a patient moves. Within this ring, this X-ray tube passes around a patient in less than a second. Detectors are located 180 degrees from the tube at all times so that X-ray data can be collected from all directions as the beam continuously passes through the patient as the tube moves around the patient. By using complex "reconstruction" algorithms and powerful computers, X-ray absorption data by anatomic location can be determined for all points within the scanned portion of a patient and an X-ray attenuation map generated for each "slice" of the patient included in each pass of the X-ray beam around the patient. This "attenuation map" can differentiate subtle electron density differences between tissues and display them as an image. Electron-density differences between tissues are demonstrated as differences in the whiteness, grayness, or blackness on an image.

Scanning on a CT machine is limited by two factors: patient girth and weight. Most CT scanners have gantry diameters of 28 inches and table weight limits on the order of 450 lb. Some manufacturers have recently developed CT scanners with gantry diameters of 35 inches and table weight limits of 680 lb. Except for the truly morbidly obese, girth issues rarely come into play. However, weight issues commonly limit who can be scanned. Radiology departments are strict with respect to monitoring patient weights as table warranties can be voided if, overweight patients are scanned and replacement CT tables cost on the order of $50,000 to $75,000, not to mention the fact that the scanner will not be clinically available until the broken table is replaced.

CT Concepts

IMAGE WINDOWS "Windowing" an image refers to making adjustments as to how a final image is viewed; this is similar to making adjustments on a TV. By adjusting window settings at a workstation (which is usually part of a picture archiving and communication system [PACS]), different tissues can be highlighted (Figs. 2-1 to 2-3). For example, when using a "brain" window, white matter and gray matter can be resolved whereas differences in fat and air cannot be demonstrated and will appear identical (Fig. 2-1b). Similarly, when using a "soft tissue" window, differences in acute hemorrhage, brain tissue, muscles, and fat can be resolved, but osseous regions cannot be evaluated (Fig. 2-1c). Windows of acquired (digital) images can be adjusted at any time even if a study is years old. Usually windows are "preset" at an imaging station, but they can always be manually adjusted using a mouse etc. "Blood" and "stroke" window images (Figs. 2-2 and 2-3) (in addition to "brain," "bone," and "soft tissue" window images) should also always be reviewed when looking at a head CT obtained on a patient with neurologic changes. Failure to review all pertinent windows can result in missing a clinically significant lesion.

HOUNSFIELD ATTENUATION Named after Geoffrey Hounsfield, one of the developers of CT, the relative density of a tissue can be measured in density/attenuation units, which are also called Hounsfield Attenuation (HA) units. The scale extends from greater than 1000

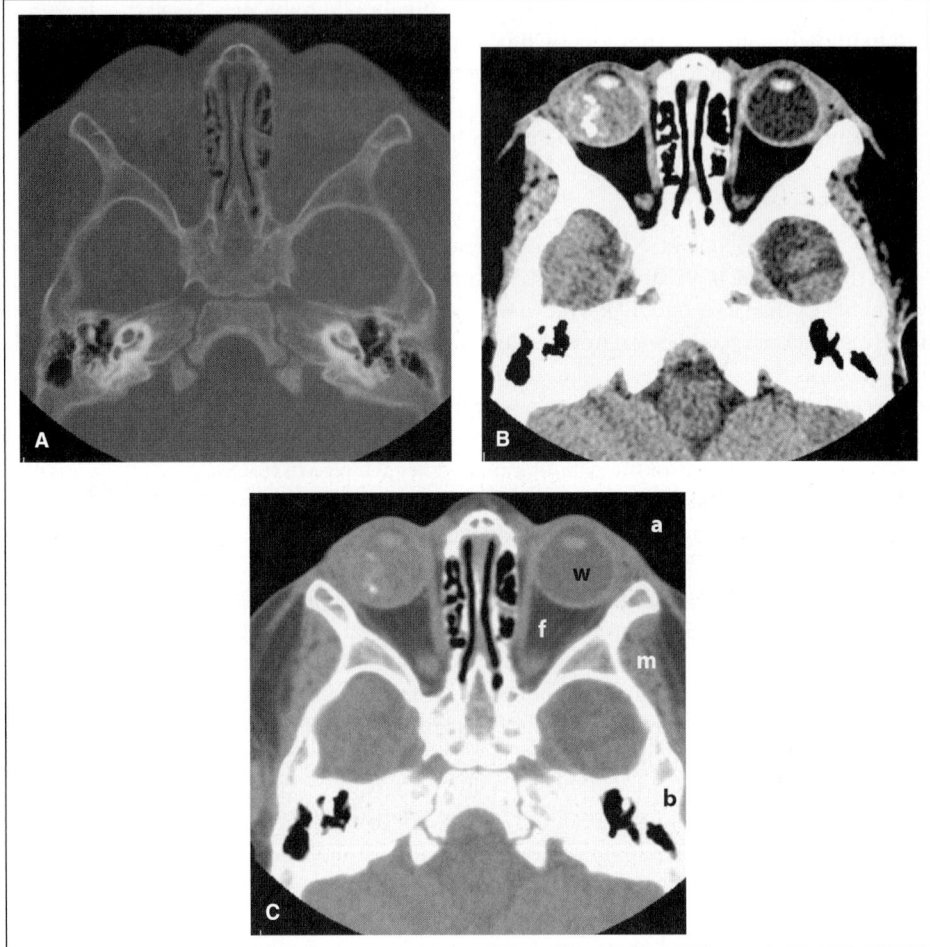

FIGURE 2-1   CT windows. (A) *Bone window images*: Exquisitely define osseous structures, but poorly delineate soft tissue and intracranial structures. (B) *Brain window images*: Best delineate brain structures, but poorly discriminate between orbital fat and air in the ethmoid air cells. (C) *Soft tissue windows*: Nicely resolve soft tissues of the face (fat, muscles, fluid), but poorly delineate osseous & intracranial structures. a = air; f = fat; m = muscles; w = water; b=bone.

(very dense structures that are white on CT scans) to less than 1000 (very low-density structures that are black on CT scan) with pure water arbitrarily defined as zero. The attenuation of tissues are well known (Table 2-2) and can be measured as "regions of interest" on any study. For example, measuring HA is one of the methods of differentiating acute blood (50–80 HA) from bone (>500 HA) as both of these tissues can appear "white" on a soft tissue or brain window CT scan (Fig. 2-2b). For actually measuring HA, there is a region of interest icon at essentially all workstations which can be selected; this results in a cursor appearing on the computer screen which when placed over a given area on an image will instantly display that region's HA.

FIELD OF VIEW   Field of view (FOV) refers to how much of a patient's body is included on each image. For example, a head FOV means the entire head will be included on each image

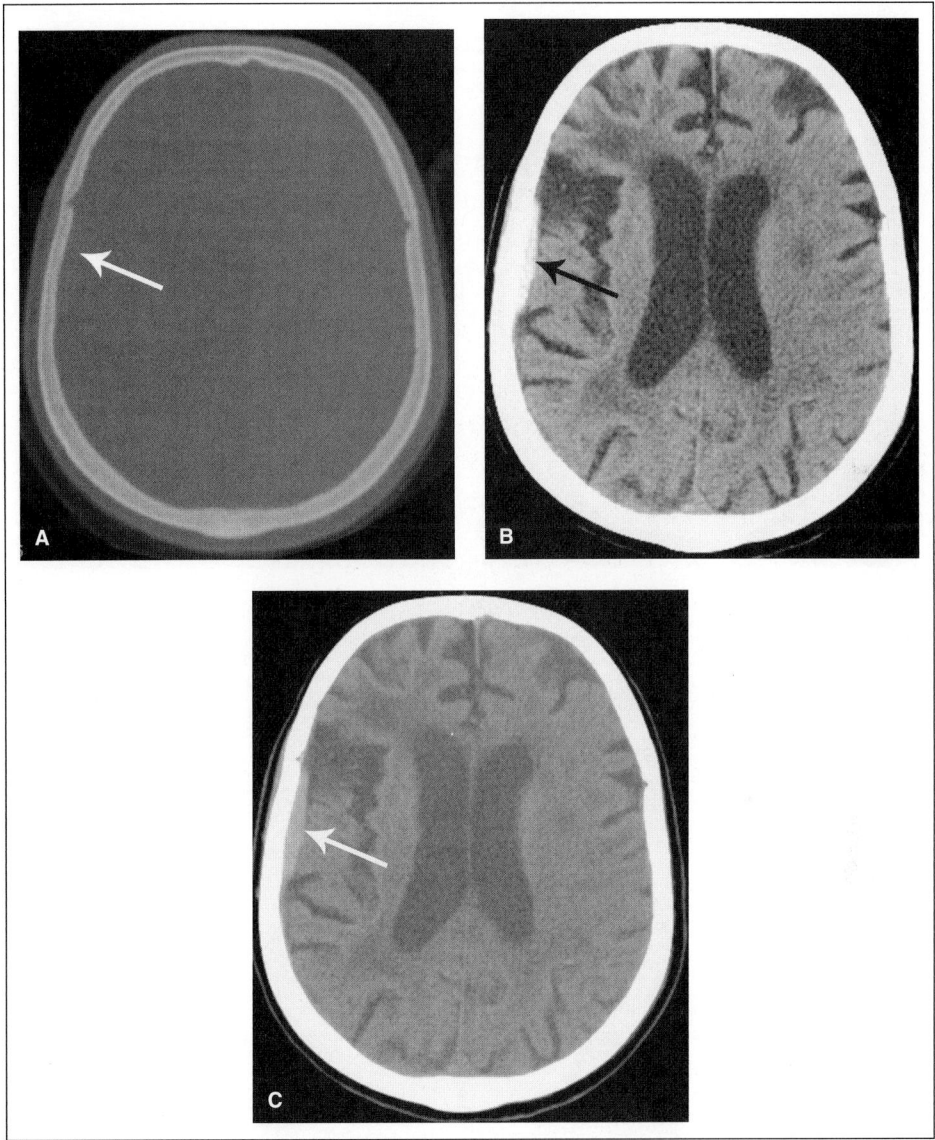

FIGURE 2-2   Value of blood windows. A small epidural hematoma (arrow) is not seen on bone window images (A), is poorly seen on brain windows (B), but is well seen on intermediate "blood" window images (C).

from the CT study while a cervical spine FOV means that only the cervical spine and immediate paraspinal regions will be included on the CT images (i.e., not the entire neck). Such targeting of a given region results in improved image quality. An FOV is set by the CT technician and is not something a requestor of an imaging study needs to specify.

INCIDENTALLY IMAGED REGIONS   When a given CT (or MR) scan is performed, areas of the body that were not intended to be scanned are often still included in the scan FOV.

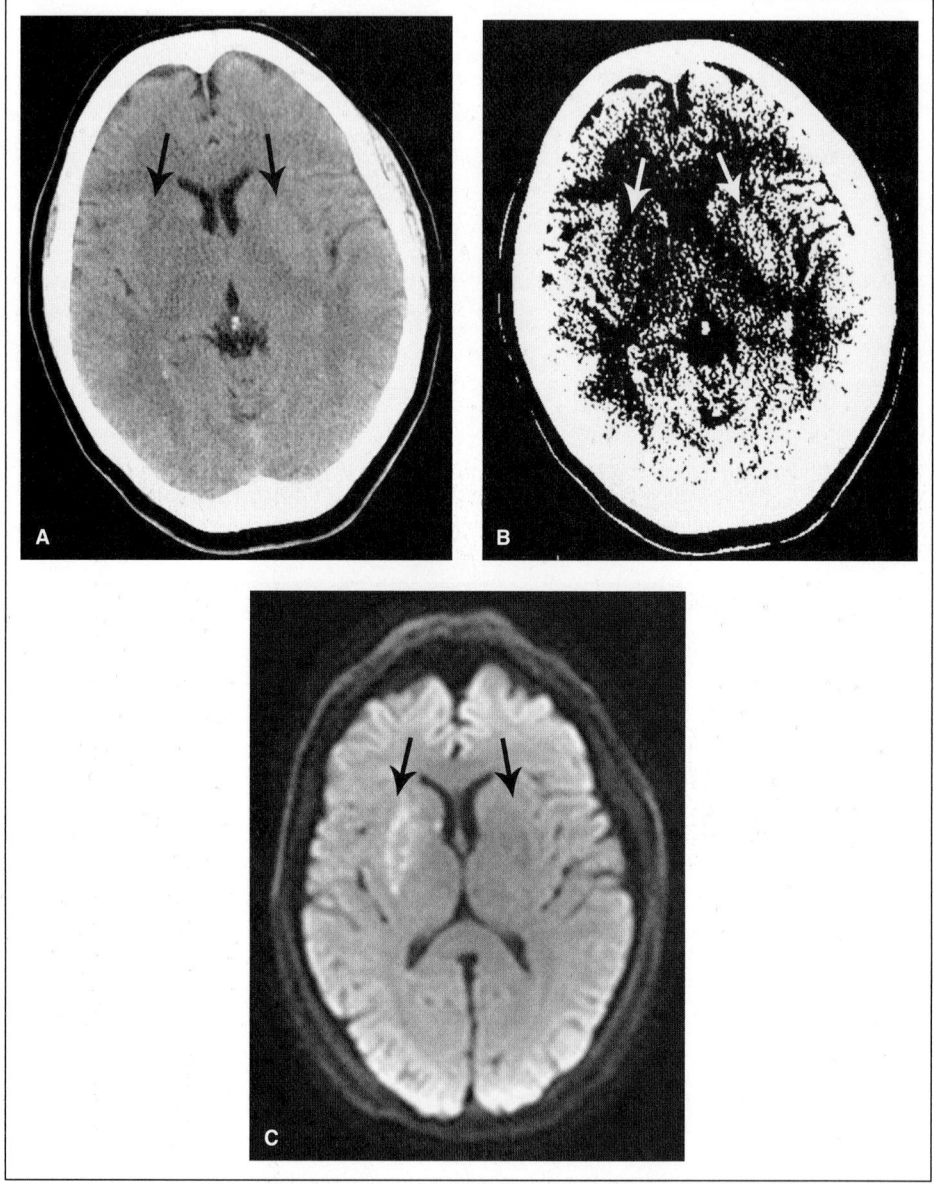

FIGURE 2-3   Value of stroke windows. Brain window images (A) poorly delineate the decreased attenuation of the right lentiform nuclei consistent with an acute ischemic event, which is better demonstrated on extremely narrow "stroke" window images (B) and is confirmed on diffusion MRI (C). Arrows show lentiform nuclei.

For example, when a chest CT is performed to rule out a pulmonary embolus or to evaluate posttraumatic changes, the thoracic spine will also be included in the scanned volume. Therefore, images of the spine can also be generated from the chest CT data and reviewed; this may sometimes result in the detection of unsuspected findings. However, as chest CT scanning parameters are suboptimal for evaluation of the spine (e.g., slice

TABLE 2-2
HOUNSFIELD ATTENUATION FOR VARYING TISSUES ON CT

Tissue	Hounsfield Attenuation
Air	< -500 HU (Hounsfield units)
Fat	-20 to -100
Water (CSF)	0 (by definition)
White matter	23–34
Gray matter	32–40
Acute hemorrhage	50–80
Mineralization	150–200
Contrast material	>500
Bone	>500

thickness is greater for most chest studies, etc.), images of the spine created from CT data obtained from a chest CT scan should not be considered equivalent to those images obtained using a dedicated spine CT scanning protocol. Similarly, evaluation of paraspinal areas on a dedicated spine CT may also yield findings (such as renal stones in a back pain patient being evaluated for vertebral column disease; splenic or liver laceration in a patient being evaluated for spinal fracture, which may require further dedicated imaging.

CONTRAST-ENHANCED SCANS As pathologic lesions can sometimes be difficult to differentiate from normal structures, CT scanning can also be performed either during or immediately after administration of contrast material through a peripheral vein. As essentially all CT contrast agents contain iodine, which is an electron-rich element, contrast material has relative high HA (and therefore appears white) on CT scans. Some of the more common indications for obtaining CT scans without or with administration of contrast material are listed in Table 2-3.

CT ANGIOGRAPHY: Arterial blood vessels can be demonstrated in a manner similar to a conventional angiogram as a CT angiogram (CTA) by taking advantage of the ability of modern CT scanners to obtain thin sections very quickly. Although there is currently no absolute consensus as to the optimal CTA scan protocol, in general, thin-section (on the order of 1–2 mm) scanning is performed while rapidly (e.g., over a 10- to 20-second interval for evaluation of cervicocranial vessels) injecting contrast material through an indwelling peripheral intravenous line.[5] Next, the obtained 100 to 200 CT sections can undergo computer processing resulting in an image of only the areas of contrast-enhanced blood (and nothing else), which can be presented as either a 2D (maximum intensity pixel [MIP]) or a 3D (volume-rendered [VR]) image (Fig. 2-4a, b)]. Aneurysms (greater than 3–4 mm in diameter), vascular dissections, and areas of narrowing or occlusion involving larger cervicocranial vessels (e.g., arteries from the level of the aortic arch to the level of the primary terminal branches of the circle of Willis vasculature) can usually be demonstrated eliminating the need for diagnostic endovascular (i.e., utilizing a catheter directly placed within blood vessels see page 47)

TABLE 2-3 ————————————————————————————

INDICATIONS FOR TYPES OF CT SCANNING

Indication for CT Scan	Noncontrast vs. Contrast-Enhanced Scanning
Rule out intracranial hemorrhage	NC
Rule out TIA/stroke[a]	NC ± CT perfusion
Rule out hydrocephalous/increasing ICP[a]	NC
Rule out shunt malfunction[a]	NC
Following trauma	NC ± reformatted images
Rule out mass (no acute symptoms)[a]	CE
Rule out arteriovenous malformation (AVM)[a]	NC & CE
Rule out infection/abscess[a]	NC & CE
Acute mental status changes (rule out acute mass, mass effect, etc.)	NC
Rule out fracture	NC with reformatted images
New onset seizure[a]	NC & CE
Rule out arterial dissection[a]	CTA
Rule out DVST[a]	CTV

NC, noncontrast CT scanning; CE, contrast-enhanced CT scanning; CTA, CT arteriography; CTV, CT venography; TIA, transient ischemic attack; ICP, intracranial pressure; DVST, dural venous sinus thrombosis.
[a]Should also consider MRI.

angiography in many patients. However, the spatial resolution of CTA (on the order of 0.35 mm/pixel) remains inferior to that of endovascular angiography (~0.15 mm/pixel).

Major intracranial venous structures (dural venous sinuses) can also be demonstrated with modern CT scanners by using a technique similar to that used for CTA, but delaying scanning so that venous structures are optimally imaged. Such CT venography (CTV)[6] can be used to assess for dural venous sinus thrombosis (DVST), invasion of dural venous sinuses by neoplasm, etc. This technique is considerably faster than MR venography (MRV) (see page 45), but is considered inferior to MRV due to contrast material administration issues, the use of ionizing radiation, and also with respect to evaluation of some venous structures located either at the skull base or in contiguity with calvaria. Also, associated intraparenchymal abnormalities such as areas of early venous ischemia are better seen on MRI. Rarely, and not reliably, high-attenuation thrombosed cortical veins can be seen on noncontrast CT scans.

CT PERFUSION Perfusion CT scanning[7] takes advantage of the fact that modern CT scanners can evaluate individual sections of the brain in less than 1 second. Contrast material is rapidly injected through a large peripheral intravenous catheter and dedicated selected sections through the brain at several locations are each scanned multiple times. From the collected data, various blood flow parameters, including mean transit time (MTT: how long it takes blood to flow into or through a portion of the brain), cerebral blood flow (CBF: the rate at which blood passes through the brain), and cerebral

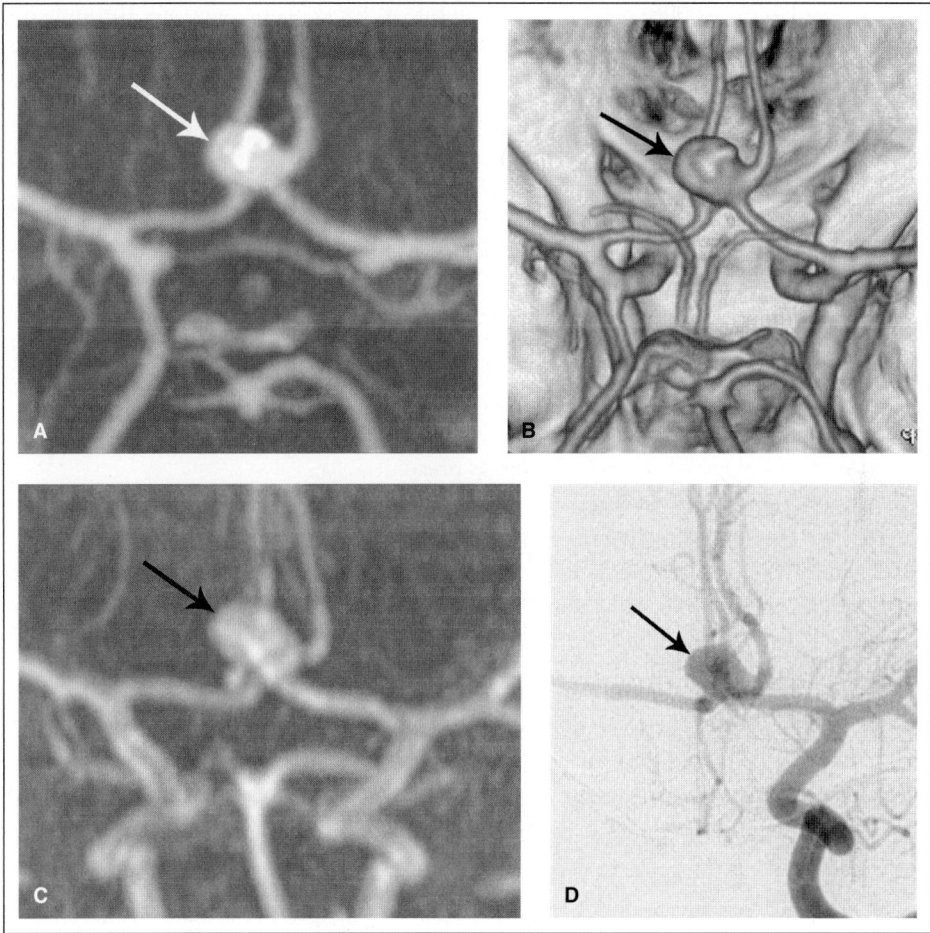

FIGURE 2-4   Anterior communicating artery aneurysm. A 1-cm anterior communicating artery aneurysm (arrows) is seen on (A) 2D CT angiography, (B) 3D CT angiography, (C) MR angiography, and (D) catheter angiography.

blood volume (CBV: the amount of blood in a section of the brain at any given time) among others, can be quantified and demonstrated as color maps.

Recent work suggests that elevated MTT reflects decreased blood perfusion of that area of the brain (which may or may not be a reversible process) and that decreased CBV below a certain threshold may represent irreversibly injured brain. It has been proposed that areas of MTT–CBV "mismatch" might identify penumbra brain that could potentially respond to aggressive therapy[7] in the appropriate clinical setting [see Chapter 5]. Such scanning may be complementary to, or have the potential to replace diffusion/ perfusion MRI (see page 46) for the evaluation of an acute "rule out stroke" patient as an entire perfusion CT takes less than 5 minutes to complete. One of the current limitations of perfusion CT using a 64-slice scanner is that only limited portions of the brain can be evaluated for each perfusion study. However, newer 256-slice CT scanners, which became available in 2008, are able to generate CT perfusion sections through the entire brain. This should make CT perfusion a more viable alternative to diffusion/ perfusion MR.

LIMITATIONS OF CT   While CT is an excellent modality for evaluating the brain, it does have certain limitations:

- "Beam-hardening" (also called Hounsfield) artifacts from scanning through both dense bone and less dense brain on a single section can result in "streak" artifacts on an image, which can limit evaluation of some regions (e.g., posterior fossa, inferior aspects of the temporal lobes, spinal canal).
- Thin lesions that appear on only one or two slices (or even between two slices) can be missed. An important example of this is nondisplaced skull fractures that happen to be oriented in the plane of section of a CT scan.
- "Partial volume artifacts" between two normal structures can result in the appearance of pathology when no pathology is present.
- Calcified blood vessels (e.g., atherosclerotic mineralization within a blood vessel wall) can mimic the "hyperdense vessel sign" of an acute intravascular thrombus.
- Some pathologic processes can take hours to days to manifest on CT (e.g., ischemic changes) and therefore may be missed if CT scanning is performed too soon after an ischemic event at a time when only an MRI scan would be positive. Similarly, a subarachnoid hemorrhage that is more than a week old might be missed on CT as the blood would have "faded" over time (Fig. 2-5).
- Finally, motion artifacts can degrade any CT image.

Magnetic Resonance Imaging

Magnetic resonance imaging (MRI) has been available for clinical use since the early 1980s. Generation of images by MRI is fundamentally different from that by conventional X-rays or CT and is much less intuitive. A full discussion of generation of MR images[8] is beyond the scope of this text but will be briefly summarized.

Conventional MRI is performed by imaging the protons in water molecules and is therefore sometimes called proton-MRI. Water molecules can be thought of as magnetic dipoles, which can "line- up" in the strong magnetic fields used for clinical MRI (e.g., 1.5 T MR machine exposes water molecules to magnetic fields 25,000 times that of the earth's magnetic field). When "lined up" in the strong magnetic field of the MR scanner, the water molecules are considered to be in their respective lowest energy states. The water molecules are then transiently perturbed with a carefully selected radiofrequency pulse, which excites some of the protons in these water molecules to a higher energy state. As the exciting radiofrequency pulse is transmitted only for a fraction of a second, after that pulse has been turned off, the excited protons return to their baseline energy state. As the protons return to their baseline energy state, they give off energy. The rate at which energy is given off is partially determined by the local magnetic environment of each proton (e.g., protons in different tissue environments give off energy at different rates). These rates can be measured and localized in 3D space resulting in an MR image.

There are 20 to 30 parameters that need to be programmed into the MR machine before each scan begins. Fortunately, standard MR scan protocols either come with the respective MR machines from the manufacturer or are set up by physicists/radiologists

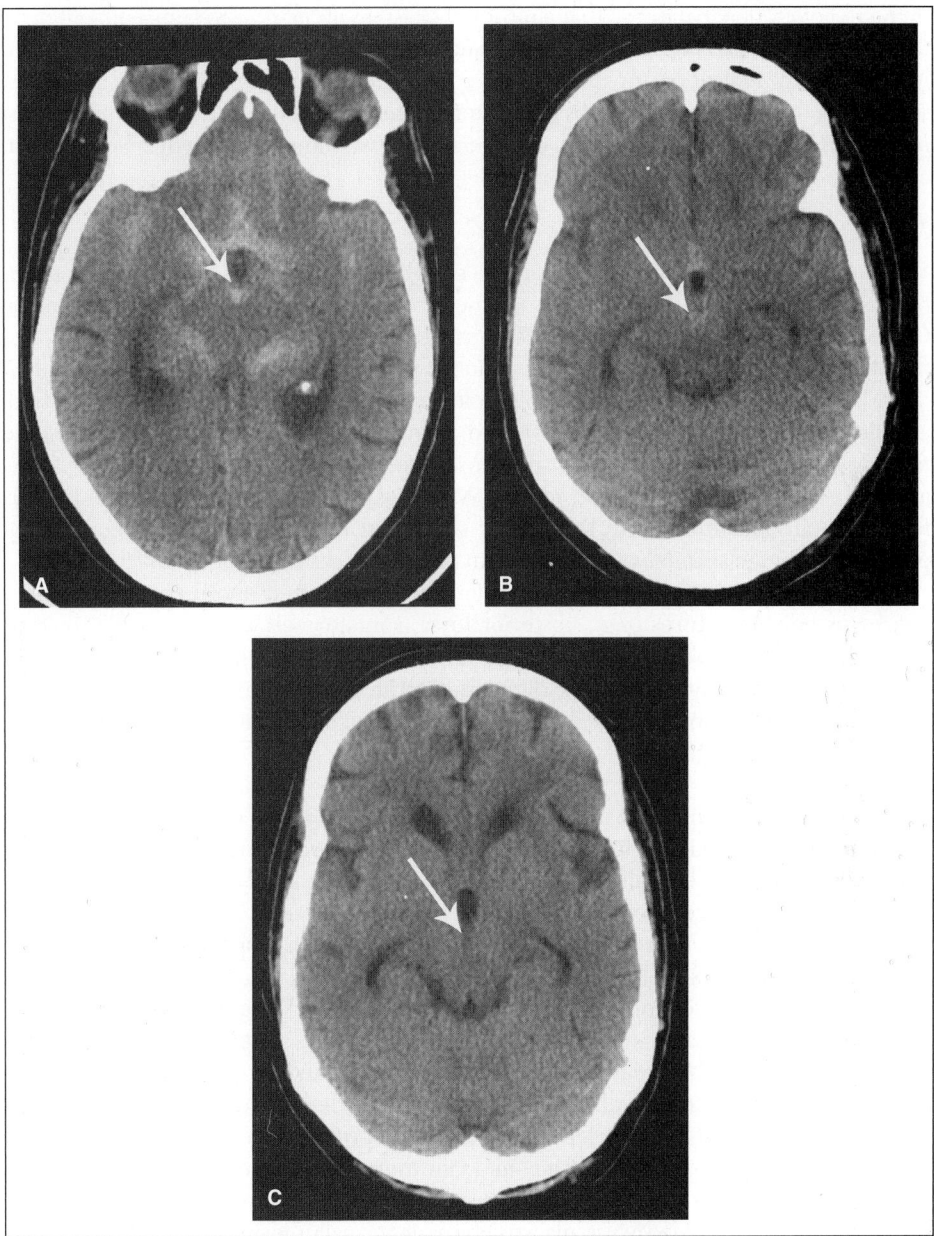

FIGURE 2-5   Fading of subarachnoid hemorrhage over time. CT of aneurysmal SAH demonstrates "fading" of SAH in the interpeduncular cistern (arrows) over time. SAH is well seen on the day of the aneurysm rupture (A), poorly seen 8 days after the bleed (B), and no longer seen 16 days after the bleed (C).

in the radiology department so that almost no decisions about how to scan a patient need to be made by a referring physician (or even the MR technologist) except for determining the clinical indication for the MR scan, determining the region of clinical interest (i.e., the body part to be scanned), determining whether the use of intravenous contrast material is warranted for the study, or determining whether MRI might be contraindicated because of indwelling foreign material.

MRI Concepts

SUPERIORITY TO CT   The major advantage of MRI over CT scanning is the greater *contrast* resolution of MRI. In other words, structures that appear similar, if not identical, on CT scans are often easily resolved on MR scans. This not only improves identification of normal structures but results in better delineation of pathologic processes (Figs. 2-6 to 2-9).

MRI can also demonstrate some physiologic processes such as water motion on both a molecular level (diffusion imaging)[9] and at macroscopic levels (cerebrospinal fluid motion)[10,11] and also the biochemical status of some tissues (MR spectroscopy).[9] The absence of ionizing radiation also renders MRI a safer test than CT. MRI can be performed in any plane unlike CT, which is somewhat limited by the need to reorient patients within the scanner to optimize scan planes.

The beam-hardening artifacts intrinsic to CT mentioned above (page 38) due to nearby osseous structures (e.g., posterior fossa, spinal canal) are not present on MR scans. Similarly, extensive CT artifacts from some indwelling materials (some spinal hardware, aneurysm clips, endovascular coils, etc.) are markedly reduced on MRI. Elimination and/or reduction of these artifacts can result in a nondiagnostic CT study becoming a diagnostic MR study.

MRI LIMITATIONS   An important limitation of MRI with respect to CT is its sensitivity to patient motion as most MR scans take minutes to acquire during which patients must remain motionless or else all acquired images will be degraded (CT scans take on the order of 1–2 seconds or less per section).

Cortical bone is much less well delineated on MR with respect to CT. Therefore, while bone marrow is well delineated on MRI, osseous fractures and certain other processes that result in some osseous pathology are poorly delineated on MRI and require CT (or plain radiography) for evaluation. Similarly, mineralization (e.g., calcification) of normal or abnormal structures is poorly delineated on MRI; in fact, abnormal mineral can result in either abnormally increased or decreased signal on T1- or T2-weighted scans or can be completely occult. Dense proteinaceous fluid collections can appear black on MRI (mimicking air) and can therefore be completely overlooked in certain regions such as the paranasal sinuses.

Normally moving blood in vascular structures or normally moving CSF in the spinal subarachnoid space can result in misleading appearances that can mimic pathology. For example, apparent "brightness" in some blood vessels on noncontrast MR scans can mimic intraluminal pathology. Normal cerebrospinal fluid motion can also result in areas of blackness within the usually white spinal subarachnoid space on T2-weighted scans mimicking subarachnoid space pathologic processes such as vascular malformations and/or cystic masses.

MRI is such a sensitive imaging tool that many clinically insignificant findings can be identified, which can potentially confuse a given clinical presentation; for example, more than half of all people beyond the age of 50 have clinically insignificant "white spots"

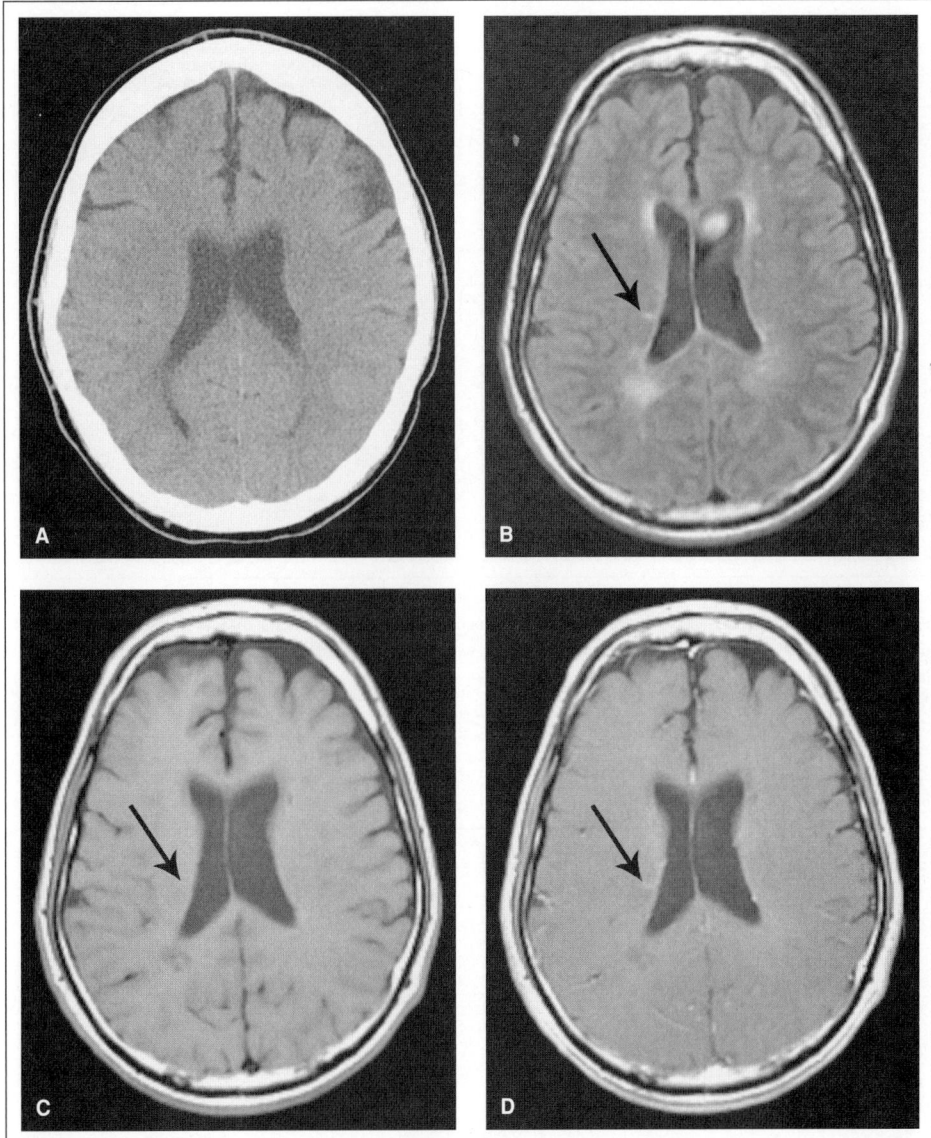

FIGURE 2-6   Multiple sclerosis—MRI better than CT. Acute deterioration in a patient with known demyelinating disease. CT (A) is normal. FLAIR MRI (B) demonstrates multiple periventricular lesions consistent with multiple sclerosis plaques. Noncontrast T1-weighted (C) and contrast-enhanced T1-weighted (D) MRI scans demonstrate an enhancing lesion (arrow) consistent with active demyelination.

(also called white matter hyperintensities [WMHs], unidentified bright objects [UBOs], chronic small vessel ischemic changes of aging, etc.) involving supratentorial white matter on T2-weighted scans,[12] which can mimic pathologic processes.

Up to 15% of patients become claustrophobic when placed within the MR scanner,[13] with a smaller percentage of those patients unable to tolerate scanning despite oral or intravenous sedation for the study. Some patients require general anesthesia to undergo MRI.

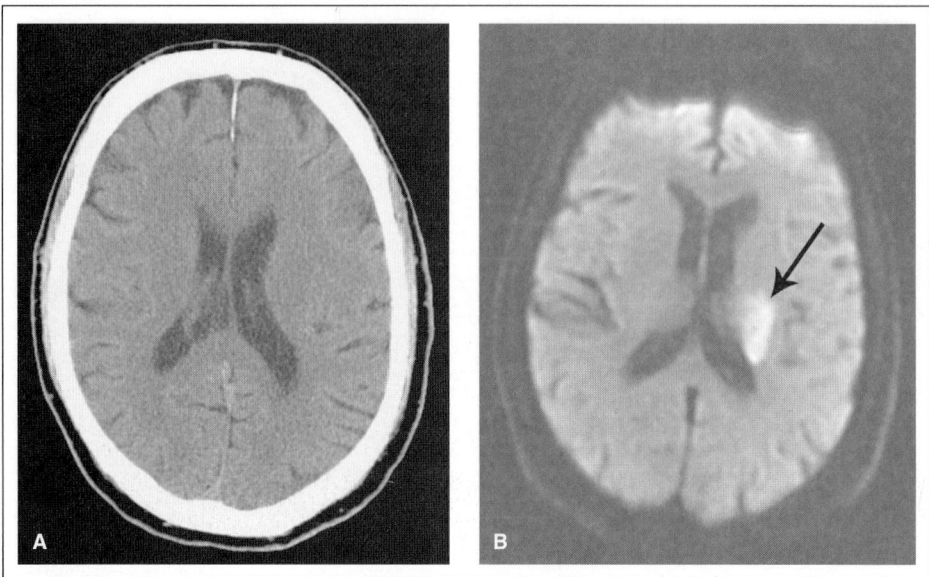

FIGURE 2-7   Acute stroke—MRI better than CT. An acute left corona radiata stroke is not seen on a CT scan obtained 2.5 hours after onset of symptoms (A), but is well seen on the diffusion MRI scan obtained 30 minutes later (B) (arrow).

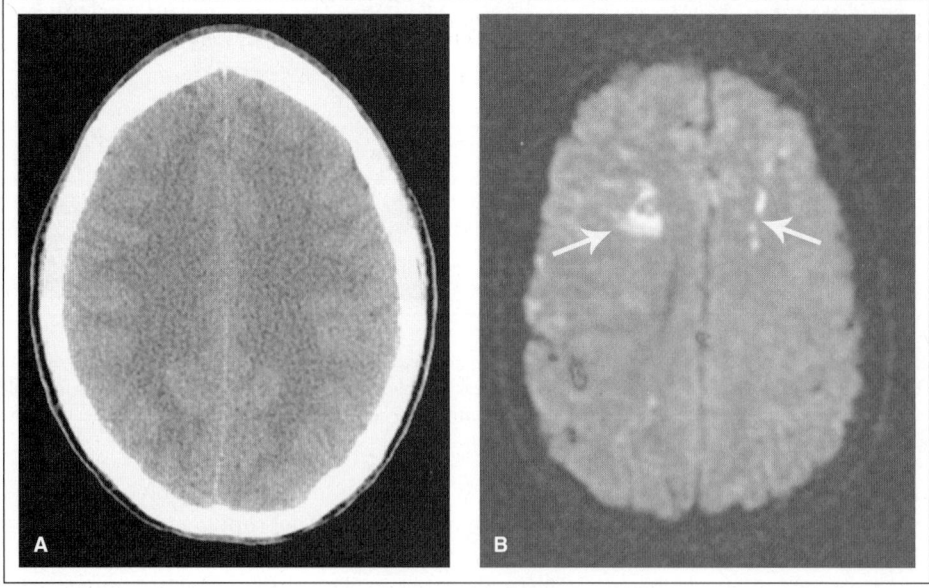

FIGURE 2-8   Diffuse axonal injury—MRI better than CT. A CT scan (A) in an unresponsive patient following high-speed MVA is normal, but diffuse axonal injury is well seen on the diffusion MRI scan (B) (arrows).

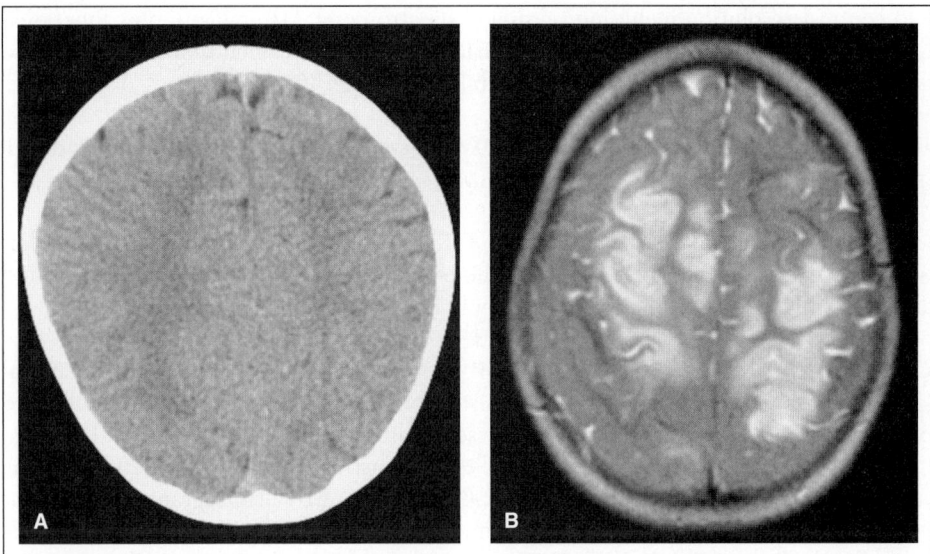

FIGURE 2-9   Encephalitis—MRI better than CT. A CT scan (A) in a febrile, clinically deteriorating 1.5-year-old child is essentially normal. T2-weighted MRI scan (B) demonstrates extensive changes of encephalitis.

While MR scanners have table weight limits less than those of CT scanners (around 350 lb), this is rarely an issue as standard MR gantry diameters are less than that of standard CT scanners (24 vs 28 in) such that it is unusual to successfully place even a 250- to 300-lb patient into a standard MR scanner. Some manufacturers have recently developed 1.5 to 3.0 T MR scanners with gantry diameters of 28 in and table weight limits of 550 lb. Some lower field strength (0.15–1.0 T) "open" MRI scanners have almost limitless weight capacities but suffer from loss of image quality at these lower magnet field strengths.

There is a long list of hardware and other implants that can be placed in situ. Similarly, there are many foreign bodies that may have accidentally or intentionally been placed inside a patient or on the skin. Many of these foreign materials have the potential to move or heat up during an MR scan potentially endangering patients. Patients need to be screened for such materials. There are several good references reviewing which foreign materials contraindicate MR scanning and specifically which materials have been tested for MR compatibility/safety.[14,15] As of 2009, a Web site that is continually updated with respect to compatibility of devices for MR is www.MRIsafety.com. In addition, even some make-up (cosmetics) and some hair products can interfere with the generation of MR images.

FIELD STRENGTH   The "field strength" of an MRI machine refers to the magnetic field within the scanner to which a patient is exposed. Almost all clinical scanners have field strengths between 0.15 T (1500 G) and 3.0 T (30,000 G). Most clinical units currently in use are in the 1.5 to 3.0 T range with the exception of some lower magnetic field strength magnets (0.5–1.0 T), which are found in open machines used for scanning severely claustrophobic or larger patients (at the price of lower image quality). In addition, in the case of 3.0 T vs 1.5 T machines, there are additional advantages beyond the increased spatial and contrast resolution including improved spectroscopy, MR angiography, functional MRI, sensitivity to contrast agents, sensitivity of diffusion imaging sequences for acute ischemic stroke, and sensitivity of susceptibility (see page 46) sequences.

FIELD OF VIEW Issues with scanning FOV are similar to those encountered with CT (see page 32).

INCIDENTALLY IMAGED REGIONS As with CT (see page 33), note should be made that when a given scan is performed, areas of the body that were not intended to be scanned are often still included in the FOV and should be reviewed.

CONTRAST-ENHANCED SCANS As with CT (see page 35), intravenous contrast material (gadolinium-based contrast agents) administration is often necessary to better delineate pathologic processes or to identify otherwise occult pathologic processes on MR scans. Contrast-enhanced scans can also be used to demonstrate "active" vs "inactive" lesions such as in demyelinating disease (Fig. 2-6), optimize MR arteriograms (MRA) and venograms (see below and page 45), perform perfusion MR (see page 46), and also sometimes for localization purposes for MR spectroscopy and/or functional MRI. Although considered a safe drug, gadolinium-based contrast agents have been associated with rare, but serious reactions, including nephrogenic systemic fibrosis (see below).

***NEPHROGENIC SYSTEMIC FIBROSIS*[16,17]** Nephrogenic systemic fibrosis (NSF) is a rare, but serious (sometimes fatal) disease that can occur days to months following the administration of a gadolinium-based contrast agent. This disease has been encountered exclusively in patients with severe renal failure (chronic kidney disease grade 4 or 5; i.e., GFR <30 mL/min).

The FDA recommends that patients with a glomerular filtration rate of less than 30 mL/min *not* be given any gadolinium-based contrast agent. Therefore, no contrast-enhanced MR imaging can be performed in this patient group unless no alternative imaging can be performed and provided that MR contrast material administration is absolutely urgently needed. If such imaging is performed, the radiologist, referring clinician, and the patient must all consent to the procedure and each must acknowledge that they understand the risks of NSF. Such consent should be documented in the patient's medical record.

***MR ANGIOGRAPHY*[18]** MR scanning protocols can be optimized to demonstrate flowing blood in one direction (e.g., cephalad), which can be used to demonstrate blood flow into the head through the arterial system. Such MRA can be used to identify vascular stenosis, occlusions, dissections, and aneurysms, often mitigating the need for endovascular angiography or CTA. While the exact sensitivity and specificity of MRA vs catheter angiography (or CTA) is unknown, if a diagnosis can be made with MRA eliminating the inherent risks (stroke) and expense of catheter angiography and eliminating the nontrivial radiation exposure associated with CT angiography, MRA can be used as an initial essentially noninvasive test to assess for intrinsic vascular pathology.

Some artifacts intrinsic to MRA can be overcome by performing scans (particularly in the superior mediastinum and neck regions) with contrast (gadolinium-based contrast agent) administration.

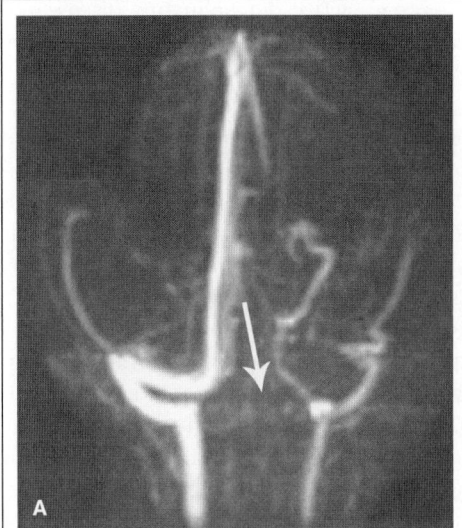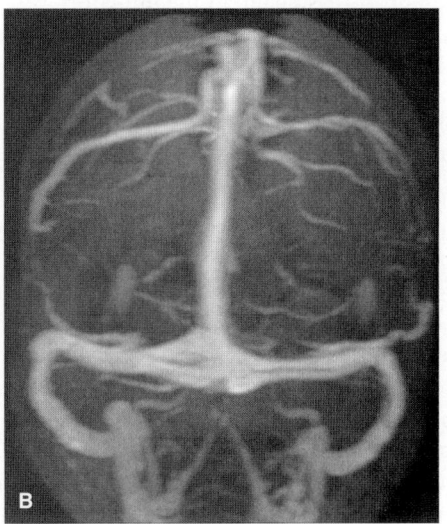

FIGURE 2-10   MR venography. Absence of the left transverse sinus on MR venography (A) (arrow) is consistent with dural venous sinus thrombosis, though confirmation with a structural MRI study was necessary as 14% of cerebral angiograms and 20% of MR venograms normally do not demonstrate a left transverse sinus. For comparison, a normal MR venogram from a patient with a patent left transverse sinus is shown (B).

LIMITATIONS OF MRA   It is recognized that the spatial resolution of MRA is less than that of endovascular catheter angiography. MRA may not even be as good as CTA with respect to image quality because not all MRA artifacts can be overcome with the use of contrast agents and the spatial resolution of MRA is slightly less than that of CTA.

MR VENOGRAPHY   MRV can also be performed using scan protocols that optimize visualization of blood flow in the direction of veins. While multiple MRV scan techniques are currently available (which are often dependent on the manufacturer of the MR machine used), contrast-enhanced "time-of-flight" MRV is currently the most useful (Fig. 2-10). It should be remembered that all MRV studies must be interpreted alongside structural MRI scans as some MRV findings may simply represent normal variant findings and not a pathologic process (as will be confirmed on the standard structural MRI scans).

DIFFUSION MR[9,19]   Diffusion MR (dMR) is an MR technique that takes advantage of the fact that MR scanners can image the (apparent) diffusion of water molecules ("Brownian motion") within tissues. Practically, areas of acute decreased ("impeded") diffusion as seen in acute ischemic events will appear bright (white) on dMR scans and usually (>95%) reflect irreversibly injured (i.e., infarcted) brain. Diffusion imaging is almost always positive within 15 minutes of an irreversible ischemic insult and will remain positive for 7 to 10 days. Beyond 1 to 2 weeks, dMR is no longer sensitive to the detection of areas of recent ischemia. Rarely, even in the presence of ischemia, dMR can initially be negative.

It should be remembered that not all areas of dMR abnormality represent ischemic change as bright (white) areas on dMR scans can also be seen in abscesses, in some tumors, occasionally in inflammatory processes (e.g., active demyelinating disease), in areas of immediate postictal brain, in posttraumatic lesions (e.g., diffuse axonal injury [Fig. 2-8]), and even in some normal variant structures (e.g., some choroid plexus cysts).

PERFUSION MR[9,19]   Similar to CT, (see page 36), MR scans can be rapidly acquired through the entire brain during administration of contrast material, and various parameters related to blood flow through the brain can be calculated and images generated. An image reflecting the overall blood flow through a given region of the brain (perfusion MR [pMR] scan) similar to perfusion CT (mean transit time [MTT] or time to peak [TTP] perfusion CT scans) can be generated. Some researchers believe that when a pMR scan is compared to a dMR scan, it may be possible to differentiate between irreversibly injured and potentially viable brain. Specifically, if a patient's pMR scan demonstrates a brain parenchymal defect that is more extensive than abnormality demonstrated in the same general region on the patient's dMR scan, the difference between the two scans may reflect the "ischemic penumbra" of brain that has not been irreversibly damaged, but might be at risk to go on to irreversible damage if left untreated (Chapter 5). Therefore, such penumbra brain might be amenable to aggressive reperfusion therapy regardless of the age of the lesion. As of 2009, this proposed approach to identifying candidates for reperfusion therapy remains unproven.

SUSCEPTIBILITY AND GRADIENT MR[9,20]   Susceptibility-weighted (SW) MR scans take advantage of differences in local magnetic field inhomogeneities. They are similar to, but more sensitive than, the currently more widely employed gradient recalled echo (GRE) MR scans. Practically, both types of scanning can sometimes reveal small areas of calcium/mineral or subacute blood (i.e., hemorrhage that is hours to days old) that may be occult on all other types of MRI scans. Such imaging may have a role in the evaluation of trauma patients when assessing for diffuse axonal injury (DAI) (Fig. 2-8) and also in patients with unexplained small intraparenchymal hemorrhages (e.g., to search for multiple cavernomas, amyloid angiopathy, etc.).

MR SPECTROSCOPY[9]   MR spectroscopy (MRS) is used to noninvasively create a chemical spectra of a given region of the brain. MRS can be used to characterize some metabolic, inflammatory, infectious, neoplastic, and degenerative disorders. While some work has been done using MRS to identify acute ischemic changes and possibly to identify an ischemic "penumbra,"[21,22] there is currently no defined role for MRS in the evaluation of patients with acute neurologic changes.

MR SUMMARY   In general, MR is better than CT for the evaluation of most central nervous system processes with the exception of assessing for acute hemorrhage or acute fractures. However, a CT scan is still sometimes obtained after an MR scan to better characterize a lesion.

However, indications for emergent MR scanning are somewhat limited (Table 2-4). So, even though MR is better than CT to detect and characterize most acute CNS processes, it does not have to replace CT (which in most emergency department settings is an easier and quicker study to obtain) to answer many emergent clinical questions that may need urgent intervention such as to assess for the presence of increasing intracranial pressure, significant shift of intracranial structures (i.e., significant intracranial

TABLE 2-4

INDICATIONS FOR EMERGENT CNS MR

Spinal cord or cauda equina compression	MRI
Arterial dissection[a]	MRI/MRA
DVST	MRI/MRV
Suspected PRES[b]	MRI
Stroke[b]	MRI, diffusion/perfusion MR, MRA
Encephalitis[b]	MRI
Child abuse[b]	MRI/MRA/MRV

DVST, dural venous sinus thrombosis; PRES, posterior reversible encephalopathy syndrome.
[a]If CTA not available or nondiagnostic, or intracranial ischemia is also of clinical concern.
[b]Relative indications for emergent MRI.

mass effects), to localize intracranial foreign material, to assess for most epidural or subdural hematomas, or to assess for soft tissue injuries. Similarly, assessment for acute encephalitis usually only requires CT scanning to rule out intracranial masses and mass effects and to make sure a lumbar puncture is safe as patient management will be determined in most cases by clinical and CSF findings and not the presence or absence of imaging findings.

Cerebral Angiography

Cerebral angiography, also called endovascular angiography, dates to the 1920s and is considered the best test for evaluation of most intrinsic vascular pathologic processes (Table 2-5). There are many excellent texts that review the technical and diagnostic aspects of this procedure.[23,24]

TABLE 2-5

INDICATIONS FOR EMERGENT CNS ENDOVASCULAR ANGIOGRAPHY

Diagnostic
Evaluation of SAH (with or without proceeding CTA/MRA)
Rule out dissection (if CTA/MRA nondiagnostic)
Rule out ongoing extravasation
Intraoperative: following aneurysm clipping, revascularization procedure, etc.
Rule out vasculitis (usually not emergent)

Therapeutic
Aneurysm treatment
Acute ischemia: thrombolysis, clot retrieval, etc.
Treatment of acute ongoing hemorrhage
Treatment of fistula, AVM (rarely performed emergently)
Dissection—sometimes emergently treated (e.g., stenting)

Most endovascular angiographic examinations are performed via an arterial puncture of a femoral artery with intra-arterial placement of a catheter, which is then fluoroscopically directed to the aortic arch and then through the great vessels (innominate [brachiocephalic], left common carotid and left subclavian arteries) into one or more of the blood vessels that directly supply the brain [carotid and vertebral arteries]. Catheters are sometimes moved intracranially for interventional management of aneurysms, arteriovenous malformations, vasospasm, fistulas, and other pathologic processes. Serial (sometimes hundreds) of X-ray images are obtained while contrast material is injected and passes through the arterial, capillary, and venous vasculature. Data is collected and presented on a computer screen. Extensive "postprocessing" of collected data can also be performed to generate additional (e.g., 3D) images.

Digital Subtraction Angiography

Digital subtraction angiography (DSA) is the current technology used for endovascular angiography. The term refers to the fact that X-ray detectors linked to computers are used to collect the imaging data and present the image on a computer screen (as opposed to on film). Cerebral angiography is performed using intra-*arterial* DSA (IA-DSA) technique. Currently, intra*venous* DSA (IV-DSA) is rarely performed for the evaluation of central nervous system vasculature.

RISKS OF CEREBRAL ANGIOGRAPHY[25]   Besides the usual risks of exposure to contrast material and radiation (which can be quite extensive during some dedicated therapeutic neurointerventional procedures), additional risks of endovascular angiography include *causing a neurologic event* (1%–3%) or death (0.1%) and causing local damage to blood vessels (particularly at the femoral arterial puncture site), resulting in either hematoma or, rarely, a dissection or a pseudoaneurysm. For the most part, these are operator-dependent issues and suggest that only a dedicated team of specialists should be performing these procedures.

Rarely intraprocedural aneurysm rupture also can occur in patients being evaluated for, or treated for, a recent aneurysm rupture. Very rarely, transient (24–48 hours) global amnesia and cortical blindness can occur related to the intra-arterial injection of contrast material. These events have been attributed to vasospasm.

Interventional Cerebral Angiography[26]

Interventional cerebral angiography refers to treating a pathologic process via an endovascular procedure (as opposed to *diagnostic* cerebral angiography, which only identifies a pathologic process that may be treated in the future either with surgery, radiation therapy, endovascular therapy, or not at all). Some processes that are treated endovascularly include aneurysms (often treated emergently), vascular malformations, dural (and cavernous-carotid) fistulas, vasospasm, focal areas of stenosis, stenting across the base of a broad-necked aneurysm to make the aneurysm more amenable to endovascular coiling, preoperative management of some vascular neoplasms, etc. Many interventional cerebral endovascular procedures need to be performed with the patient under general anesthesia.

Myelography[27]

Myelography is a procedure performed to visualize the subarachnoid space of the spinal canal and any pathologic process that encroaches upon, or is within, the subarachnoid space. This procedure has largely been replaced by MRI over the past 20 years, but still has occasional specific indications.

A myelogram is performed by injecting a specific (see page 50) nonionic contrast agent into the thecal sac (subarachnoid space) via a fluoroscopically guided lumbar puncture or a fluoroscopically guided lateral neck (C1-2) puncture. By changing patient positioning to optimize the effects of gravity, the intrathecal contrast material can be moved throughout the spinal canal subarachnoid space and plain radiographs are then obtained visualizing the portion of the spinal canal of clinical interest. The spinal cord and intrathecal portions of nerve roots can be indirectly visualized as normal filling defects within the thecal sac. Intrathecal pathologic processes, which are separate from the spinal cord and nerve roots, will be completely outlined. Extrathecal processes encroaching on the thecal sac will also be identified as contour deformities of the thecal sac. Essentially every myelogram is immediately (within 1–2 hours) followed by a CT scan to better characterize any pathologic process suspected from the myelogram.

Indications for Myelography

As mentioned above, MRI has essentially replaced myelography, particularly for the evaluation of acute onset of neurologic symptoms including pain, radiculopathy, and myelopathy. However, there are instances when myelography is indicated on an emergent basis (Table 2-6).

If symptoms of *acute* spinal cord or cauda equina dysfunction such as in posttraumatic, neoplastic, or inflammatory settings are present and MRI is not available or is contraindicated, myelography followed by CT scanning should be expeditiously performed (Chapter 5). With the exception of the very rare instance of multiple distinct lesions compressing structures in different regions of the spinal canal simultaneously, myelography followed by CT scanning will identify any lesion compressing intracanalicular structures at least as well as MRI.

In patients with spinal hardware that is MR compatible, the clinical region of interest may still be obscured by MR-related artifact from the hardware necessitating performance of myelography followed by CT scanning. Finally, in the immediate postoperative period, new neurologic symptoms may require myelography followed by CT scanning for

TABLE 2-6 ———————————————————————————————————
INDICATIONS FOR EMERGENT MYELOGRAPHY

Spinal cord compression
- If MR not available or contraindicated (e.g., pacemaker)
- If patient body habitus and/or weight precludes MRI
- If internal hardware obscures region of interest on MRI

Patient clinically too unstable for MRI[a]

To assess for CSF leak[a]

Immediate (within several days) postoperative spinal cord/nerve symptoms (MR can be misleading)[a]

"Nondiagnostic" MRI[a]

[a]Relative indications.

evaluation as these patients may have misleading MR scans (i.e., MR scans might suggest spinal canal pathology, which actually represents only expected postoperative change).

Risks/Limitations of Myelography

The use of iodinated contrast material and exposure to ionizing radiation are risks of myelography that are eliminated when MRI is performed. Myelography is invasive as it requires placement of a spinal needle (and contrast material) within the thecal sac. When placed in the lumbar region, needle placement can cause "decompression" below the level of a spinal cord compression, which can result in exacerbation of a patient's spinal cord compression symptomatology.

Even when performing the CT scan after a myelogram, imaging planes are limited in comparison to MRI and characterization/delineation of a pathologic process by CT is usually inferior to MRI due to the inferior contrast resolution of CT, as described above (see page 40).

Myelographic Contrast Agents—Comment

Currently, only certain water-soluble, nonionic iodinated contrast agents are used for myelography (i.e., injected into the subarachnoid space for any reason). Most contrast agents (e.g., even some of the water-soluble, nonionic iodinated contrast agents) are actually contraindicated for injection into the thecal sac. In our opinion, the preferred iodinated contrast agent for myelography is Iohexol (Omnipaque, Amersham Health, Ireland) in a concentration of $\leq$300 mg%, though package inserts should always be consulted.

Ultrasound[28,29]

Ultrasound (US), also called sonography, uses nonionizing electromagnetic radiation to visualize intracorporeal structures including blood vessels. Its main advantages are the lack of any known associated risks (e.g., US does not use ionizing radiation and rarely if ever requires any sort of a contrast agent), portability (particularly important when evaluating acutely ill neonates in an ICU setting), real-time capabilities (for intraoperative use, evaluation of moving structures such as a fetus, the heart, or blood flow), painless nature of the examination, and low cost. It is limited by the necessity of an "acoustic window" (need for a direct route for the US "beam" to access the region of interest without having to pass through intervening osseous or gaseous structures) and relatively low-contrast resolution.

As most bones block US waves, the intracranial compartment can rarely be evaluated in most patients. Exceptions include (a) neonates where fontanelles are still open, (b) intraoperative evaluation of intracranial structures while the overlying calvaria are temporarily absent, (c) some patients through the squamosal portion of the temporal bone (which can be quite thin and allow at least some sound waves to pass through), and (d) through the temporal bone suture regions where flow velocities of the circle of Willis region blood vessels can sometimes be assessed (see page 51).

In the neck, the carotid arterial bifurcation region can usually be assessed with US, but overlying structures preclude evaluation of the mediastinal portion of the common carotid arteries, the mid and distal cervical internal carotid arteries, the skull base portion of the internal carotid arteries, and the thoracic inlet, foraminal transversarial, and intracranial portions of the vertebral arteries.

In the spine, intracanalicular structures cannot be assessed because of overlying vertebral osseous structures. However, intraoperatively (i.e., when posterior spinal osseous structures have been removed), the spinal cord and other spinal canal structures can be evaluated.

Indications for Ultrasonography

For the evaluation of acute neurologic changes in neonates (and fetuses), US is ideal as open fontanelles in neonates act as "acoustic windows" for sonographic examinations. Acute intracranial pathologic processes such as hemorrhage, hydrocephalous, ischemia, some masses, mass effects for whatever reason, and major dural venous sinus thrombosis can often be delineated. US is portable, causes less pain, and does not use ionizing radiation which makes it an ideal imaging tool for evaluating this patient population.

US can be used emergently to evaluate the globe and other intraorbital regions for intraocular pathology including evaluation of the retina (in the setting of trauma) and the orbit as a whole for masses (e.g., retroocular hematoma) or intravascular abnormalities (as might be manifest as reversed flow in an ophthalmic vein in the setting of an acute cavernous-carotid fistula), and even to search for small orbital foreign bodies.

US can be used for the evaluation of patients with TIA, stroke, or other neurologic symptoms[30–32] to assess for intravascular pathology in the neck. It has been used to assess morphology, flow, and plaque density in those portions of the carotid circulation in the neck amenable to evaluation. Areas of vascular narrowing, occlusion, abnormal flow, and/or dissection can sometimes be detected, but evaluation for such pathologic processes with US remains inferior to CTA, MRA, and endovascular angiography as the entire course of cervical vessels cannot be directly assessed with US owing to limited acoustic access. Even if delineated on US, the extent of a lesion or the detection of tandem lesions is often not possible. However, it should be noted that abnormal flow velocities or frank reversal of flow, when detected on US, can be important in the acute evaluation of the cervical vasculature with respect to localizing a potential pathologic process for further evaluation.

While Doppler US can be used to attempt to evaluate flow direction and velocity of *intracranial* vasculature (usually of the vessels of the circle of Willis and the proximal terminal intracranial branches of the circle of Willis) to assess for vasospasm, vascular occlusion, or flow reversal, the significance and reproducibility of such findings remains controversial.

Finally, while emboli from the heart can also be a cause of acute neurologic changes, and the heart is well evaluated with US (to assess for abnormal cardiac motion, valvular disease (e.g., endocarditis), and/or intracardiac thrombi), such evaluation is rarely performed on an emergent basis.

Nuclear Medicine

Nuclear medicine imaging studies involve intravenous injection of a radioactive agent into the body and then using special cameras to identify regions of the body where the injected agent collects. A full range of acute and chronic pathologic processes can be detected using these techniques.

There are essentially no nuclear medicine imaging techniques that are used for the evaluation of acute neurologic changes. The one potential emergent radionuclide study with neurologic indications is a "brain death" perfusion scan. A radiopharmaceutical (usually technectium-99m HMPAO) is injected through a peripheral vein and imaging over the head and neck regions is performed approximately 10 minutes later. If no blood flow (i.e., no radioactivity from the injected agent) is detected in the region of the head, a diagnosis of brain death may be made. Such a test may be necessary on an emergent basis in the setting of the need for timely harvesting of organs for potential transplantation.[33]

SPECIAL TOPICS IN EMERGENT NEUROIMAGING

Mental Status Changes

The differential diagnosis of mental status changes is long and does not always require imaging for evaluation. However, once the decision to image has been made, the type of imaging to be performed is dependent on the primary clinical concern.

Stroke

As of 2009, in the emergent setting, if an ischemic stroke is of clinical concern, the only *imaging* test required is a CT scan to assess for hemorrhage or a nonischemic cause of symptoms. Because 15%–20% of patients with suspected ischemic stroke are actually experiencing other nonischemic intracranial pathologic processes (tumor, infection, hemorrhages not related to ischemia, etc.), such a CT scan usually can rule out these other processes.

The role of head imaging in the setting of a suspected ischemic stroke is further discussed in Chapter 5. For at least the near future, CT will probably remain the emergent imaging modality of choice as CT scans are usually easier to obtain than MR scans, it is easier to monitor a sick patient in a CT area than in an MR area, and CT is currently faster than MR for what is considered a complete evaluation of these patients.

Finally, even though current patient management with respect to the potential use of thrombolytic agents in acute stroke patients is based on the NINDS and subsequent studies (see Chapter 5), which require acute noncontrast CT scanning as the *only* required neuroimaging evaluation, many acute care settings currently have more extensive acute stroke imaging protocols in place, which are directed at identifying either (a) an ischemic penumbra (which may eventually prove to be an indication for aggressive interventional management regardless of the time interval from onset of symptoms) or (b) a large vessel occlusion that might be amenable to endovascular clot retrieval or aggressive local (i.e., intra-arterial) thrombolysis beyond the currently approved FDA therapeutic window for intravenous thrombolytic therapy. Such protocols might include (a) a noncontrast CT followed by a perfusion CT followed by a CTA or (b) a gradient MRI, followed by *d*MRI/*p*MRI, which is followed by an MRA to assess for the presence of acute hemorrhage, an ischemic penumbra, and/or a large blood vessel compromise, respectively, in both protocols.

COMMENT: TREATMENT OPTIONS FOR ACUTE ISCHEMIC STROKE Treatment of acute ischemic stroke with systemic intravenous thrombolysis within 3 hours of onset of patient symptoms has been shown to result in absolute improvement in patient clinical outcome at 3 months and such therapy has had FDA approval for over 10 years.[34] This therapeutic window may soon be extended to 4.5 hours by the FDA.[35] In fact, in 2009, the American Heart Association and the American Stroke Association both endorsed a 4.5 hour treatment window for the use of intravenous tPA in the appropriate acute stroke patient group (see page 134). Local intra-arterial therapy with direct injection of a thrombolytic agent into a clot within an intracranial vessel performed beyond the 3-hour window has also been shown to be of some value,[36] but as of 2009 has not yet been approved by the FDA. Finally, mechanical thrombectomy[37] to achieve vascular recanalization after the accepted 3-hour intravenous thrombolytic therapeutic window was approved by the FDA in 2004 but remains controversial as no randomized control studies with respect to the use of such mechanical devices have yet to be performed.

Therefore, there are multiple therapeutic options available with respect to the management of these patients and such management currently depends on multiple factors, including the experience of the supervising physician in managing acute stroke patients, the interval since onset of symptoms, the imaging identification of an associated large vessel thrombus, the availability of an endovascular neurointerventional team, etc.

Dural Venous Sinus Thrombosis

Dural venous sinus thrombosis (DVST) within a major dural venous sinus blocks egress of blood from the brain, which can result in (venous) ischemia, infarction (often hemorrhagic), and death.

DVST can be evaluated with MR (MRV) (Fig. 2-10) or CT (CT venography).[6] Both imaging modalities utilize intravenous contrast administration, though a less sensitive noncontrast MR technique is also available. MR has the added advantage of being more sensitive than CT to associated intraparenchymal venous ischemic lesions and does not use ionizing radiation.

Cortical venous thrombosis (CVT) is a difficult imaging diagnosis to make, as the normal pattern of cortical venous structures is variable. Occasionally, abnormal increased density on CT or abnormal signal on MR within a cortical vein can suggest CVT.

There is no consensus as to whether CTV or MRV should be used to assess for cortical or dural venous sinus thrombosis. While both are considered sensitive for the detection of dural venous sinus thrombosis (eliminating the need for catheter angiography), disadvantages of both techniques exist. MRV suffers from flow artifacts, the need for contrast material, the need for carefully timed scanning during contrast administration, and the relatively poor delineation of associated *hemorrhagic* strokes, while CTV is associated with the use of ionizing radiation, the need for carefully timed contrast material administration, and potential difficulties in delineating high-attenuation contrast material from nearby high-attenuation calvarial structures. Currently, contrast-enhanced MRV is somewhat preferred because of its high sensitivity and the ability to obtain simultaneous MRI to assess for associated parenchymal brain injuries (i.e., venous infarctions).

Intracranial Mass Effect

Intracranial mass effects can be due to any space-occupying lesion including tumors, infections, hematomas, hydrocephalus for any reason, focal or diffuse cerebral edema associated with a pathologic process, etc. Significant mass effects can almost always be detected on a noncontrast CT scan, though sometimes artifacts intrinsic to CT scanning can limit evaluation of some intracranial regions (e.g., inferior middle cranial fossa, posterior fossa). It should be noted that a normal-appearing CT does not definitely rule out increasing intracranial pressure (e.g., 10% of comatose patients following TBI have increased intracranial pressure and normal head CT scans[38]).

Imaging findings of increasing intracranial pressure on CT include diffuse cerebral edema as manifest by loss of gray matter and white matter differentiation, effacement of sulci, and effacement of the CSF spaces (cisterns) at the base of the brain (e.g., suprasellar cistern) or around the brainstem (e.g., perimesencephalic cistern). The ventricles may be small/effaced when the primary cause of the increased intracranial pressure is cerebral edema. However, the ventricles may be disproportionately enlarged (with the other above-described findings of increasing intracranial pressure unchanged) with associated periventricular decreased attenuation ("transependymal migration of CSF") when acute enlargement of the ventricular system is the cause of the increasing intracranial pressure. When intracranial mass effects are local, one or more herniation syndromes (e.g., transtentorial, uncal, subfalcine, cerebellar tonsillar) may also be present.

Inflammation/Infection

If clinically suspected, treatment of a potential intracranial infectious/inflammatory process is often initiated regardless of imaging findings. However, a noncontrast CT is often obtained to assess for increasing intracranial pressure before a lumbar puncture is performed as CT is at least 90% sensitive for detecting increasing intracranial pressure. Rarely, to increase clinician confidence, an emergent MR study may also be necessary to confirm a clinical impression (Fig. 2-9).

Seizure

As reviewed in Chapter 12, the differential diagnosis of a patient presenting with a seizure is extensive and sometimes does not require any emergent neuroimaging. When emergent imaging evaluation of the intracranial compartment is deemed necessary, non-contrast CT scanning is usually performed to assess for acute increasing intracranial pressure, hemorrhage, mass, mass effect, etc. In some patients, an MR study will follow on a nonemergent basis to more completely evaluate the intracranial compartment (assess for more subtle structural abnormalities, etc.).

Nontraumatic Subarachnoid Hemorrhage (Suspected Aneurysm)

CT can detect as little as a few milliliters of acute subarachnoid hemorrhage (SAH), but can miss much larger amounts of subacute (more than 1-2 weeks old) SAH as such SAH will no longer appear hyperdense (Fig. 2-5). Once an acute SAH has been identified on a noncontrast CT scan (or by a nontraumatic lumbar puncture), further evaluation to rule out a ruptured aneurysm or vascular malformation (AVM) with additional emergent imaging is usually performed. While *diagnostic* endovascular cerebral angiography remains the most sensitive test (approaching 100%) for the detection of aneurysms/AVMs, whether such angiography needs to be performed emergently (or at all in the age of CTA/MRA) is controversial (see Chapter 8).

It is recognized that CTA/MRA regularly misses aneurysms smaller than 3 to 4 mm in diameter. As a screening test, missing such small aneurysms is probably acceptable because the rupture rate for previously unruptured aneurysms less than 10 mm in diameter is on the order of 0.05% annually.[39] However, as the rerupture rate for recently ruptured aneurysms (on the order of 30% within 1 month of initial rupture) is independent of the size of the recently ruptured aneurysm (i.e., small aneurysms rebleed at a rate similar to larger aneurysms), neither CTA nor MRA should be considered adequate for definitively ruling out an aneurysm in the setting of acute SAH. Therefore, while CTA and MRA can comfortably rule in an aneurysm, they cannot rule out an aneurysm and, as such, SAH in the setting of a negative CTA/MRA study requires further evaluation with formal endovascular angiography in a timely manner.[5] Similarly, CTA/MRA evaluation for incremental unruptured aneurysms (i.e., identifying additional unruptured aneurysms in a patient with a ruptured aneurysm already identified on CTA/MRA) is not currently acceptable and also suggests that formal endovascular angiography is necessary in this patient population, though not necessarily on an emergent basis.

In a patient without documented SAH, but with other clinical signs and symptoms that suggest the possibility of an intracranial aneurysm, or, in the setting of SAH, if endovascular angiography is not immediately available, CTA is preferred over MRA for the evaluation of a suspected aneurysm because (a) CTA is a faster study, (b) it is easier to monitor sick patients in a CT scanner than in an MR scanner, (c) less patient cooperation is required for CTA, (d) CTA is associated with fewer artifacts than MRA, (e) there is better evaluation of aneurysm morphology (particularly the neck) with CTA, and (f) there is better assessment of nearby intracranial (osseous) structures with CTA, which can be important in planning a surgical approach.

Nonaccidental Trauma (Child Abuse)[40]

Neonates and small children with a clinical history suspicious for nonaccidental trauma may be imaged for both medical and legal reasons. At a minimum, when imaging is performed, a skeletal survey (including skull imaging in at least two planes) is performed. If there is any suspicion for an intracranial injury, a noncontrast head CT should also be performed. (Note is made that even if a head CT has already been performed, the skull X-ray portion of the skeletal survey should still be performed as linear, nondisplaced calvarial fractures can sometimes be identified on skull radiographs that cannot be seen on either the "scout" images for the CT scan or the axial images from the CT scan.) Often, if clinical suspicion persists, an elective head MRI is then performed to assess for further evidence of multiple intracranial injuries occurring at different points in time and to better assess the extent of injuries.

Trauma—Head

Head injuries are almost always evaluated with a head CT (Chapter 10) to assess for associated hemorrhage, intracranial and extracranial soft tissue injuries, and fractured bones. With the exception of suspected nonaccidental trauma (child abuse; see above), there is no role for plain radiographs in the evaluation of head injuries. Dedicated maxillofacial, orbital, temporal bone and/or skull base CT imaging (i.e., different field of view, usually thinner sections, multiplanar scanning, etc., in comparison to standard head CT scanning) can also be performed as necessary. Significant (i.e., associated with mass effects that might warrant emergent treatment) epidural hematomas (Fig. 2-11), subdural hematomas (Fig. 2-12), intraparenchymal hemorrhages, and/or intraventricular hemorrhages will be adequately delineated on noncontrast CT scans. Occasionally, some of these lesions will need further characterization emergently with MRI (e.g., in regions where CT scanning can be limited by artifact, such as the more caudad portion of the posterior fossa). However, emergent MRI for evaluation of immediate posttraumatic intracranial injuries is usually not necessary. Finally, occasionally, delineation of diffuse axonal injury (DAI) may be clinically important; MRI is the best test for detection of DAI lesions (Fig. 2-8).

Similar to searching for aneurysms, CTA and MRA can be used to search for posttraumatic cervicocranial vascular dissections (see page 59).

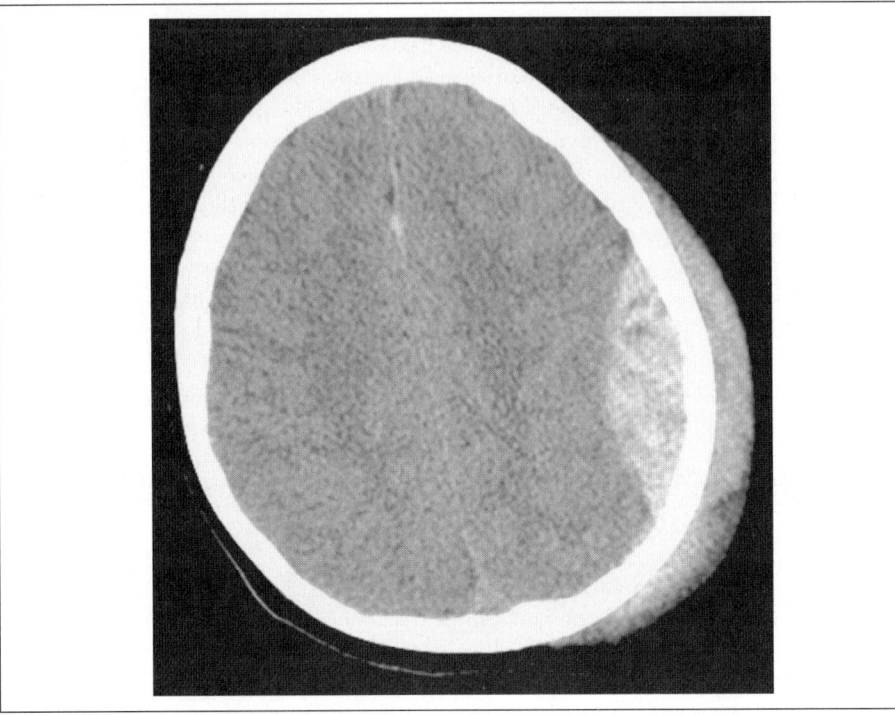

FIGURE 2-11   Epidural hematoma. An acute high-attenuation lenticular epidural hematoma with mass effect on contiguous brain is seen on a noncontrast CT scan. Soft tissue swelling of structures superficial to the calvaria consistent with recent trauma is also seen.

Trauma—Spine[41]

In some patients with spinal trauma, no imaging is necessary as the spine can be "cleared" clinically (see page 272 and Table 10-10). In patients with trauma who cannot have their respective spines cleared clinically and therefore require imaging evaluation, the 2008 American College of Radiology Appropriateness Criteria (ACRAC) for Suspected Spine Trauma states that the sensitivity of plain radiography for cervical spine injury is 52%.[42] The detection of spinal injury by plain radiographs is greater than 50% in the thoracic and lumbar spinal regions in some series. However, even if apparently normal on plain radiographs, certain regions of the spine (e.g., C1 and C2, the cervicothoracic junction, lumbosacral junction, sacrum) are suboptimally evaluated with plain radiographs and can require further evaluation with CT scanning. Similarly, unresponsive and/or altered state of consciousness patients who cannot be examined clinically and/or who cannot describe areas of pain or tenderness should be evaluated with CT.

The 2008 ACRAC for Suspected Spine Trauma also states that the sensitivity of CT for cervical spine injury is approximately 98%.[42] Therefore, it appears that patients with a low likelihood of fracture can be completely evaluated with plain radiographs. Finally, almost all spinal fractures identified on plain radiographs should be further characterized with CT as additional fractures both contiguous and noncontiguous to the known fracture may be found (which are often occult on plain radiographs).

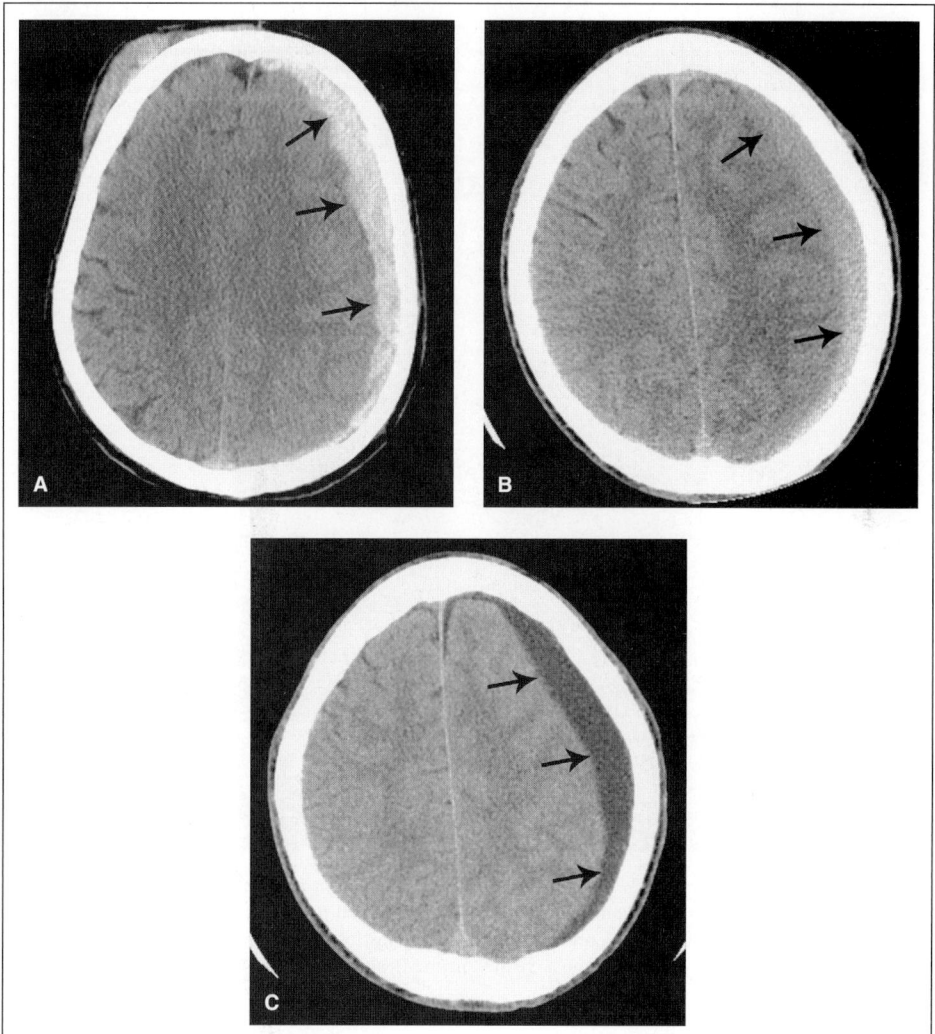

FIGURE 2-12   Subdural hematomas. Typical subdural hematomas are crescentic (arrows). They demonstrate attenuation greater than brain in the acute stage (A), are similar in attenuation to brain in the subacute stage (B), and demonstrate attenuation less than brain in the chronic stage (C).

Carefully performed thin section (1.5- to 2.0-mm section thickness) helical CT scanning with sagittal and coronal reformatted images will identify essentially all spinal fractures. It should be recognized that the imaging work-up of patients with spinal trauma or suspected spinal trauma is an evolving paradigm; this paradigm may progress in the future to the point of requiring CT in all cervical spinal trauma patients if CT scanning is available regardless of plain radiographic findings.

If significant spinal misalignment is identified on plain radiographs or reformatted CT scans, or there are concerning spinal cord or cauda equina neurologic findings (regardless of the findings on plain radiographs or CT scans), emergent spinal MRI

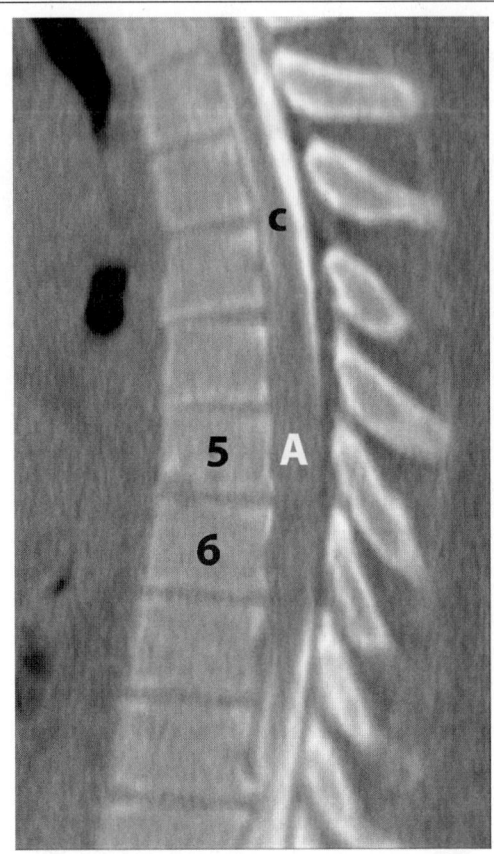

FIGURE 2-13 Abscess compressing spinal cord. A reformatted sagittal postmyelogram CT image in a patient with loss of the ability to walk over the previous 12 hours demonstrates compression of the spinal cord by an epidural abscess. This 355-lb patient was too large to fit in an MR scanner. 5 = T5 vertebral body; 6 = T6 vertebral body; c = spinal cord; A = abscess.

should also be performed to assess for associated intracanalicular injuries such as epidural hematoma, traumatic disc herniation, or frank cord/cauda injury. Note is made that intracanalicular (spinal cord and spinal canal) injuries cannot be ruled out on a noncontrast CT. As mentioned earlier, if MRI is indicated, but not available, further evaluation of the spinal canal and its contents with myelography followed by CT scanning can be performed (Fig. 2-13).[43] Finally, the need for emergent surgical intervention may sometimes take precedence over obtaining CT or MR imaging.

Ligamentous injuries can be missed on static plain radiographic and CT studies. The best test for assessing for significant spinous ligamentous injury is lateral flexion/extension plain radiography, which may not be possible in the immediate posttraumatic period (e.g., posttraumatic cervical myofascial spasm may prevent adequate flexion/extension imaging for 1–2 weeks following trauma). While ligamentous injuries are well delineated on MR imaging, MR scans appear to significantly overestimate the prevalence of significant ligamentous injury.[42,44,45]

Suspected Cervicocranial Vascular Dissection

Cranioverterbral vascular dissection is often due to trauma, which can be major or trivial in degree. Dissections can also be seen in various medical diseases and may even be spontaneous. There are advantages and disadvantages of different imaging techniques for the detection of dissections. US can only directly evaluate the cervicocranial vasculature through limited acoustic "windows" and therefore cannot evaluate the full extent of blood vessels. MRI/MRA, while excellent for delineating intramural hematomata, is limited by the direction and the magnitude of blood flow (i.e., blood vessel narrowing or occlusion can be over/underestimated) and is also limited by areas of mineralization (e.g., calcium-related) artifacts. Endovascular angiography is an invasive test that shows only luminal contour abnormalities and does not directly demonstrate intrinsic vessel wall hematomas. CTA can also be limited by calcified lesions, radiation dose, the use of contrast material, and "timing" issues with respect to the administration of the required contrast material.

Currently, while still controversial,[46,47] on the basis of its relative ease of scheduling, shorter scan times, higher spatial resolution, relative lack of artifacts and good reproducibility, CTA can be considered the imaging examination of choice for the initial evaluation of suspected cervical carotid/vertebral dissection, with MRI/MRA and/or endovascular angiography reserved for problem solving if the CTA is not diagnostic. If associated intracranial ischemia is of clinical concern, MRA/MRI could be performed as the initial study.

Acute Myelopathy (Rule Out Spinal Cord Compression)

As discussed further in Chapter 5, the major concern when a patient presents with a rapidly progressing myelopathy is that there is an acute spinal cord compression due to neoplasm, infection (abscess), or trauma. Although the differential diagnosis of acute myelopathy also includes transverse myelitis and spinal cord infarction, clinically differentiating these pathologic processes from frank spinal cord compression can be difficult in the acute setting and therefore rapid evaluation of these patients is also necessary.

Emergent imaging of the entire spinal canal with MRI to assess for a compressive lesion (and any additional occult non-compressive lesions particularly in the case of metastatic disease, lymphoma, etc.) is necessary in this patient group (Fig. 2-14). Contrast-enhanced scans should also ideally be performed to assess for extent of disease and/or carcinomatous meningitis that might otherwise be missed. If MRI is not available or contraindicated, emergent myelography followed by CT scanning (myelography/CT) can be performed (Fig. 2-13). Myelography/CT will not miss a lesion compressing the spinal cord that an MRI study would identify. In fact, MRI can sometimes be confusing as it can demonstrate incidental insignificant lesions (e.g., bulging discs, moderate degenerative central spinal stenosis, postoperative changes) that can mimic significant acute pathology.

Acute Back Pain

As discussed further in Chapter 15, 50% of patients who have acute onset on new uncomplicated back pain (e.g., new back pain without myelopathy, radiculopathy or weakness in a patient who also has an otherwise uncomplicated past medical history) will feel better within 2 weeks. In 80%–90% of these patients, symptoms will resolve within

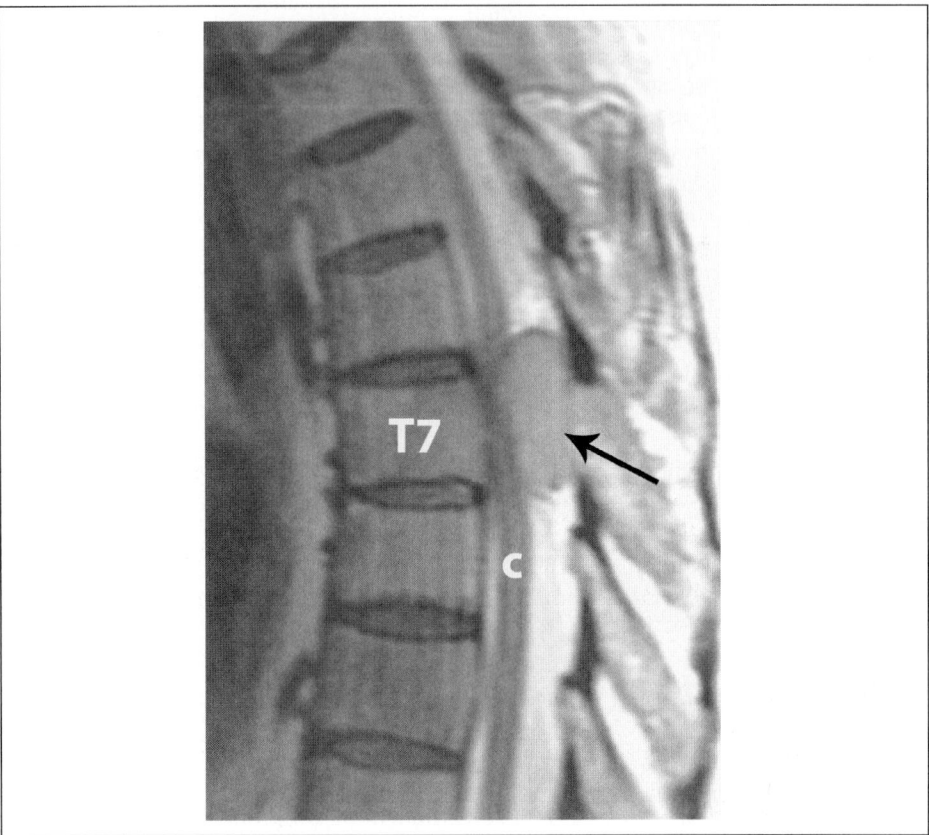

FIGURE 2-14   Metastatic lesion compressing spinal cord. Epidural T7 level small cell lung carcinoma metastasis (→) compressing the midthoracic spinal cord is seen on a sagittal T2-weighted MRI. T7 = T7 vertebral body; c = spinal cord.

3 months.[48] Therefore, in this patient group, no imaging should be considered until at least 8 weeks of symptoms have not responded to conservative therapy.

Patients with new onset back pain with risk factors (i.e., "red flags") for significant spinal pathology should be evaluated in a more urgent manner (see Chapter 15).

When imaging is indicated, ideally, the initial test should be an MRI examination as it yields more information than other imaging examinations without using ionizing radiation. Plain radiographs are of limited value as they cannot demonstrate most spinal pathologic processes that encroach on the distal spinal cord, cauda equina, or exiting nerve roots. They do not demonstrate intracanalicular processes. Even for intrinsic osseous abnormalities, plain radiographs are limited as 30%–75% of the internal architecture (calcium) of a vertebra must be replaced by a pathologic process for that process to manifest on plain X-rays.[49]

Other imaging tests can be used as adjuncts to MRI. CT scanning may be necessary to rule out fractures. Dynamic plain radiography (e.g., lateral flexion and extension X-rays) can be used to assess spinal stability. On a nonemergent basis, nuclear scintigraphy, discography, and angiography can also be considered to further characterize some pathologic spinal processes.

Finally, it should be remembered that many abnormalities on imaging have no clinical correlate. For example, approximately 25% of myelograms, 33% of CT scans, and 40% of MR scans of the lumbosacral spine will reveal abnormalities in asymptomatic individuals with these numbers being even greater in elderly populations.

Appearance of Blood Products in the Central Nervous System

Intracranial blood has a specific appearance on both CT & MRI, which demonstrates reproducible changes over time.

Computed Tomography[50]

The appearance of intracranial blood on CT, and its evolution over time, is somewhat dependent on the location of the hemorrhage—subarachnoid, subdural, epidural, intraventricular, or intraparenchymal. In a nonanemic patient, an acute intracranial hemorrhage demonstrates increased attenuation (whiteness) for about 1 to 2 weeks on CT scans (Fig. 2-12a), assuming the hemorrhage is not rapidly resorbed (as is often the case for SAH). Next, as residual cellular and proteinaceous elements of the hemorrhage are metabolized, hemorrhage resorption continues, and also some hemodilution effects by water absorbed by the subacute clot occur (and assuming that there is no rehemorrhage into the initial area of bleeding), the attenuation of the hemorrhage gradually decreases so that usually within 1 to 3 weeks (but possibly as long as 4–5 weeks depending on the size and hemoglobin concentration of the initial hemorrhage) the bleed can demonstrate attenuation similar to brain (i.e., will become "isodense" to brain) (Fig. 2-12b). After this period, with further dilution and absorption of cellular/proteinaceous elements, the original area of hemorrhage will appear darker than brain ("hypodense" to brain) (Fig. 2-12c). After several months, the attenuation of any residual non-resorbed intraparenchymal or extra-axial blood products will appear similar to that of cerebrospinal fluid.

Mass effect associated with a hemorrhage can initially increase within hours to days of the initial hemorrhage as the new clot absorbs water from surrounding tissue. This mass effect resolves as clot resorption occurs.

The "fading" of extravasated blood on CT scans with time can be problematic when evaluating a patient with subacute symptoms, particularly in patients with SAHs. Specifically, if a patient reports a clinical history suggestive of an acute SAH occurring days to several weeks earlier (see Chapter 8), a CT scan might not reveal any abnormality in the subarachnoid space as subarachnoid blood could be difficult to identify as it might not still be present having been first diluted by CSF and then resorbed because of the rapid turnover of CSF in the subarachnoid space, or, even if present, it would no longer demonstrate high attenuation (Fig. 2-5). MRI, particularly the FLAIR scanning sequence, is excellent for delineating such residual subacute SAH. Therefore, while CT is the best test for identifying *acute* SAH, MRI is a better test for identifying any residual *subacute* SAH that could be missed on CT.

As mentioned above, as normally all intracranial and spinal CSF completely "turns over" approximately four times a day, it is not surprising that over a period of days to several weeks, a SAH could be completely resorbed without any residual CT findings. However, when a hemorrhage is in the subdural region, chronic low-attenuation hemorrhage (i.e., chronic subdural hematoma) may persist for years. Finally, intraparenchymal and intraventricular hemorrhages also tend to be resorbed over weeks to months such that very little residual abnormal fluid (and therefore no abnormality on CT) and no mass effects will remain in the region of the original bleed after several months.

Acute extra-axial blood (e.g., subdural or epidural hemorrhages in particular) when relatively thin and located adjacent to osseous structures can be difficult to differentiate from the contiguous overlying bone as both will demonstrate high attenuation (appear white) on CT scans. As described earlier, the use of appropriate CT "blood" windows can alleviate this problem (Fig. 2-2).

Anemic patients may not demonstrate high-attenuation bleeds on CT even in the acute period. Therefore, an acute intracranial hemorrhage in an anemic patient (hemoglobin on the order of 8–10 g/dL) can appear isodense on an initial CT scan mimicking an older (i.e., subacute several weeks old) bleed.[51]

Magnetic Resonance[52,53]

The appearance of extravascular blood products on T1- and T2-weighted MRI evolve rapidly over time (Table 2-7) as (a) blood proteins (hemoglobin) within extravasated blood cells are metabolized from oxyhemoglobin to deoxyhemoglobin to methemoglobin, (b) cell wall breakdown results in the local environment of methemoglobin changing from intracellular to extracellular within weeks, and (c) extracellular blood breakdown products are eventually metabolized to hemosiderin. The appearance of each of these metabolites over time has a distinct appearance on MRI and this appearance can be used to determine the age of a hemorrhage (or if hemorrhages of different ages are simultaneously present) (Fig. 2-15), which can be of clinical significance.

Like CT, the appearance of intracranial blood on MR and its evolution over time is similar regardless of the location of the hemorrhage—subarachnoid, subdural, epidural, intraventricular, or intraparenchymal, assuming the blood products have not been severely diluted by CSF or frankly resorbed. Again, when a hemorrhage is subdural, chronic fluid collections may persist for years while intraparenchymal, subarachnoid, and intraventricular hemorrhages tend to be resorbed over time such that, with the exception of sometimes identifying some residual abnormal decreased signal in the region of the previous hemorrhage (representing hemosiderin staining of macrophages that retain this resorbed metabolized blood breakdown product), on MR scans, little abnormality and no mass effect will remain in these areas after several months.

TABLE 2-7

MRI APPEARANCE OF CNS BLOOD PRODUCTS OVER TIME[53]

Time After Bleed	Hemoglobin (Hb) State	MRI Signal	
		T1-Weighted	T2-Weighted
0–6 hours	Oxyhemoglobin	↔	↑
6 hours to 3 days	Deoxyhemoglobin	↔↓	↓↓
3 days to a week	metHb (intracellular)	↑↑	↓↓
Weeks	metHb (extracellular)	↑↑	↑↑
Months	Hemosiderin/ferritin	↔↓	↓↓

metHb, methemoglobin; ↔, isointense to brain; ↑, hyperintense to (whiter than) brain; ↓, hypointense to (darker than) brain.

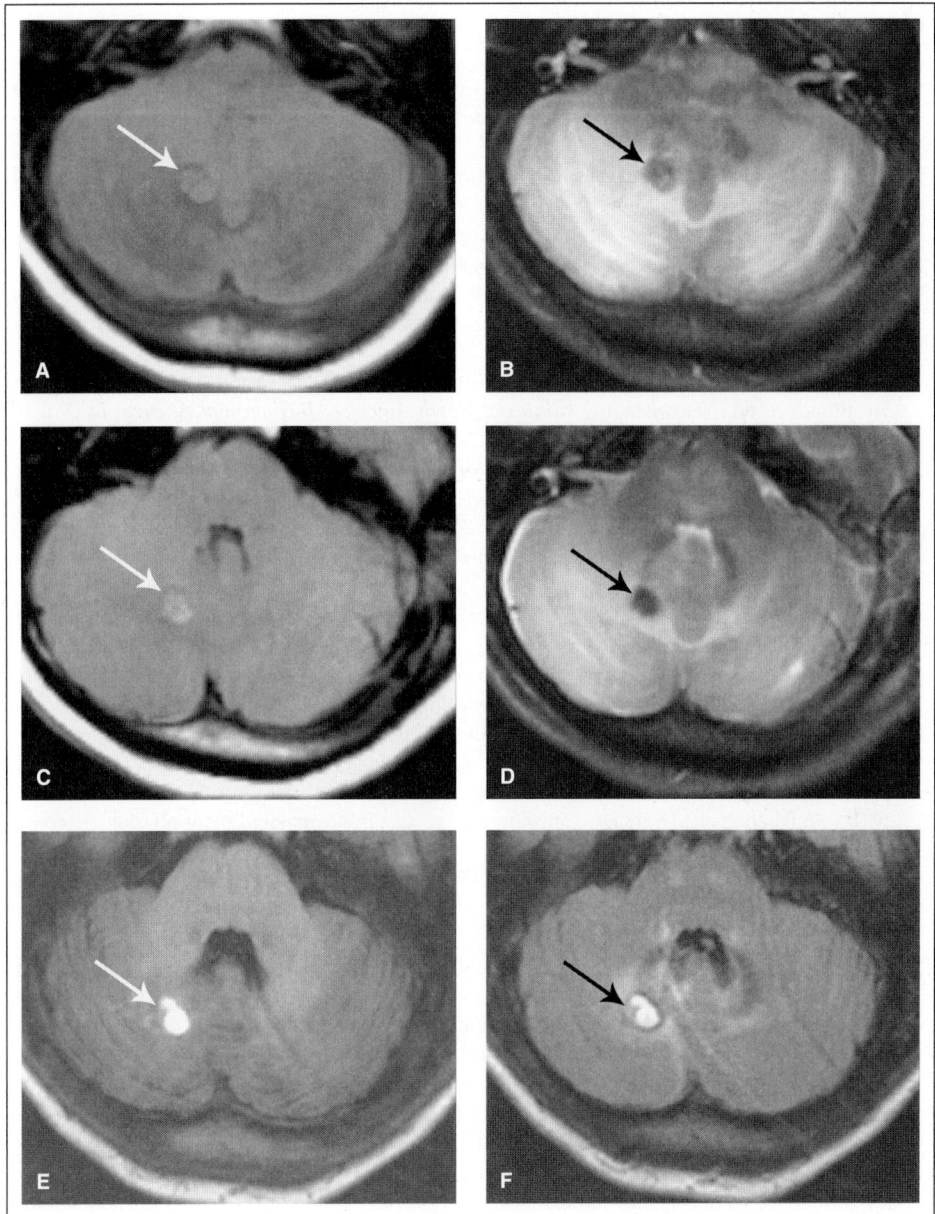

FIGURE 2-15 Evolution of cerebral blood products over time on MRI. A 2-day-old right cerebellar intra-parenchymal hemorrhage demonstrates intermediate signal on a T1-weighted MR scan (A) and decreasing sig-nal on the T2-weighted MR scan (B) due to the presence of intracellular deoxyhemoglobin. Two days later (4 days after the initial hemorrhage), the lesion demonstrates increasing signal on the T1-weighted scan (C) and decreas-ing signal on the T2-weighted scan (D) consistent with intracellular methemoglobin. Finally, 10 days later (14 days after the initial hemorrhage), the lesion demonstrates increasing signal on the T1-weighted scan (E), and also on the T2-weighted scan (F) consistent with extracellular methemoglobin. The age of an intracranial hemorrhage can be inferred by its imaging characteristics.

REFERENCES

1. Goodenough DJ. Tomographic imaging. In: Beutel B, Kundel HL, Van Metter RL, eds. *Handbook of Medical Imaging*. Washington, DC: SPIE Press; 2000:532. *Physics and Psychophysics;* Vol 1.

2. Cohan RA, Kaufman RA, Myers PA, Towbin RB. Cranial CT in the abused child with head injury. *Am J Roentgenol*. 1986;146:97-102.

3. Holmes JF, Akkinepalli R. Computed tomography versus plain radiography to screen for cervical spine injury: a meta-analysis. *J Trauma Inj Infect Crit Care*. 2005;58:902-905.

4. Sundgren PC, Philipp M, Maly PV. Spinal trauma. In: Thurnher MM, ed. *Neuroimaging Clinics of North America: Spinal Imaging: Overview and Update*. Philadelphia: Elsevier; 2007:73-85.

5. Bracard S, Anxionnat R, Picard L. Current diagnostic modalities for intracranial aneurysms. In: Biondi A, ed. *Neuroimaging Clinics of North America: Intracranial Aneurysms*. Vol 16. Philadelphia: Elsevier (Saunders); 2006;391-411.

6. Selim M, Caplan MR. Radiologic diagnosis of cerebral venous thrombosis. In: Caso V, Agnelli G, Paciaroni M, eds. *Handbook on Cerebral Venous Thrombosis*. Basel, Switzerland: Karger Publishing; 2008:96-111.

7. Hoeffner EG, Case I, Jain R, et al. Cerebral perfusion CT: technique and clinical applications. *Radiology*. 2004;231:632–644.

8. Stark DD, Bradley WG, eds. *Magnetic Resonance Imaging*. 3rd ed. St Louis, MO: Mosby; 1999:1-306.

9. Grossman RI, Yousem DM. Techniques in neuroimaging. In: Grossman RI, Yousem DM, eds. *The Requisites: Neuroradiology*. 2nd ed. Philadelphia: Mosby; 2003:1-35.

10. Enzmann DR, Pelc NJ. Normal flow patterns of intracranial and spinal cerebrospinal fluid defined with phase-contrast cine MR imaging. *Radiology*. 1991;178:467-474.

11. Yamada S, Miyazaki M, Kanazawa H, et al. Visualization of cerebrospinal fluid movement with spin labeling at MR imaging: preliminary results in normal and pathophysiologic conditions. *Radiology*. 2008;249:644-652.

12. Cajade-Law AG, Cohen JA, Heier LA. Vascular causes of white matter disease. In: Edwards MK, ed. *Neuroimaging Clinics of North America: White Matter Diseases*. Philadelphia: Saunders; 1993;361-377.

13. Murphy KJ, Brunberg JA. Adult claustrophobia, anxiety and sedation in magnetic resonance imaging. *Magn Reson Imaging*. 1997;15:51-54.

14. Shellock FG. *Reference Manual for Magnetic Resonance Safety, Implants, and Devices:* 2008 ed. Los Angeles, CA: Biomedical Research Publishing Group; 2008.

15. Shellock FG, Spinazzi A. MRI safety update 2008: part 2, screening patients for MRI. *AJR Am J Roentgenol*. 2008;191:1140-1149.

16. Shellock FG, Spinazzi A. MRI safety update 2008: part 1, MRI contrast agents and nephrogenic systemic fibrosis. *AJR Am J Roentgenol*. 2008;191:1-11.

17. Thomsen HS. Nephrogenic systemic fibrosis: a serious late adverse reaction to gadodiamide. *Eur Radiol*. 2006;16:2619-2621.

18. Rubin GD, Rofsky NM, eds. *CT and MR Angiography: Comprehensive Vascular Assessment*. Philadelphia: Lippincott Williams & Wilkins; 2009.

19. Moseley ME, Butts K. Diffusion and perfusion. In: Stark DD, Bradley WG, eds. *Magnetic Resonance Imaging*. 3rd ed. St Louis, MO: Mosby; 1999:1515-1538.

20. Tong KA, Ashwal S, Obenaus A, et al. Susceptibility-weighted MR imaging: a review of clinical applications in children. *Am J Neuroradiol*. 2008;29:9-17.

21. van der Zijden JP, van Eijsden P, de Graaf RA, Dijkhuizen RM. ^{1}H/^{13}C MR spectroscopic imaging of regionally specific metabolic alterations after experimental stroke. *Brain*. 2008; 131:2209-2219.

22. Gillard JH, Barker PB, van Zijl PCM, Bryan RN, Oppenheimer SM. Proton MR spectroscopy in acute middle cerebral artery stroke. *Am J Neuroradiol.* 1996;17:873-886.

23. Osborn A. *Diagnostic Cerebral Angiography*. 2nd ed. Philadelphia: Lippincott Williams & Wilkins; 1999.

24. Morris P, ed. *Practical Neuroangiography*. 2nd ed. Baltimore: Williams & Wilkins; 2006.

25. Morris P. Complications of cerebral angiography. In: Morris P, ed. *Practical Neuroangiography*. 2nd ed. Baltimore: Williams & Wilkins; 2006:63-75.

26. Hurst RW, Rosenwasser RH, eds. *Interventional Neuroradiology*. New York: Informa Healthcare (CRC Press); 2008.

27. Castillo M. Myelography. In: Castillo M, ed. *Neuroradiology Companion: Methods, Guidelines, and Imaging Fundamentals*. 3rd ed. Philadelphia: Lippincott Williams & Wilkins; 2005:16-20.

28. Ma OJ, Mateer JR, Blaivas M. *Emergency Ultrasound*. 2nd ed. New York: McGraw Hill; 2008.

29. Zwiebel W, Pellerito J, eds. *Introduction to Vascular Ultrasonography*. 5th ed. Philadelphia: Elsevier (Saunders); 2005.

30. Chernyshev OY, Garami Z, Calleja S, et al. Yield and accuracy of urgent combined carotid/transcranial ultrasound testing in acute cerebral ischemia. *Stroke.* 2005;36:32-37.

31. Arnold M, Baumgartner RW, Stapf C, et al. Ultrasound diagnosis of spontaneous carotid dissection with isolated Horner syndrome. *Stroke.* 2008;39:82-86.

32. Johnston DCC, Goldstein LB. Clinical carotid endarterectomy decision making: non-invasive vascular imaging vs angiography. *Neurology.* 2001;57:2012-2014.

33. Karcioglu O, Ayrik C, Erbil B. The brain-dead patient or a flower in the vase? The emergency department approach to the preservation of the organ donor. *Eur J Emer Med.* 2003;10:52-57.

34. The National Institute of Neurological Disorders and Stroke rt-PA Stroke Study Group. Tissue plasminogen activator for acute ischemic stroke. *N Engl J Med.* 1995;333:1581-1587.

35. Hacke W, Kaste M, Bluhmki E. Thrombolysis with Alteplase 3 to 4.5 hours after acute ischemic stroke. *N Engl J Med.* 2008;359:1317-1329.

36. Furlan A, Higashida R, Wechsler L, et al. Intra-arterial pro-urokinase for acute ischemic stroke: the PROACT II study: a randomized controlled trial. *JAMA.* 1999;282:2003-2011.

37. Smith W, Sung G, Saver J, et al. Mechanical thrombectomy for acute ischemic stroke: final results of the multi-MERCI trial. *Stroke.* 2008;39:1205-1212.

38. Mayer SA, Chong JY. Critical care management of increased intracranial pressure. *J Intensive Care Med.* 2002;17:55-67.

39. International Study of Unruptured Intracranial Aneurysms Investigators. Unruptured intracranial aneurysms—risk of rupture and risks of surgical intervention. *N Engl J Med.* 1998;339:1725-1733.

40. Hornor G. Physical abuse: recognition and reporting. *J Pediatr Health Care.* 2005;19:4-11.

41. France JC, Bono CM, Vaccaro AR. Initial radiographic evaluation of the spine after trauma: when, what, where, and how to image the acutely traumatized spine. *J Orthop Trauma.* 2005;19:640-649.

42. Daffner RH, Hackney DB, Dalinka MK, et al. Expert panel on musculoskeletal and neurologic imaging. *Suspected Spine Trauma* [Online publication]. Reston, VA: American College of Radiology (ACR); 2007. http://www.guideline.gov/summary/summary.aspx?doc_id=11597. Accessed November 7, 2009.

43. Quint D. Indications for emergent MRI of the central nervous system. *JAMA.* 2000;283:853-855.

44. Sliker CW, Mirvis SE, Shanmuganathan K. Assessing cervical spine stability in obtunded blunt trauma patients: review of the medical literature. *Radiology.* 2005;234:733-739.

45. Daffner R, Hackney D. ACR Appropriateness criteria on suspected spine trauma. *J Am Coll Radiol.* 2007;4:762-775.

46. Provenzale JM. MRI and MRA for evaluation of dissection of craniocerebral arteries: lessons from the medical literature. *Emer Radiol.* 2009;16:185-193.
47. Vertinsky AT, Schwartz NE, Fischbein NJ, et al. Comparison of multidetector CT angiography and MR imaging of cervical artery dissection. *Am J Neuroradiol.* 2008;29;1753-1760.
48. Andersson GB. Epidemiological features of chronic low-back pain. *Lancet.* 1999;354:581-585.
49. Hamaoka T, Madewell JE, Podoloff DA, Hortobagyi GN, Ueno NT. Bone imaging in metastatic breast cancer. *J Clin Oncol.* 2004;22:2942-2953.
50. Scotti G, Terbrugge K, Melançon D, Bélanger G. Evaluation of the age of subdural hematomas by computerized tomography. *J Neurosurg.* 1977;47:311-317.
51. Smith WP, Batnitzky S, Rengachary. Acute isodense subdural hematomas: a problem in anemic patients. *AJR Am J Roengtenol.* 1981; 136:543-546.
52. Gomori JM, Grossman RI, Goldberg HI, Zimmerman RA, Bilaniuk LT. Intracranial hematomas: imaging by high-field MR. *Radiology.* 1985;157:87-93.
53. Bradley WG. Hemorrhage. In: Stark DD, Bradley WG, eds. *Magnetic Resonance Imaging.* 3rd ed. St Louis, MO: Mosby; 1999:1329-1346.

3

INITIAL EVALUATION
OF A NEUROLOGIC
COMPLAINT

BASIC PRINCIPLES

Evaluation of the patient with an acute neurologic complaint requires a carefully focused clinical history and physical examination. In the emergency department or outpatient setting, there is not much time for a full classic evaluation. Patients must be seen expeditiously and decisions made rapidly. The general neurologic examination done electively in a neurologist's office is simply not appropriate for most emergency settings. The goal of the emergency neurologic evaluation is to identify rapidly progressive or life-threatening processes that cannot wait for more leisurely evaluation. No one can review all aspects of a patient's medical history or perform a full general and neurologic examination each time a patient is seen. The neurologic examination needs to be focused. When time is limited, the three key items in a neurologic examination are as follows: hear them talk, watch them walk, and look at their eyes. These three simple acts can evaluate much of the nervous system and will be the guide to a more detailed neurologic evaluation. If the physician can keep these three basic principles—hear them talk, watch them walk, and look at their eyes—in mind, the vast majority of diseases with active physical manifestations will be detected.

The fundamental question as to what should and should not be included in the evaluation of any given patient's specific neurologic complaint in an acute care setting has never been fully delineated and remains up to the discretion of the individual physician. Increased patient loads have resulted in physicians reevaluating the value of the need to perform certain neurologic testing in every patient. This chapter will focus on what may be considered the most useful and least productive parts of the classic neurologic examination.

Most of a neurologic evaluation can be performed by simple observation. There are four major ways in which the nervous system can manifest pathology. Ablative or deficiency problems will present with a lack of ability of the nervous system to perform a specific function. This may mean destruction or functional impairment of specific nervous system tracts. Inability to move an extremity following a hemispheric infarction is an example of this

TABLE 3-1

SUMMARY OF NERVOUS SYSTEM RESPONSE TO DISEASE

Disease	Type of Loss	Example
Ablative	Interruption of nervous tract or inability to initiate a specific activity	Paralysis following a cerebral vascular lesion
Irritative phenomena	Overabundance or abnormal nervous system discharge	Major motor seizure
Release phenomena	Inability to control initiated activities	Hyperreflexia and spasticity
Compensation	Integration of various other nervous system functions to adjust for other nervous system deficits	Circumduction of a paralyzed limb

phenomenon. An irritative phenomenon indicates that a specific tract is intact but that either increased normal impulses or abnormal impulses are being transmitted. The most graphic example of an irritative phenomenon is a major motor seizure. Release syndromes indicate that the nervous system has lost the ability to coordinate control and/or temper various activities once they have been initiated. The hyperreflexia and spasticity seen in patients with upper motor neuron lesions or the motor rebound phenomena seen in patients with cerebellar disease are illustrative of the release phenomena. Compensation phenomena are seen throughout the nervous system. The body adjusts its approach to solving specific problems by compensating for deficits. The head tilt seen in ocular nerve palsies and the circumduction of a paretic limb are examples of the compensation phenomena.

Careful attention to these four major manifestations of nervous system disease during history taking and the physical examination is important to making a diagnosis (Table 3-1).

History

The historical features of a potential pathologic neurologic process are important to the understanding of the disease and need to be elucidated when obtaining a neurologic history. Manner of onset, duration of the symptoms, and exacerbating or mitigating factors of any symptoms should be reviewed. Current concomitant illnesses, medications, and previous similar episodes are also important aspects of history taking. Recent travel may also be of importance.[1]

Some general concepts about neurologic disease can be stated. The pace of onset and progression of symptoms help delineate the disease process involved.[1]

1. *Rapid onset:* Vascular disease generally presents with a rapid onset, and the maximum deficit is usually manifested almost immediately.[1,2] A major hemorrhage or cerebral infarction may result in a very large functional deficit, which tends to improve with time. Multiple small cerebral infarctions also can result in a rapid

TABLE 3-2

SUMMARY TIME COURSE OF NEUROLOGIC PROBLEMS

Time Course	Neurologic Diseases
Seconds to minutes	Vascular
Minutes to hours	Metabolic
Hours to days	Metabolic or infection
Days to weeks	Infection; tumor; compressive masses
Months to years	Slow tumors or degenerative disease

onset of more minor neurologic symptomatology; with each new infarction, symptoms can progress reflecting involvement of greater areas of the brain. A transient ischemic attack (TIA) should be considered the forerunner of a stroke. At least 10% of strokes are preceded by TIA in the 3 months before the stroke; 33% in the 3 years before a stroke.[1] TIAs initially present with maximal deficit and then clear without any neurologic residual within a few minutes to a few hours.[2]

2. *Slow onset—variable course:* Degenerative disease and neoplasms are disease entities that generally follow a mildly undulating but overall downhill course, usually in the order of months and sometimes years. They are generally not associated with sudden acute changes in neurologic status, but tend to be unrelenting in their symptomatology.[3]

3. *Variable onset—changing rapidly from symptomatic to asymptomatic:* Multiple, anatomically unrelated areas of varied symptoms and signs along with and fluctuating physical examinations are an example of this phenomenon. Such a course is often seen in demyelinating disease, such as multiple sclerosis.[4]

4. *Rapidly reversible diffuse process:* Transient reversible neurologic processes are those that affect the central nervous system (CNS) through compromise of the supply of oxygen or nutrients to the CNS or involve chemical substances that may depress or otherwise alter neurologic function. These processes, such as toxic ingestions, hypoglycemia, hypokalemia, or uremia generally result in diffuse nonfocal alterations of the central or peripheral nervous system that improve with resolution of the underlying problem. In the case of hypoglycemia, focal findings can occur and may represent a false localizing sign.

In the urgent or emergent settings, elicited clinical history must be specifically targeted toward the chief complaint of the patient (Table 3-2). It is important that for each chief complaint, positive and negative information pertinent to potential differential diagnoses be obtained from the patient (Table 3-3).

PHYSICAL EXAMINATION

The nervous system can be altered by pathology involving any organ system of the body.[3] The foundation of a proper neurologic examination is a careful physical examination.[4] Consider framing the complaint/examination in the context of the general approach when you enter the room, e.g., body position; then determining symmetric versus asymmetric, central versus peripheral.

TABLE 3-3

SPECIFIC HISTORICAL FEATURES IN NEUROLOGIC DISEASE

Chief Complaint	Historical Features
Coma or altered mental status	History taken from family and friends, etc.; trauma, drugs, alcohol, seizure history, kidney disease, heart disease, previous episodes
Stroke (acute lateralized deficit)	General neurologic history; area of maximum deficit; time course; previous episodes; cardiovascular disease; diabetes; drug usage
Seizures	History obtained from witnesses; the current antiepileptic medications, other medication and drug usage; other metabolic diseases; present length of time unconsciousness; approximate rate and pattern of recovery; presence of single or multiple seizures; history of trauma or other underlying conditions
Headaches	Basic headache history; current mode of onset; location, duration, pulsations; associated weakness, numbness, visual problems, nausea, vomiting; relationship to food intake; time of year; activity loss of consciousness; trauma; medications
Minor head trauma	Nature and type of trauma, loss of consciousness, specific focal symptoms, generalized systemic symptoms
Dizziness	Rate of onset, duration, exacerbating factors; presence of sensation of movement, presence of sensation of fainting; visual, auditory changes; nausea, vomiting; drug history, medications; current illnesses
Syncope	General medical conditions; medications and drug usage; activity at the time of syncopal episode; length of loss of consciousness; presence or absence of seizure activity; presence of pulses; heart rate during the episode; previous episodes
Double vision, blindness	General medical conditions; current medications, drugs or concomitant neurologic disease; bilateral or unilateral change in vision; type of loss (i.e., peripheral, central, total); patient's usual visual status; trauma; current infection; other related neurologic symptomatology; pain

Vital Signs

Appropriate vital signs are important and should be reviewed. The nervous system can be dramatically altered by inadequate cardiac output, e.g., from arrhythmias or shock.[3,5] Likewise, hypertension in extreme cases can severely alter neurologic function. Extremes of temperature, either hyperthermia or hypothermia, can markedly affect mental status and general nervous system functioning. Arrhythmias may be associated with or be the result of acute vascular events affecting the nervous system. Relatively small changes in oxygen saturation in previously compromised pulmonary patients can negatively affect mental status.

General Physical

Evaluation of a neurologic complaint may require special attention to selected aspects of the general physical examination.[6] Examination of the head and neck, paying particular attention to bruises and palpable areas of tenderness or deformity, is important in cases of suspected trauma. General examination of the limbs and trunk may give clues about the possibility of trauma or underlying disease. The cardiac examination may be extremely useful in a patient complaining of intermittent weakness, dizziness, or focal deficits.

Lateral tongue biting, when present, has a high association with a recent major motor seizure.[7]

NEUROLOGIC EXAMINATION

The emergency neurologic examination will not be the same as the examination performed in a neurologist's office. It should be tailored so that the examining physician may arrive at the underlying diagnosis in the most judicious manner. Modifications of the neurologic examination will be required depending on the chief complaint of the patient. The basic underlying examination points (hear them talk, watch them walk, look at their eyes) are still valid. They form the core of the neurologic examination.

Mental Status

Mental status examination is generally carried out while the history is being obtained.[4] A full formal mental status examination is usually not required in the emergency setting for most chief complaints. The manner in which a patient understands and answers questions and is concerned and involved with his or her own chief complaint is the best general assessment of mental status.[8] Many patients who appear "normal" are quite compromised and at a minimum an assessment of orientation should be performed when a more complete and detailed mental status examination is required. A common approach to follow is based on the mnemonic "Jim A. Motsig."[9] This mnemonic mixes the neurologic and the psychiatric mental status examinations. These two distinct pathways—organic and psychiatric—must be kept separate to be able to distinguish encephalopathy from dementia or acute psychiatric deterioration.

J (Judgment)—Tested by problem solving and situational analysis, i.e., "How would you find your way if you were lost in a city?"

I (Intelligence)—Depending on the patient's previous level of education and functioning, i.e., choice of words, general vocabulary, problem-solving ability. This is not a true test of intelligence, which is impossible to test in an emergent setting, but more an assessment of expected function.

M (Memory)—Three types: instantaneous memory (the ability to repeat back something said within the past minute); short-term memory (remembrance of events that have taken place within the past few hours or days); and past memory (what is remembered from the patient's more remote past). Memory is dependent on attention, so attention must be assessed before memory.

A (Affect)—The patients' basic response to the disease process. Are they appropriate to the current clinical situation? Are they indifferent to a severe functional deficit? Or, are they inappropriately upset and/or anguished over essentially no problem?

M (Mood)—Is the patient appropriately angry or sad in the context of ongoing events?

O (Orientation)—To time, person, place.

T (Thought processes and content)—What thoughts are preoccupying the patients? Do they have unusual or bizarre delusions about their disease processes?

S (Speech)—Presence of aphasia, dysphasia, dysarthrias. Rate and cadence of speech are important.

I (Insight)—Does the patient have any understanding of his or her disease process and its relation to the current clinical situation?

G (Grooming)—Can the patient dress appropriately and care for his or her body in an appropriate manner?

The key to the mental status examination is in evaluating the story the patient is telling. Orientation to time and place as well as being able to relate the historical events of the illness is the core to understanding the patient. If there are two areas of mental status that stand out above all others in importance, it is the general level of alertness of the patient and their speech and language.[3,6,10] Not only does speech test the inventory of cortical function with regard to language, but also incoordination of such output may reflect a dysarthria. In testing memory it is good to remember that different types of memory are processed in different parts of the brain. Remember that remote memory may be well maintained in patients who have transient global amnesia, who may have little or no memory of what has happened over the last few days. Likewise, patients can have excellent memory of their past life and yet cannot remember three objects assigned to them to recall over a period of 5 minutes. Such deficits may indicate an inability to form or imprint new memory. The general level of wakefulness, the speed and smoothness of speech, and their participation and involvement with their own health care should also help guide a clinician in determining whether further mental status evaluation is required. In no other area is expansion or contraction of a focused examination as important as in these cortical evaluations.

The goal of mental status testing is to rapidly determine whether a more complex, detailed evaluation is required. Excellent tests of general functioning, besides just listening to the patient talk, include simple yet sensitive indicators of patient performance. The first of these is three-object retention. Simply retaining the memory of three dissimilar objects over the period of the evaluation is a good general indicator of the patient's cortical function. An excellent combination test is one that involves three separate parts: right–left orientation, crossing the midline of the body, and movement without the aid of vision. The patient is asked to remember three separate commands and not to begin them until all parts have been given. The patient is then asked to close the eyes, take the right thumb and touch the left ear, and then stick out the tongue. This deceptively simple maneuver tests multiple areas of the cortex. In general, a patient who can perform a three-part test with crossing the midline motor activities, without the use of visual input, has reasonable alertness and mental status functioning. Such testing can give the emergency physician an indication as to whether the patient can function in an outpatient setting.

In patients who seem to perform basic tests well, the use of double-linked but unrelated questions can be useful in sorting out fine and more subtle cortical problems. If a patient is asked a question such as, "do you walk to work or do you carry your lunch?" they must recognize that these two questions are unrelated. If they are unable to do so, more detailed mental status testing may be required. This type of question is best used in the patient who seems just minimally slow in their responses or just mildly confusional.[4]

In patients with bizarre thought disorders, the actual neurologic functioning in terms of speech and memory retention may be intact and yet thinking may actually be deranged. A provocative question such as "do helicopters eat their young?" will occasionally provoke bizarre responses from patients suffering from major thought disorders. Such bizarre responses would then require a psychiatric evaluation.

It may be useful to ask patients about major psychotic symptoms. If there is concern that the patient may be "hearing voices," it is perfectly reasonable to specifically ask the patient about this. Any crisis that can be brought out in the relatively controlled acute care setting can be better handled than allowing the condition to go undiagnosed and untreated. Agitated patients in psychotic states frequently wish to discuss symptoms that are troubling them.

Assessment of speech is essential in the evaluation of a patient's mental process. It is important to remember that speech is processed at multiple levels in the brain including reception (auditory), understanding, initiation, and mechanical production. Lesions along any part of these brain pathways can result in abnormal speech.[11,12] Whether we are conscious of it or not, we test speech on every human being with whom we interact. Speech has a cadence and a rhythm. Abnormalities in the usual rhythmic flow of speech should be noted. The rate of speech and word-finding abilities are also essential elements of the communication process.

In testing speech, it is important to understand that the patient may have only a hearing difficulty.[4] If the patient does not initially respond to an examiner, asking questions in a louder, more direct voice or with the patient having a full view of the examiner's lips may increase responsiveness. Asking simple yes/no questions and then expanding to more complex questions should be performed if the patient seems to have communication difficulties. The spontaneity of speech is also important. For a patient who is carrying on normal conversation with rapid, well-articulated speech, it is generally unnecessary to test any other specific areas. Fluent speech generally means that the motor system is intact. Unusually paraphasic or meaningless speech can be indicative of a Wernicke's type aphasia. Assessment of the aphasias/dysphasias is outlined in Figure 3-1.

The terminology in abnormalities of speech is often confusing. The term *aphasia* should be reserved for a lack or absence of speech. Dysphasia is a term used to indicate any disorders of speech involving understanding, thought, or word finding.[4,6,7] The term *Broca's aphasia* is often synonymous with expressive aphasia and is a motor initiation

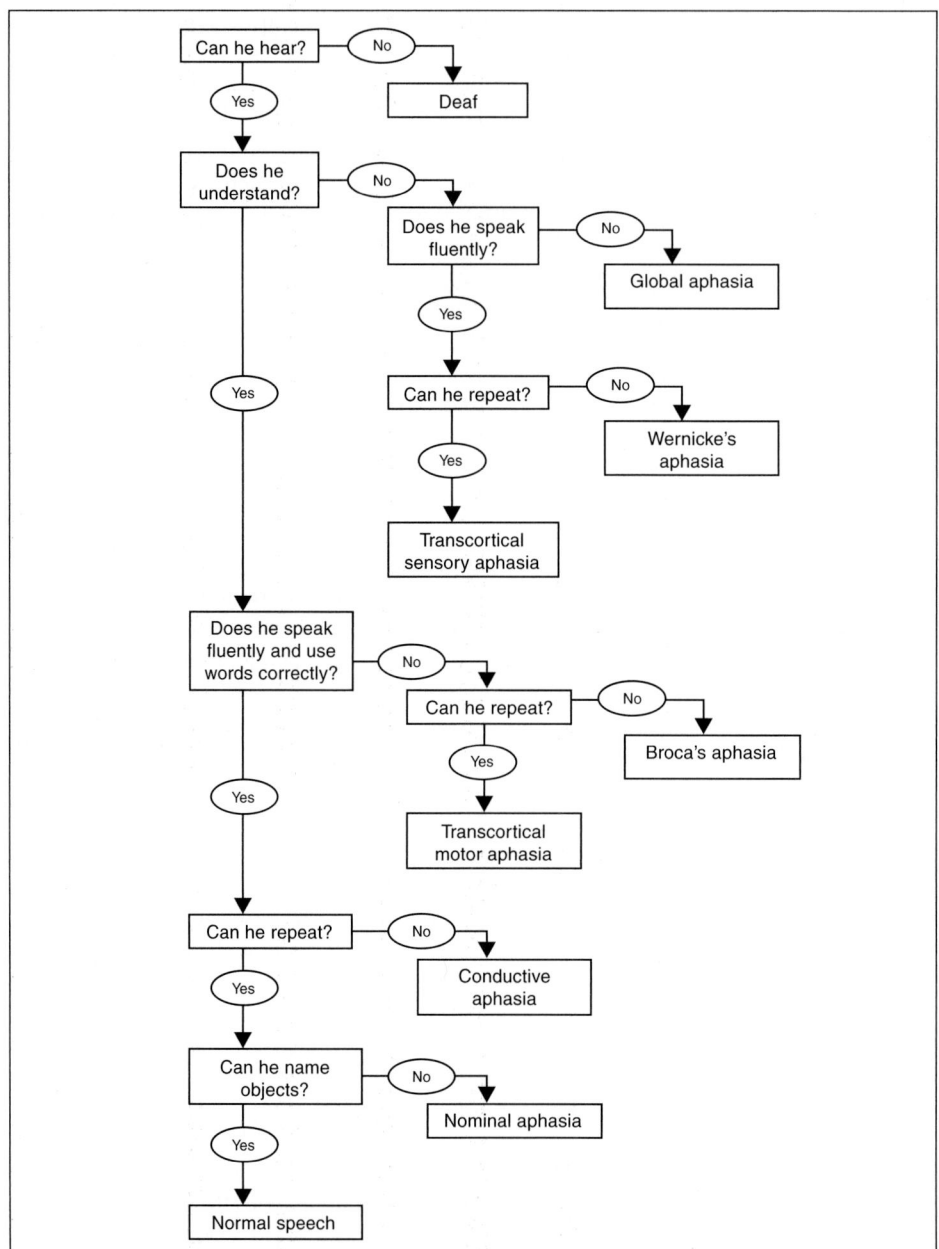

FIGURE 3-1   Flow chart for aphasia.   (Adapted from Fuller G, Gale M. *Neurological Examination Made Easy.* 2nd ed. London: Churchill Livingstone; 1999, with permission.)

problem. These patients understand what is being said to them and asked of them but have difficulty initiating the motor aspects of speech. Wernicke's aphasia is a receptive type of aphasia, in which patients can produce speech and often produce a meaningless or gibberish type speech because they have difficulty in processing incoming information and cannot monitor their own speech patterns.[11,12] Nominal aphasia is the term used when patients have difficulty in finding specific words. Patients suffering from this problem may have difficulty naming the parts of a watch or the specific parts of a pen and yet understand how the instrument should be used. These difficulties are often due to dysfunction of secondary word-association areas, which are usually in the dominant hemisphere. Conductive aphasia generally involves the arcuate fasciculus. Such patients will be able to listen intently and may be able to initiate speech, but they have considerable difficulty in repetition of speech, though comprehension and output is preserved.

There are variants of the various speech abnormalities. Transcortical sensory aphasia is a Wernicke's type aphasia with preserved repetition. Transcortical motor aphasia is a Broca's type aphasia with preserved repetition but inability to initiate one's own speech.

Dysphonia is an abnormality in the actual production of the volume of speech. If this seems to be of clinical concern, one can ask the patient to cough. Assuming that the laryngeal mechanisms are normal, a normal coughing sound should be produced. A cough that lacks an explosive start, occasionally referred to as a bovine cough, can be found with vocal cord paralysis. If the patient is asked to sustain a sound by saying the letter "E" for a long period and cannot do this, the possibility of myasthenia gravis should be considered (see Chapter 6). Further testing for myasthenia gravis may be required.

Dysarthrias are problems in the actual motor coordination of speech. Repeating difficult phrases (Peter Piper picked a peck of pickled peppers) may be extremely difficult for a patient who cannot coordinate motor movements. The rhythm of such speech is usually abnormal, and slurring of words is common. Such dysarthrias can be either a chemical problem, such as that induced by alcohol intoxication, or be related to other disease processes such as multiple sclerosis, hereditary ataxias, or stroke. Delayed speech with difficulty in word formation as well as articulation can be seen in extraparaneural dysarthria and in a disease such as Parkinson's. Figure 3-2 outlines the evaluation of dysarthria.

Cranial Nerves

For a summary of cranial nerve evaluation, see Table 3-4.

I. Olfactory nerve: Difficult to test in an emergency department or outpatient setting; usually not of value in making a specific diagnosis. Testing of this system is so complex that it is to be considered a research level process and is rarely helpful in the emergency setting.

II. Optic nerve: Examined with funduscopy and assessment of visual acuity, and pupillary response. The second cranial nerve is actually an extension of the diencephalon of the brain, and the optic nerve heads are the only places in the body where the brain is directly visible. The optic nerve is tested by the amount of light received in areas of the visual fields in which the light is sensed and is the first essential element in processing light. The light reflex, both directly and consensually, may be tested. Visual fields are tested through confrontational field testing. Such testing is done with simultaneous finger movement in the four principal quadrants of vision, which is usually sufficient (see Chapter 9).

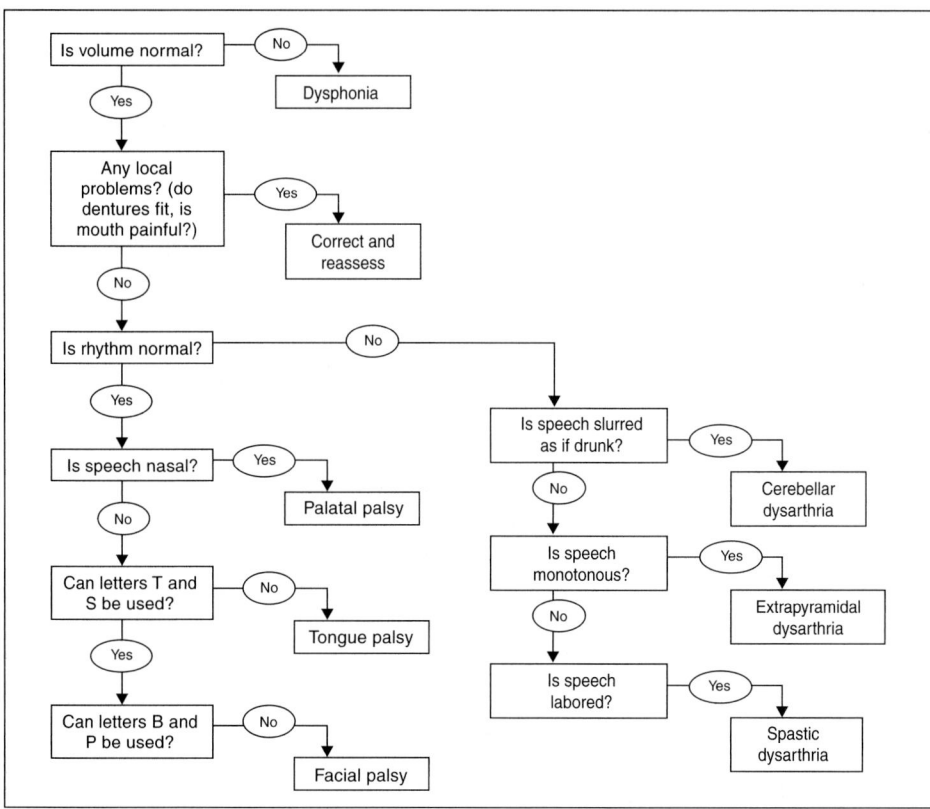

FIGURE 3-2   Flow chart for dysarthria.   (Adapted from Fuller G, Gale M. *Neurological Examination Made Easy.* 2nd ed. London: Churchill Livingstone; 1999, with permission.)

Confrontation testing of visual fields is required only when a cortical lesion is suspected or a specific complaint of partial visual loss is voiced by the patient. The swinging flashlight test (the Marcus-Gunn pupil) may indicate abnormalities in optic neurotransmission (see Chapter 9).

III. Oculomotor nerve: Somatic motor function is checked by extraocular movements in conjunction with nerves IV and VI (see Fig. 9-1). All extraocular muscles, except for the superior oblique and lateral rectus, are innervated by cranial nerve III. Parasympathetic fibers that travel with the third cranial nerve and then extend to the midbrain are tested through the pupillary reflex arc in conjunction with the second cranial nerve.

IV, VI. Trochlear and abducens nerves, respectively: Cranial nerves IV and VI are tested in conjunction with cranial nerve III during evaluation of extraocular movements (Fig. 3-3) Cranial nerve IV innervates the superior oblique muscles and thus aids in pulling the eye medially and downward. The sixth cranial nerve innervates the lateral rectus muscle and is involved in all abduction movements of the eye globe. All other extraocular muscles are innervated by the third cranial nerve.

V. Trigeminal nerve: Motor function of this nerve (third division of cranial nerve[5]) is tested by assessing the strength of several of the muscles of mastication (e.g., the masseter and

TABLE 3-4 ────────────────────────────────────

SUMMARY OF SCREENING CRANIAL NERVE EXAMINATION

Nerve	Testing	Comments
Cranial nerve I: olfactory nerve	None	An advance made, not routine
Cranial nerve II: optic nerve	Pupils, gross visual fields	Field testing only if history suggestive of cortical lesion, visual complaint
Cranial nerve III: oculomotor nerve	Extraocular movements	Best rapid test of the brainstem
Cranial nerve IV: trochlear nerve		
Cranial nerve V: trigeminal nerve	Facial sensation— mastication muscles	Three divisions of the nerve
Cranial nerve VI: abducens nerve		
Cranial nerve VII: facial nerve	Facial muscles	Other division of VII *not* generally tested
Cranial nerve VIII: auditory nerve	Gross hearing— tuning fork tests	Finer tests of hearing not done unless symptoms related to hearing or brainstem
Cranial nerve IX: glossopharyngeal nerve	Stimulated swallowing	If patient is swallowing normally and handling secretions
Cranial nerve X: vagus		
Cranial nerve XI: accessory nerve	Shoulder shrug— sternocleidomastoid function	Rarely tested unless brainstem complaint
Cranial nerve XII: hypoglossal nerve	Tongue strength	No formal testing unless abnormal speech or brainstem complaint

pterygoid muscles). The masseter muscle is tested by asking the patient to forcefully close his or her jaw. The pterygoid muscles are tested by asking the patient to move his or her jaw from side to side. The sensory portions of the fifth cranial nerve, which include all three divisions of the nerve, are tested by assessing fine touch to the face and the corneal reflex (Fig. 3-4). When postnuclear pathology is suspected, all three divisions of the nerve need to be tested separately.[13]

VII. *Facial nerve:* The motor function of this nerve is tested by observing movement of the facial musculature. Facial innervation has both crossed and uncrossed fibers except near the mouth. Therefore, lesions affecting the seventh cranial nerve fibers above the

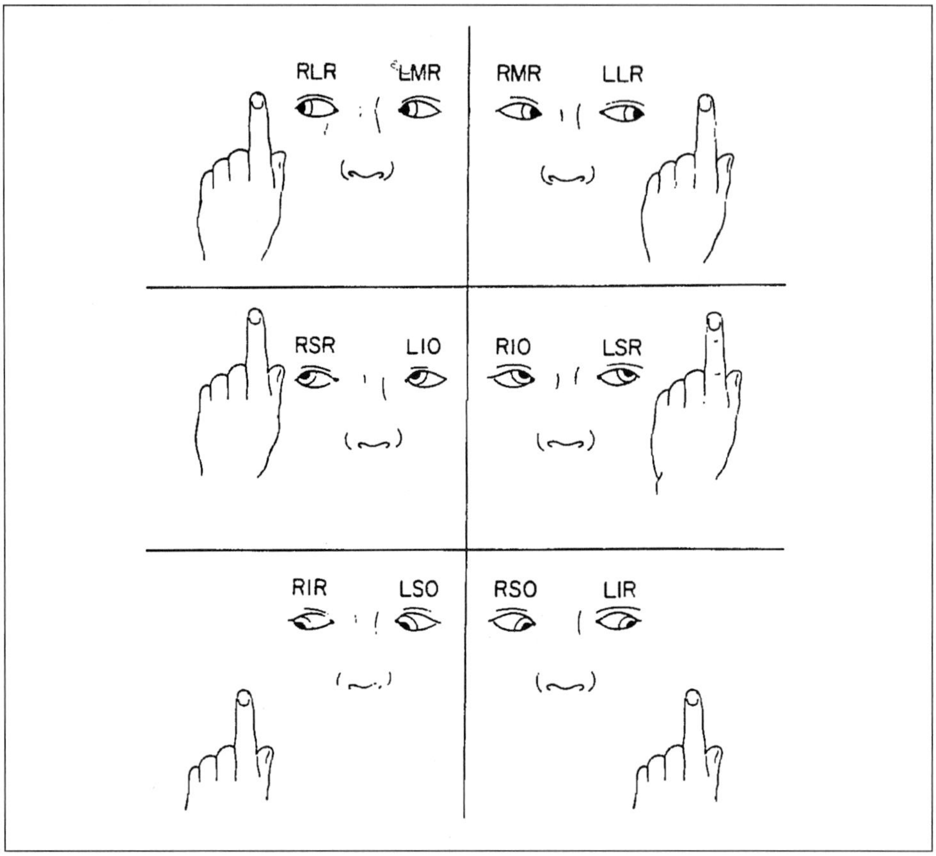

Abbreviation	Muscle	Nerve
LR	lateral rectus	VI CN
SO	system oblique	IV CN
IO	inferior oblique	III CN
MR	medial rectus	III CN
SR	superior rectus	III CN
IR	inferior rectus	III CN

FIGURE 3-3 **Extraocular movement testing.**   (From Simpson J, Magee K. *Clinical Evaluation of the Nervous System.* Ann Arbor, MI: Overbeck; 1970, with permission.)

level of the seventh nerve nucleus in the brainstem will result in only minimal facial dysfunction. Lesions of the seventh nerve that affect the nerve distal to its nucleus will result in facial hemiparesis.

VIII. Acoustic (Vestibulocochlear) nerve: The acoustic portion of this nerve is tested by assessing the gross speech reception threshold and by the discrimination of sounds. Tuning fork tests are utilized to determine the location (conduction vs sensorineural) of a

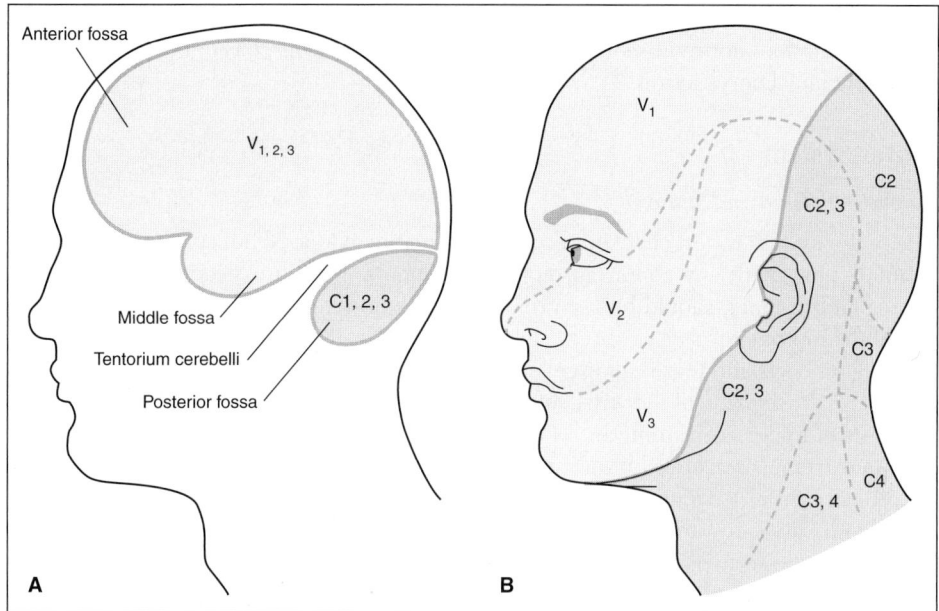

FIGURE 3-4   Innervation of pain-sensitive intracranial compartments (A) and corresponding extracranial sites of pain radiation (B). The trigeminal (V) nerve, especially its ophthalmic (V_1) division, innervates the anterior and middle cranial fossae; lesions in these areas can produce frontal headache. The upper cervical nerve roots (especially C2) innervate the posterior fossa; lesions here can cause occipital headache.   (Reproduced with permission from Simon R, Greenberg D, Aminoff M. *Clinical Neurology*. 7th ed. New York: McGraw-Hill; 2009.)

hearing deficit within the ear proper and in the temporal bone including the middle ear cleft, along the acoustic portion of the eighth cranial nerve, or more centrally. Tuning fork testing is rarely needed in the acute care setting. The Weber test determines lateralization of sound. It is performed by striking a tuning fork and placing it in the center of the top of the head. If the sound lateralizes to one specific side, this is the side with a conduction deficit (i.e., middle ear or more lateral). The Rinne test compares air conduction with bone conduction.[1] This test is performed by striking the tuning fork and then placing it on the mastoid bone located behind the ear (to assess bone conduction) and comparing it with the sound heard by placing the tuning fork near the auditory canal itself (to assess air conduction). If bone conduction is greater than air conduction, the patient has a conductive hearing loss. Unless there is a specific brainstem- or hearing-related complaint, formal testing of hearing is not generally required.

IX, X, and XI. Glossopharyngeal, Vagus, and Spinal Accessory cranial nerves, respectively: These cranial nerves are not generally tested on a screening neurologic examination because of a lack of lateralization and specificity. A patient who is speaking and swallowing normally and does not have a brainstem type of complaint does not need individual testing of these nerves. These nerves are usually specifically tested only if there are other indications of brainstem or posterior fossa involvement.

XII. Hypoglossal nerve: This nerve is tested by examining for deviation of the tongue on voluntary tongue protrusion. The tongue deviates toward the side of the weakness or nerve involvement. A patient who is speaking normally and who does not have a twelfth nerve lesion, does not require formal testing. On rare occasions, local disease may mimic a twelfth cranial nerve lesion.[14,15]

Motor System

Cerebellum, Gait, and Station

The motor system is best checked through observation. General bulk of the musculature is noted along with any abnormal motor movements. Both gross movements, such as chorea and tremors, should be recorded as well as fine muscle fasciculations. The best test of the motor system is to observe how the patient uses muscles for normal activities. Walking on heels and toes is an excellent test to assess strength in the lower extremities. Handgrip, dorsiflexion of the wrist, and abduction of the arms at the shoulders are excellent tests of upper limb strength.

An extremely sensitive but nonspecific test for motor system dysfunction is to assess for pronator drift.[6,3,10] Patients are asked to hold their upper extremities in front of themselves with palms upward and then to close their eyes and attempt to maintain this position. There are four possible responses to a pronator drift test. If, when the eyes are closed, the arms remain outstretched without any deviation for 10 seconds, the test should be considered normal. This would indicate no difference in the outflow tracts of the two major motor tracts.

In the event of involvement of a motor tract (and without the aid of the visual system to correct imbalances), the limb on the affected side will slowly drift downward, and the hand will begin to pronate. This can be an extremely sensitive check on the motor system and is often positive much earlier than detected on confrontational strength testing.

The third possible response is observed when one arm elevates and the fingers seem to move in a searching manner in space. This generally does not reflect a motor system problem. It represents a problem with spatial orientation. When the patient is forced to maintain a stationary position and is unable because of the lack of compensating visual input then it is almost always due to a lesion in the parietal lobe.

The fourth possible response is that of impersistence. This is typically seen in demented patients. If a patient is asked to extend the arms and then close the eyes, they have difficulty maintaining this position for any period of time without visual input. It can be extremely frustrating to the examiner, who may initially confuse this response with noncooperation. Motor impersistence is associated with frontal lobe disease and concomitant dementia.

Strength in the motor system should be graded on a 0 to 5 scale with 0 representing not even a flicker of movement and 5 representing normal strength. The best test of both coordination and strength is to watch the patient walk or complete some other motor task.

Tone in the motor system is best tested passively by moving the arms at the elbows (and the legs at the knees) through a range of motion without assistance from the patient. Movement "hesitations" and cogwheel-type limitations with generally increased tone or spasm may be noted.

Specific tests for cerebellar coordination include finger-to-nose testing of the upper extremities and heel-to-shin testing of the lower extremities. These maneuvers test the lateral cerebellar hemispheres. Midline cerebellar structures are tested by having patients sit on the side of the bed or stand, and see if they can maintain their position without using their arms or utilizing assistance from the examiner. Tandem walking (i.e., heel-to-toe walking) is also an excellent test of central or midline cerebellar functions. Rapid alternating movement testing can be performed to further evaluate or confirm equivocal findings.

An important differential diagnostic point in evaluating the motor system is to decide whether a lesion represents an upper motor neuron or lower motor neuron abnormality. Upper motor neuron lesions refer to involvement of the nervous system centrally from the level of the cerebral cortex to synaptic connections within the anterior horn cells in the spinal cord, usually at the level that a nerve leaves the spinal cord. Lower motor neuron lesions refer to involvement of nerves as they leave the spinal cord (not when they leave the spinal canal) and then extend through a peripheral nerve to their respective target muscle. The important differences between upper and lower motor neuron lesions are summarized in Table 3-5.

Sensory System

Sensory testing is the least accurate and generally the least reproducible portion of the neurologic examination. It is essentially subjective being dependent on patient responses. Both dorsal column and lateral spinothalamic tract functions should be tested.[9]

TABLE 3-5

DIFFERENTIATION BETWEEN UPPER AND LOWER MOTOR NEURON WEAKNESS

Parameter	Upper Motor Neuron[a]	Lower Motor Neuron[b]
Type and distribution of weakness	Lesions in brain: "pyramidal distribution," i.e., distal, especially hand muscles, and weaker extensors in arm and weaker flexors in legs Lesions in cord: variable, depending on location	Depends on which lower motor neurons involved: which segments, roots, or nerves
Tone	Spasticity: greater in flexors in arms and extensors in legs	Flaccidity
Bulk	Slight atrophy of disuse only	Atrophy may be marked
Associated reflexes	Accentuated reflexes; Babinski sign present	Absent or diminished; no Babinski sign
Fasciculations	No	Possible

[a] Synonyms: pyramidal tract, corticospinal tract, corticobulbar tract.

[b] Synonyms: anterior horn cell, ventral horn cell, somatic motor portions of cranial nerves, final common pathway.

Dorsal column functions include vibration and position sense, which are assessed by use of a tuning fork or by graded movement of the joints of the extremities. It is important to record how far proximally one must evaluate a patient's extremities to identify the extent of abnormality of these functions.

The lateral spinothalamic tracts transmit temperature and pain sensation. These tracts should also be assessed by evaluating from distal to proximal regions of the extremities and then up the trunk of the body. If a patient can feel pain/temperature appropriately distally, more proximal testing is unnecessary unless a specific area of numbness has been described by the patient. It should be remembered that the innervation of the lower extremities (L_1–S_2) does not arise from the most distal segments of the spinal cord. The most distal spinal cord segments (S3–S5) innervate the anus and genitalia. Therefore, examination of the genitalia and perirectal areas evaluates the most distal portions of the spinal cord. These distal segments are usually not evaluated unless there is a specific complaint relative to the regions they innervate or that there is a suspected lower spinal cord or cauda equina lesion.

If a patient expresses concern over a specific area of sensory loss, the patient should specifically delineate the region and then it should be specifically tested by the examiner. A sensory level may be found in patients who have a spinal cord injury.

In the emergency department or other acute care setting, it is important to recognize specific patterns of sensory loss. Lesions involving specific nerve roots or specific peripheral nerves must be differentiated from central nervous system involvement (Fig. 3-5). Table 3-6 summarizes these specific sensory patterns.

Cortical localization and interpretation of sensation can be tested by assessing for extinction of double simultaneous stimuli (DSS). A sensitive indicator for parietal lobe dysfunction is if stimuli, which are simultaneously administered to the same region of both sides of the body, cannot be distinguished. The appreciation of stimuli presented on symmetrically opposite areas of the body requires normal parietal lobe function.

If only one stimulus is perceived, the parietal cortex on the opposite side from the nonperceived stimulus may be involved. Such parietal extinction also holds true for visual stimuli. For example, appreciation of fingers in the various visual fields presented separately but denied when presented simultaneously is pathognomonic for visual extinction from parietal lobe disease.

The Romberg test assesses input from a combination of neural systems. This test is performed on a standing patient with the feet together, the arms at the sides, and the eyes open. The Romberg test evaluates cerebellar integration of visual, sensory, and vestibular inputs with respect to orientation in space. If the patient remains steady with the eyes open, the systems can be assumed to be essentially intact. If the patient then becomes unsteady once the eyes are closed, it means that the position sense from the extremities is not reaching the central nervous system. This is not a cerebellar problem but more likely a spinal cord (dorsal column) or peripheral nerve sensory problem.

REFLEXES

Tendon reflexes (Table 3-7) are relevant only when compared from side to side or compared between the upper and lower extremities, and lesions above and below the foramen magnum. Tendon reflexes are usually assessed at the ankles, knees, forearms,

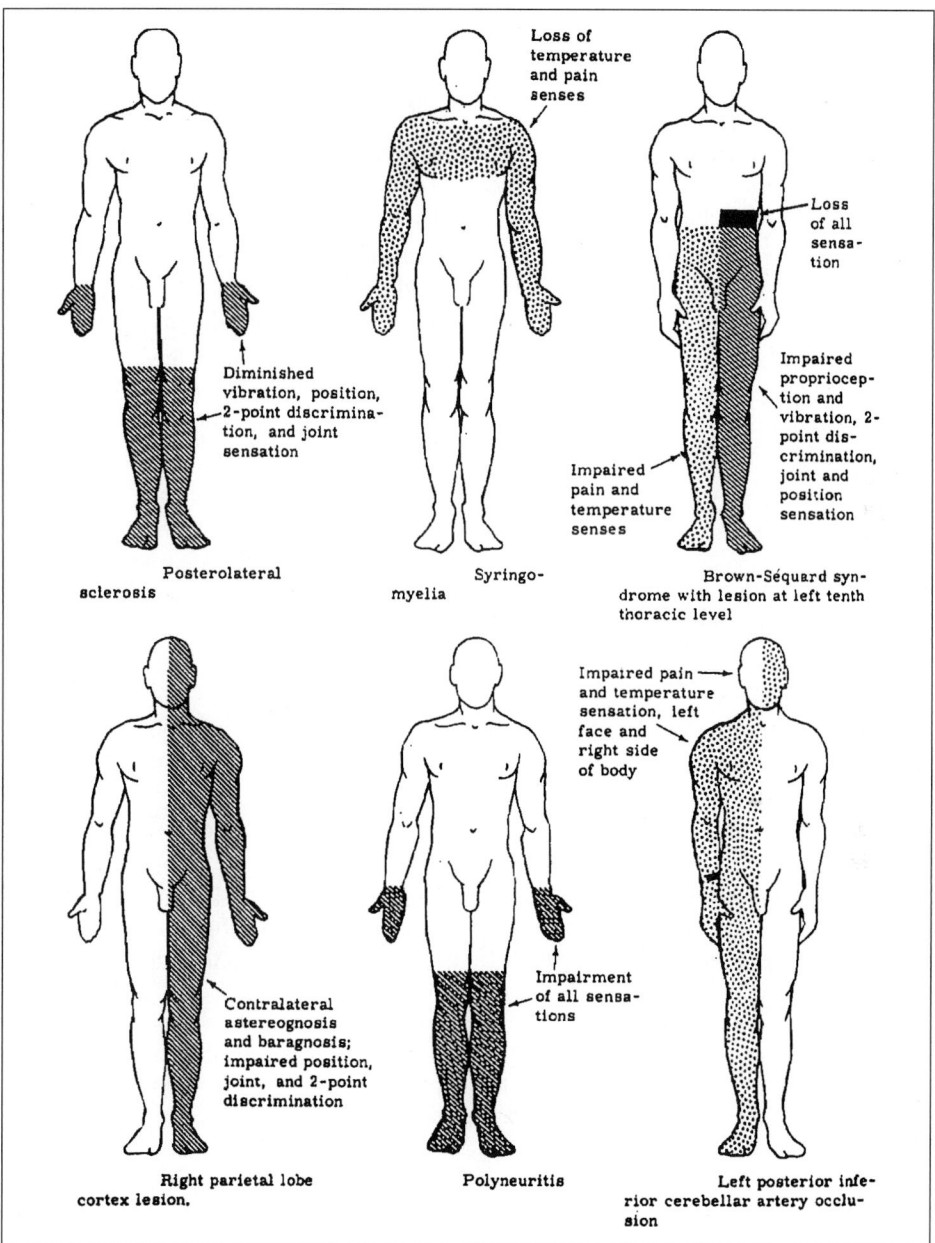

FIGURE 3-5   **Principal patterns of sensory loss.**   (From Chusid J. *Correlative Neuroanatomy and Functional Neurology.* 14th ed. Los Altos, CA: Lange; 1970, with permission.)

TABLE 3-6

ANATOMIC CORRELATES OF SENSORY LOSS PATTERNS

Pattern of Loss	Anatomic Location
Specific dermatomal segment	Involvement of isolated nerve root or roots
Specific peripheral nerve	Structural lesion involving isolated peripheral nerve or vascular compromise to the nerve
Diminished vibration and position in the limbs	Lesion of the dorsal columns in the spinal cord
Loss of temperature and pain across or in the arms and shoulders in a capelike distribution	Central cord syndrome: trauma or syringomyelia; developmental
Loss of all sensation below a specific vertebral level	Complete spinal cord transection
Loss of vibration and proprioception on one side; loss of pain and temperature on the opposite side of the body below a specific level	Brown-Sequard syndrome with hemisection of the spinal cord
Complete loss of sensation on one side of the body including head neck, trunk, and extremities	Central nervous system located, above the upper brainstem and internal capsule region
Loss of all sensory modalities on distal limbs	Peripheral neuropathy of the arms and legs from any cause
Impairment of sensory modality on one side of the face and the opposite side of the neck and body	Involvement of uncrossed facial fibers and crossed body fibers in the middle to lower brainstem or multiple lesions

TABLE 3-7

PRIMARY REFLEXES

Reflex	Roots Involved	Muscles Involved
Jaw jerk	Fifth cranial nerve	Masseter and pterygoids
Ankle jerk	S1–S2	Gastrocnemius
Knee jerk	L3–L4	Quadriceps
Biceps	C5–C6	Biceps
Brachioradialis	C5–C6	Brachioradialis
Triceps	C7–C8	Triceps

and elbows. The absolute magnitude of any reflex is not as important as its respective symmetry. Reflexes are usually graded on a 0 to 4+ basis; 4+ reflexes indicate clonus or some type of sustained uninhibited reflex function. A zero reflex indicates that the reflex was not elicited. In examining tendon reflexes, it may be necessary to divert the patient's attention if there is any suspicion that concentration is affecting the results.

Regressive reflexes (reappearance of primitive reflexes which are usually lost as the central nervous system matures) indicate some degree of loss of inhibition by the central nervous system on reflex arcs. A positive Babinski's sign is nonspecific but denotes some decreased upper motor neuron influence. Regressive reflexes in the head and neck area include such findings as snouting, sucking, rooting, and the presence of the palmomental reflex. The presence of these reflexes usually indicates longstanding cortical disease and lack of frontal lobe inhibition of these more primitive reflex activities.

AUTONOMIC NERVOUS SYSTEM

Testing the autonomic nervous system is extremely complex and is usually not required in the urgent care setting. Certain autonomic functions with regard to vision are reviewed in the chapter on pupillary abnormalities (Chapter 9). The overall functioning of the autonomic nervous system requires input from multiple areas. Therefore, blood pressure, heart rate, general vascular tone, sweating, etc., are all affected by multiple systems and various forms of pathology.[16] More complete testing of the autonomic nervous system can be performed on a nonemergent basis.

EXAMINATION MODIFICATIONS FOR SPECIFIC COMPLAINTS

Just as the neurologic history has important information that can be obtained specific to any given patient's chief complaint, the neurologic physical examination may be similarly modified to accommodate individual patient symptoms. Pertinent neurologic examination modifications based on the patient's presenting complaint are summarized in Table 3-8.

Specific examination techniques and grading systems have been developed to enhance communication and reproducibility of results between various examiners over time. The two that are currently in use are the Glasgow Coma Scale (see Table 10-1) and the National Institutes of Health Stroke Scale (see Table 5-4). The Glasgow Coma Scale (GCS) has limitations at the higher end of neurologic performance. There can be patients with scores of 15 (the highest possible on the scale) who are not neurologically normal.

It is, however, an accepted standardized method of following a patient's clinical condition and is useful in statistical analysis of head-injury patients.

The National Institutes of Health Stroke Scale (NIHSS) is used, among other things, in the decision-making process for the considerations of the use of thrombolytic therapy in acute stroke patients. Examinations performed both before and after CT scanning are compared as a part of current inclusion criteria (see discussion of thrombolytic therapy in stroke in Chapter 4).

TABLE 3-8

NEUROLOGIC EXAMINATION FOR SPECIFIC CHIEF COMPLAINTS

Presenting Signs; Symptoms	Additional Examinations to Be Considered
Confusion; delirium	Formal mental status testing; aphasia; regressive reflexes
Flat affect	Evaluation of thought content and pathologic reflexes (snouting, sucking, grasping)
Blurred, dimmed, or absent vision	Visual acuity and light perception; funduscopic examination; slit lamp and swinging flashlight examination (see Marcus Gunn pupil, Chap. 9); visual fields, optokinetic nystagmus; intraocular pressure red glass testing
Headache	Careful palpation of head and neck structures for meningismus and funduscopic evaluation
Focal weakness	Systemic testing of nerve roots and/or peripheral nerve involved in the area of motor and sensory loss and hemispheric testing
Nonfocal weakness	Test for muscle fatigue including lid lag and pronator drift and stress tolerance
Dizziness	Orthostatic vital signs, positional testing: Nylen-Barany test and cardiac examination
Stupor, coma	Best level of consciousness, respiratory pattern; Doll's eye movements or caloric testing; pupillary responses, motor responses, and posturing; decorticate, decerebrate, flaccid
Neurotrauma	Coma: go directly to coma protocol Awake: perform limited examination until cervical spine properly evaluated Most important: check for bilaterality of motor functioning, level of consciousness, and attentiveness
Back pain without direct trauma	Straight leg raising sign, anal tone, or perianal sensation

Summary

The directed neurologic examination can and should be both effort efficient and time efficient. Concentrating an evaluation on simple indicators of mental status, motor activity, and upper brainstem cranial nerves and such testing of upper brainstem nerve function will yield the greatest benefit for time spent by an examiner. The neurologic examination needs to be modified based on the patient's presenting complaints and various positive findings in the examination itself. The overall mental status and the patient's ability to function or not are still the best indications that a more detailed examination is required.

REFERENCES

1. Acheson J, Hutchinson EC. The natural history of focal cerebral vascular disease. *Q J Med.* 1971;50:15.
2. National Institute of Neurologic Cerebrovascular Disease and Stroke. A classification and outline of cerebral vascular diseases. Ad hoc committee report. *Stroke.* 1976;6:594-616.
3. Haerer A, DeJong RN. *The Neurologic Examination.* 5th ed. New York, NY: Lippincott-Raven; 1992.
4. Aminoff M, Greenberg D, Simon R. *Clinical Neurology.* 6th ed. New York, NY: Lang Medical Books/McGraw-Hill; 2005.
5. Bannister R, Brain W. *Brain and Bannisters' Clinical Neurology.* 7th ed. New York, NY: Oxford University Press; 1992.
6. Henry G. Emergency neurological examination. In: Tintinalli J, ed. *A Study Guide in Emergency Medicine.* 4th ed. New York, NY: McGraw-Hill; 1996:1005.
7. Benbadissr A et al. Value of tongue biting in the diagnosis of seizures. *Arch Intern Med.* 1995;2:2346.
8. Mungas D. In-office mental status testing: a practical guide. *Geriatrics.* 1991;446:54-58, 63, 66.
9. Denny-Brown D. *Handbook of Neurological Examination and Case Recording.* Cambridge, MA: Harvard University Press; 1965.
10. Fuller G. *Neurological Examination Made Easy.* 2nd ed. Edinburgh, UK: Churchill Livingstone; 2000.
11. Geschwend N. Language and the brain. *Sci Am.* 1972;226:76-83.
12. Geschwend N. The organization of language and the brain. *Science.* 1970;170:940.
13. Shunklande WE. The trigeminal nerve. Part I: An overview. *Cranio.* 2000;218:238-248.
14. Silvester KC, Barnes S. Adenoidcystic carcinoma of the tongue presenting as a hypoglossal nerve palsy. *Br J Oral Maxillofac Surg.* 1990;28:122-124.
15. Felix JK, Schwartz RH, Myers GJ. Isolated hypoglossal nerve paralysis following influenza vaccination. *Am J Dis Child.* 1976;130:82-83.
16. Ravits JM. Autonomic nervous system testing. *Muscle Nerve.* 1997;20:919-937.

4

ALTERED STATES OF CONSCIOUSNESS AND COMA

The maintenance of consciousness is the most important function of the central nervous system. Alterations of consciousness are common in clinical practice, accounting for 5% of emergency department visits.[1] Despite its obvious importance and the frequency of its clinical disorders, it remains difficult to define consciousness precisely. A practical operational definition is that consciousness is the meaningful awareness of one's self and one's environment. It is important to recognize that an individual's state of consciousness is not directly observed; physicians infer the quality and content of a patient's consciousness by observing his or her responses to internal or external stimuli. Some movements or apparent responses by patients, such as involuntary or reflex movements, may appear to imply conscious awareness where none exists. Conversely, the absence of responses may imply impaired consciousness in a patient who is actually fully awake and aware, for example, in a patient paralyzed with a neuromuscular blocking agent.

Conscious awareness depends on the integrated function of large portions of the brain and brainstem, so any alteration of consciousness is a sensitive indicator or disturbed brain function. Because of the sensitivity of consciousness to even minor alterations of brain function, even relatively benign and reversible processes such as drug intoxication or the postictal confusion following a seizure may cause major alterations of consciousness. Since altered consciousness is frequently the earliest sign of an evolving brain lesion, prompt recognition and assessment may provide an opportunity for intervention before permanent injury occurs. The task of the acute care physician is to promptly recognize and evaluate alterations of mental function and to distinguish relatively benign processes from more malignant ones. Early recognition of benign conditions can avoid the expense and potential risks of unneeded diagnostic or treatment measures. Early recognition and management of malignant conditions offers the best chance for a good outcome. The importance of clinical assessment cannot be overemphasized as the correct diagnosis can be made in more than 50% of patients from the history and physical examination.[1]

TERMINOLOGY AND DEFINITIONS

As a clinical discipline, neurology is well known for the apparent mystery of its methods and the obscurity of its terminology, and this is especially true as regards the assessment of consciousness and its alterations. It is helpful to think of consciousness as having two components—arousal and "content." Arousal is roughly synonymous with wakefulness and implies the ability to perceive external or internal stimuli; content refers to the capacity to process the perceived stimuli and to mount some coherent response. Of course, this distinction is somewhat artificial. It is easy to imagine a patient with normal or even heightened arousal with impaired content of consciousness (as in a patient with acute delirium), but it is meaningless to consider the assessment of content in a patient who cannot be aroused. In reality, most clinical disorders of consciousness involve disturbances of both arousal and content to varying degrees.

Disorders of Arousal

Patients with disorders of arousal appear to be drowsy or asleep. Sleep, of course, is a normal state of decreased arousal from which an individual can be readily awakened to full consciousness. Abnormal states of diminished arousal are grouped under the general (and very imprecise) term obtundation and are indicated more specifically by the terms lethargy, stupor, and coma.

Lethargy is a condition from which an individual can be aroused with stimulation. When awakened, patients typically displays diminished awareness of themselves or their surroundings and when left undisturbed, they once again fall asleep.

Stupor is a condition of decreased awareness from which an individual can be aroused only with vigorous stimulation; even when most fully aroused, the person is unable to interact in a meaningful way with the environment or the examiner. Such individuals may groan to noxious stimuli or utter a few words, but cannot carry on a meaningful conversation or respond appropriately to questions or commands. Left undisturbed, they immediately go back to sleep.

Coma is a condition of diminished arousal from which an individual cannot be aroused even with vigorous or noxious stimulation. Any responses to noxious stimulation tend to be stereotyped and reflexive rather than purposeful.

It is evident that there is no clear distinction among the states of lethargy, stupor, and coma; rather, these states overlap one another and patients may move from one state to another as their clinical situation evolves. Because of the imprecision of these terms, they are best avoided in clinical practice. It is more precise and more useful to specify the specific stimuli required to arouse the patient and the specific level of function the patient could achieve when most fully aroused.

Disorders of Content

Many of the clinical conditions that cause substantial alteration of the content of consciousness are associated with impairment of arousal as well. There are a few situations in which even quite profound alterations of content are accompanied by apparently normal arousal or even apparent hypervigilance. Two of these, dementia and delirium, are quite common in the emergency department (ED); the third, the vegetative state, is very uncommon in the ED.

Dementia is characterized by impairments of memory, executive functions, and the ability to think logically and coherently, so that affected patients are unable to respond appropriately to their surroundings. The process is usually gradual in onset and progression rather than acute or subacute as in delirium (see *Delirium*). Arousal is preserved, at least until quite late in the course, and patients remain awake and alert. They may be able to respond quite appropriately to simple stimuli, greetings, etc., but are less able to respond to more complex questions, commands, or situations. Patients with very profound dementia, such as those at the end stage of a disorder such as Alzheimer disease, or as the result of a severe head injury, may be virtually mute or immobile, unable to respond at all, and yet apparently awake and alert.

Delirium is characterized by impairment of the ability to think logically and clearly, and to respond appropriately to internal or external stimuli. It is a very common problem, affecting from 10% to 25% of elderly patients admitted to the hospital, but is frequently overlooked.[2-4] The onset is often quite abrupt (as distinct from the gradual onset of dementia) and a patient's level of arousal may range from mild lethargy through dramatic agitation and hypervigilance. Patients may be calm and quiet, or agitated and combative, with fever, tachycardia, and sweating, and frequent fluctuation from one state to another, often at intervals of only a few minutes. They are highly distractible and may appear to be responding to multiple internal and external stimuli; auditory and visual hallucinations are frequent. The classic syndrome of delirium tremens is familiar to most ED physicians, but delirium may complicate a wide variety of medical conditions and may be caused by a wide variety of drugs and toxins. It is especially likely to occur in patients with underlying impairment of mental function such as Alzheimer disease or other chronic dementia, prior head injury or stroke, etc.[5,6]

The so-called *vegetative state* is characterized by the presence of arousal responses mediated by brainstem reflexes without any evidence of conscious awareness. It is not commonly encountered in the acute care setting, but more often occurs in persons with severe brain injury who survive the initial insult. These patients typically present acutely with unresponsive coma; with prolonged survival they recover their brainstem reflexes but do not regain conscious awareness. They exhibit primitive brainstem reflexes to stimulation, such as eye opening, pupillary light reflexes, reflex eye movements (see "Eye Movements") but have no purposeful responses to questions or commands. They do not orient toward the examiner or follow a visual target and exhibit no sign of conscious awareness. The diagnosis of the vegetative state may be difficult and often requires multiple examinations and prolonged observation.

Disorders That May Mimic Impaired Consciousness or Coma

There are several uncommon conditions in which patients with normal mental status may be misdiagnosed as having impaired consciousness or coma. It is important that these conditions be correctly identified to prevent unnecessary diagnostic studies and to facilitate appropriate treatment. When there is any doubt about a patient's state of consciousness, it is best to behave as though the patient were fully awake and alert. An incautious remark or painful procedure can cause enormous harm in a patient who appears unconscious but who is actually fully awake.[7]

The *locked-in state* is a rare syndrome most often seen in patients with a lesion (most often a stroke) affecting the ventral pons. The descending motor tracts are interrupted leaving the patient without any voluntary movement of the face, the pharynx, or the body. Since the lesion is below the midbrain centers for vertical eye movements, upgaze and downgaze are preserved, but lateral eye movements may be impaired or abolished. Because of bilateral facial paralysis, patients are unable to close their eyes. Unable to speak and unable to move except to look upward, these persons can be mistaken as unconscious even though they may be fully alert to all that is going on around them, including the remarks and comments of physicians and other caregivers. The clue to the diagnosis is spontaneous eye-opening in an apparently unresponsive patient; the ability of the patient to look upward on command confirms the diagnosis. A similar situation (but without the vertical eye movements) may be seen in patients treated with neuro-muscular blocking agents. Such patients are often treated with sedatives, but it may be difficult or impossible to tell that their sedation was inadequate or has worn off, and they may be fully alert but unable to move or respond.

Psychogenic unresponsiveness is another unusual syndrome in which patients are unresponsive to external stimulation, including painful or noxious stimulation. These individuals may appear to be either awake or asleep. Despite their lack of any voluntary responses, careful examination will reveal normal reflex responses (ocular fixation, opto-kinetic nystagmus, nystagmus on caloric testing, protective reflexes), which suggest conscious awareness. Assessment of these patients is discussed in Chapter 11.

PATHOPHYSIOLOGY OF ALTERED CONSCIOUSNESS

Normal conscious awareness depends on the integrated function of the ascending reticular activating system (ARAS) in the upper brainstem and the cerebral hemispheres. As a rule of thumb, normal function of at least one hemisphere is enough to maintain consciousness. Accordingly, substantial alteration of consciousness implies a disorder affecting either the ARAS or both hemispheres. Either structural lesions or toxic/metabolic derangements may result in impairment or loss of consciousness. Figures 4-1 and 4-2 illustrate a variety of focal structural lesions of the brainstem and cerebrum, some affecting consciousness and some not. Note that only brainstem lesions affecting the midline structures of the upper pons and the midbrain are associated with coma; lesions confined to the lower pons or the medulla, or unilateral lesions typically do not cause coma. Unilateral lesions affecting one hemisphere (such as stroke) do not cause coma, even if quite large. Conversely, even small bilateral lesions of the hemispheres (e.g., bilateral lesions of the thalamus) may cause coma.

Disorders of the ARAS

The ARAS is a complex system of nuclei and fiber tracts extending from the cervical spinal cord through the brainstem to the thalami. The portions of the ARAS in the upper pons and the midbrain are primarily responsible for maintaining the cerebral hemispheres and cortex in a state of readiness to respond to and process internal or external stimuli. During sleep, the cerebral cortex is unresponsive to stimulation; the ARAS maintains surveillance of internal and external environment and can arouse the cortex as necessary. Disorders of arousal, therefore, imply either failure of the ARAS or inability of the cortex to respond to stimulation. The ARAS may be affected directly by intrinsic

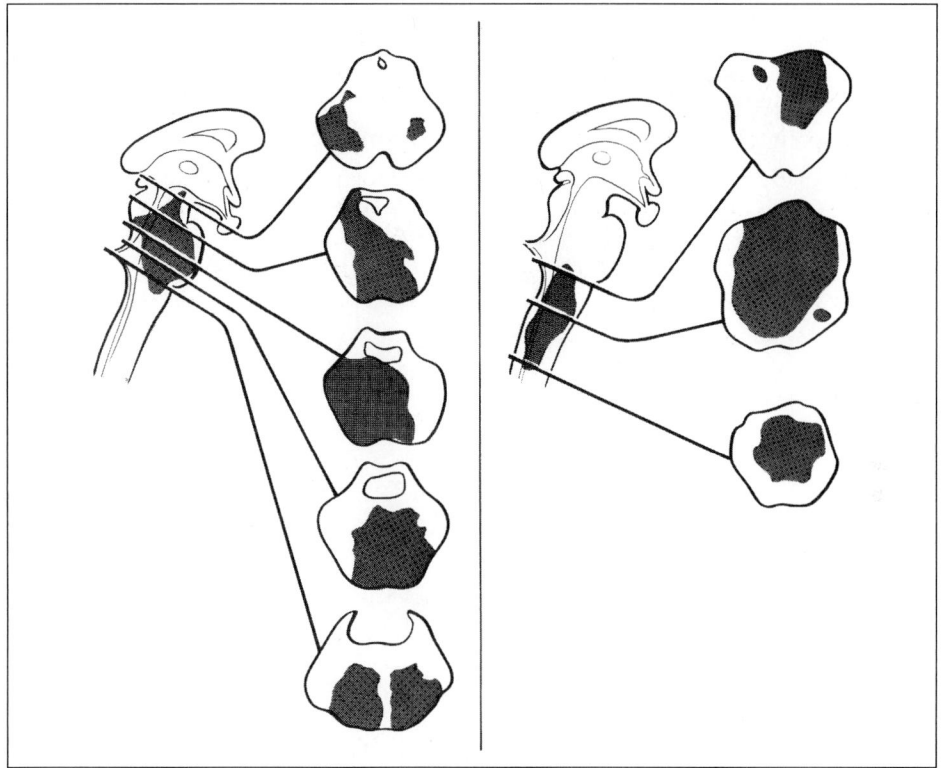

FIGURE 4-1   **Brain lesions not causing sustained coma.**   (From Posner JB, Saper CB, Schiff N, Plum F. Plum and Posner's Diagnosis of Stupor and Coma. New York: Oxford University Press, 2007, Fig. 1-9, p. 30, with permission.)

structural lesions or toxic/metabolic processes, or indirectly by mass effect from lesions in the supratentorial or infratentorial compartments of the cranium.

Because of its relatively small size, the ARAS may be affected by small structural lesions intrinsic to the brainstem such as ischemic stroke or hemorrhage. Head trauma may produce shearing or torsional forces on the upper brainstem resulting directly in failure of the ARAS.

Although the ARAS is relatively resistant to toxic and metabolic insults, severe derangements may result in ARAS failure. Examples include severe hypothermia, severe drug intoxication, or severe hypoxia or ischemia.

Mass lesions in the supratentorial compartment may result in herniation of the supratentorial contents downward through the tentorium with compression of the ARAS. Potential causes for the lesions include extra-axial fluid collections such as epidural or subdural hematomas, intracerebral hematomas, neoplasms, and infectious lesions (such as brain abscesses). Cerebral edema from stroke, encephalitis, trauma, or severe metabolic insults, etc., may also result in brain herniation. Hydrocephalus from obstruction of ventricular drainage may have a similar effect.

Mass lesions or swellings in the infratentorial compartment can result in direct compression of the upper brainstem and even upward herniation of the posterior fossa structures through the tentorium (Fig. 4-3).

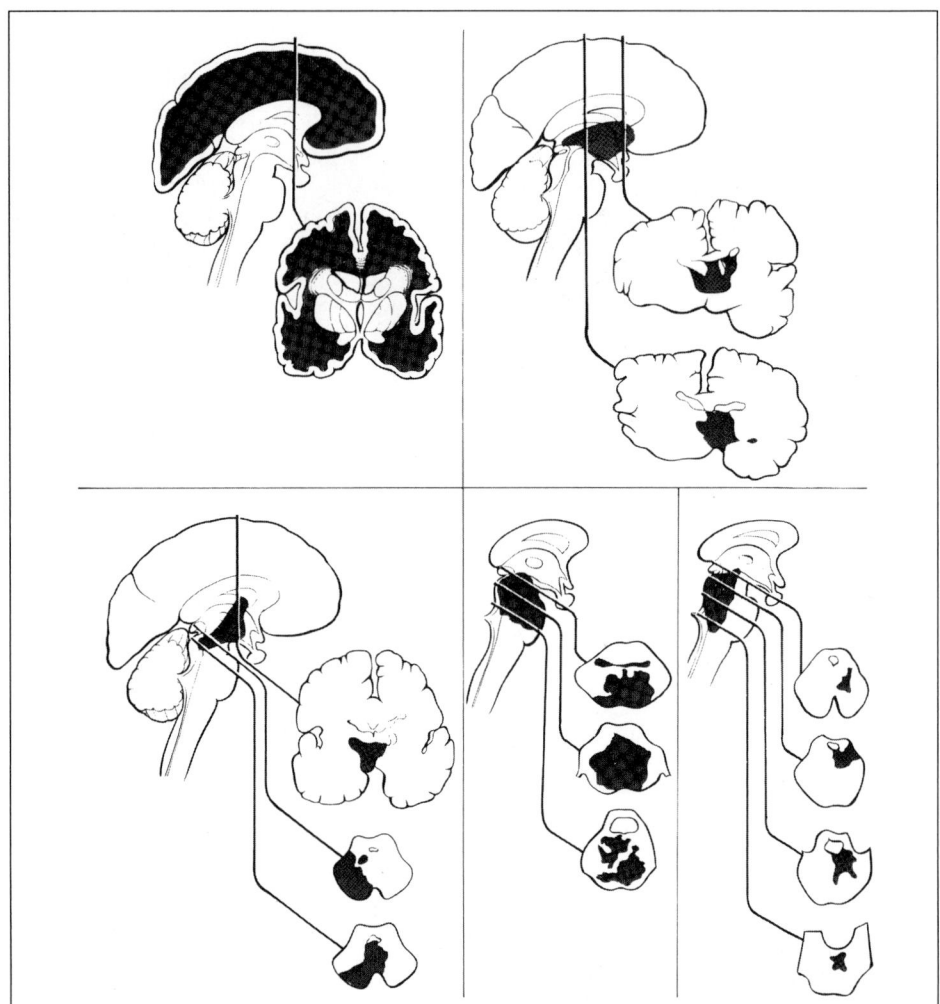

FIGURE 4-2   **Brain lesions causing sustained coma.**   (From Posner JB, Saper CB, Schiff N, Plum F. Plum and Posner's Diagnosis of Stupor and Coma. New York: Oxford University Press, 2007, Fig. 1-8, p. 28, with permission.)

Disorders of the Cerebral Hemispheres

Focal or unilateral lesions of the cerebral hemispheres do not generally cause profound alterations of consciousness. As noted above, alteration of consciousness may result when both cerebral hemispheres are affected. In clinical practice, this most commonly occurs as the result of toxic or metabolic processes that affect the brain diffusely. Other important potential causes include infection (meningitis or encephalitis), seizure activity, or increased intracranial pressure.

Toxic/metabolic encephalopathies may result from an enormous array of potential causes. Perfusion failure (cardiac arrest or severe hypotension), profound hypoxemia, hypo- or hyperglycemia, renal or hepatic failure, electrolyte abnormalities, and intoxication

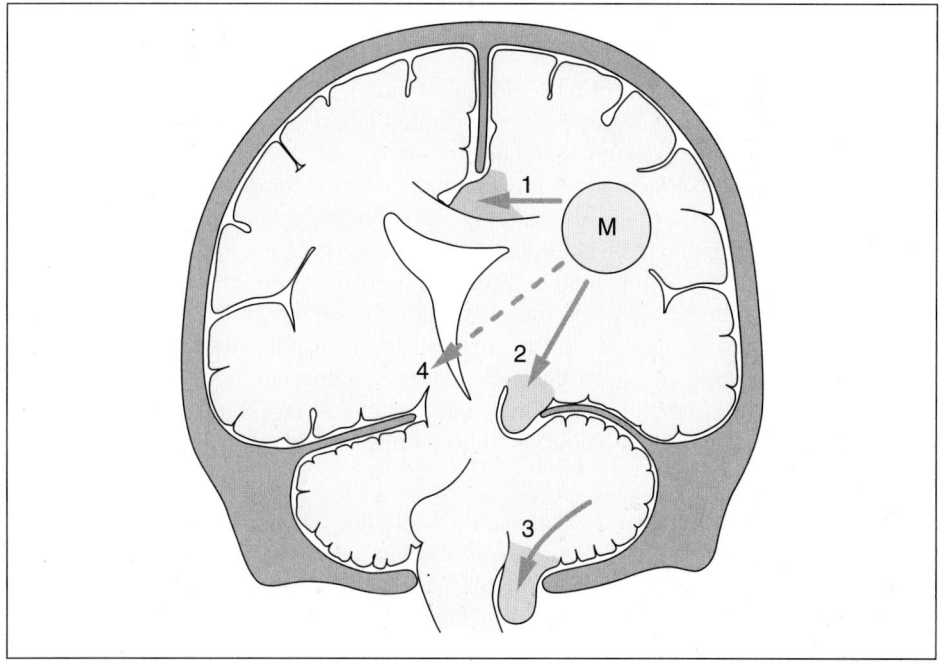

FIGURE 4-3 Schematic depiction of brain herniations between dural compartments. Transfacial (1) transtentorial uncal-parahippocampal (2) cerebellar tonsillar (3), and horizontal (4), causing Kernohan-Woltman notch phenomenon M = mass. (Reproduced with permission from Ropper A, Samuels M. *Adams and Victors' Principles of Neurology*. 9th ed. New York: McGraw-Hill; 2009.)

with licit or illicit drugs may all result in impairment or loss of consciousness. The clinical picture may range from mild confusion through severe delirium or from mild lethargy through profound coma. A similar clinical picture may result from intracranial infections (meningitis and encephalitis) or subarachnoid hemorrhage.

Seizures may cause impairment or loss of consciousness; when motor or behavioral phenomena are present, seizures are easily recognized. However, seizures may be unaccompanied by any abnormal movements or only by very subtle movements, which can be easily overlooked. Either generalized or partial seizures may be followed by a postictal period of diminished consciousness that may persist for many hours (Chapter 12).

Increased intracranial pressure may result from a variety of causes. Obstruction of the normal pathways of cerebrospinal fluid (CSF) drainage by mass lesions, blood, or other causes may lead to acute hydrocephalus. Cerebral edema may result from infection, electrolyte abnormalities, trauma, and other causes. Mass lesions (e.g., intracerebral hemorrhages, tumors, subdural, or epidural hematomas) may all cause increases in intracranial pressure with diminished consciousness or coma. Diminished consciousness is more likely to result from acute increases in intracranial pressure; in chronic disorders such as idiopathic intracranial hypertension (pseudotumor cerebri) or slowly growing mass lesions, even substantial increases in intracranial pressure may not affect consciousness.

INITIAL ASSESSMENT

The classic stepwise approach in most clinical situations is to first obtain a history, then perform a physical examination, obtain any needed laboratory or imaging studies, and finally establish a working diagnosis and initiate management. A patient in coma or with other severe alteration of mental status presents special problems. A reliable history may be unobtainable and the physical examination may be very limited. More important, altered consciousness should be considered a medical emergency, and leisurely contemplation of the situation is often not a realistic option. Instead, the physician must rapidly assess the situation and must often initiate empiric management while the assessment proceeds. Nonetheless, it is crucial to proceed in an orderly manner. A systematic approach nearly always takes less time and yields more information than a more haphazard approach. In most cases, a thorough assessment can be accomplished in a few minutes. The initial assessment should seek to accomplish several goals urgently and more or less simultaneously:

1. Recognize and manage immediately life-threatening conditions.
2. Establish the baseline level of consciousness and neurologic impairment.
3. Establish a differential diagnosis of likely causes of the patient's condition.
4. Initiate treatment and definitive diagnostic study.

Assessment of Vital Signs

The first step, of course, is to assess and manage the patient's vital functions—the classic "ABCs" of emergency medical care; this includes an immediate serum glucose determination.

Adequate oxygenation and ventilation are priorities. The airway should be secured, by intubation if needed, both to ensure adequate oxygenation and to prevent aspiration. Although observation of the pattern of respiration is of only limited practical value in localizing lesions causing alterations or loss of consciousness, the respiratory pattern should be observed, whenever possible, prior to any intervention. The presence of spontaneous respiration implies at least some preservation of brainstem function. Rhythmic regular respiration (e.g., Cheyne-Stokes respiration, spontaneous hyperventilation) implies intact brainstem function. Lesions of the pons may result in apneustic breathing, characterized by a prolonged pause (inspiratory cramp) after each inspiration. An irregular or chaotic pattern (Biot's breathing) implies a lesion at the lower pons or medulla and warns of impending respiratory failure.[8]

Adequate perfusion should be ensured. Shock should be managed aggressively, and cardiac arrhythmias should be monitored and treated as indicated. Hyper- and hypotension should be considered to have a nonneurologic cause until proved otherwise. In general, acute hypertension should not be treated urgently unless there is some other indication for such treatment (e.g., myocardial ischemia), or if true hypertensive encephalopathy is the likely diagnosis (see "Hypertensive Encephalopathy").

A rectal temperature should be obtained. Very high or very low temperatures may be either the cause of the patient's obtundation or the result of some other process. Very high temperatures may result from sepsis, from heat stroke, or from the neuroleptic malignant syndrome; very low temperatures may result from overwhelming sepsis or, more commonly, from environmental exposure. Vital signs should be monitored closely and reviewed regularly by the physician.

Obtaining the History

Depending on the clinical situation, obtaining a history may have to be deferred until after initial assessment and stabilization of the patient. It is important to remember, however, that even a very limited clinical history may vastly simplify the process of diagnosis. Although the patient is often unable to supply reliable information, witnesses may be able to describe the onset and progression of the patient's clinical symptoms. They may be aware of recent or chronic medical illnesses such as AIDS, diabetes, or heart disease, or of previous episodes of altered consciousness. Specific questions about alcohol or drug use or possible recent trauma should be asked. Witnesses should be assured that all information is confidential and will not be shared with law enforcement officers, family members or friends, or others without due process. Wallet cards, pill bottles, or medical alert tags may all yield helpful information.

Neurologic Examination

Once the vital functions are secured, a brief neurologic examination should be done to assess the patient's actual level of function, to begin the process of diagnosis, and to establish a baseline against which subsequent examinations can be compared. The neurologic examination of patients with impaired consciousness must be tailored to the patient's ability to cooperate. A useful initial neurologic examination can be carried out in only a few minutes if the physician concentrates on the essentials; a more detailed examination, if needed, can be accomplished later.

Assessment of Mental Status

The first step is to assess the patient's actual level of consciousness. The patient should be observed carefully for any spontaneous movements. Does he or she maintain a normal supine posture? Are the eyes open or closed? (If the eyes are open, the patient may be awake, even if unresponsive.) The patient should be addressed (by name if known) and the response observed. If the patient responds to voice, the ability to respond appropriately to questions or commands should be assessed. If there is no response to voice, response to touch and finally to noxious or painful stimuli should be assessed. Note that an adequate noxious stimulus need not be painful. Gentle pressure on the sternum, the clavicles, or other bony prominences will often suffice. If more painful stimuli are required, vigorous pressure on the same areas is appropriate.

It is important to avoid any risk of actual injury to the patient; twisting nipples, squeezing testicles, and other potentially dangerous maneuvers should not be performed. In patients with suspected cervical spinal cord injury, some stimulus above the neck (such as firm pressure on the mastoid process or over the supraorbital notch) should be tried. Note any sign of purposeful responses and also note whether responses are bilateral or limited to one side. Note any posturing or any change in pulse, blood pressure, or respiration in response to stimulation. In recording the results, note the specific stimuli used and describe the patients' response. This provides a useful baseline to which later examinations can be compared, even by another physician. Terms such as "lethargy," "stupor," or even "coma" are too imprecise to be very reliable and should be avoided. In patients with head trauma, the Glasgow Coma Scale may be used (see Chapters 3 and 10), but the scale is less helpful in most of the other clinical conditions which can cause altered mental function in the ED. Once it is established that the patient has altered mental status or coma, the next step is to determine if the cause is more likely a disorder of the cerebral hemispheres or of the ARAS. As noted earlier, preservation of arousal suggests a lesion of the hemispheres while coma may result from a lesion of the ARAS or of both hemispheres.

Examination of the Eyes

The important functions of those parts of the upper brainstem most concerned with maintenance of consciousness can be reliably assessed by a brief but careful examination of the eyes. Intact functions of the pupils, eyelids, and eye movements imply intact function of the relevant portions of the upper brainstem and ARAS, and suggest that the alteration of consciousness or mentation is more likely due to a lesion affecting the cerebral hemispheres.

Fundus Examination

The presence of papilledema suggests raised intracranial pressure of at least several hours' duration or longer; unfortunately, the absence of papilledema does not indicate normal intracranial pressure. Likewise, spontaneous pulsations of the retinal veins, when present, imply normal pressure. However, the pulsations may be difficult to observe, especially in a busy ED setting, and are often absent in supine patients, so the absence of venous pulsations is of no diagnostic significance. Retinal and preretinal hemorrhages are commonly seen and have a very extensive differential diagnosis.[9] In patients with subarachnoid hemorrhage, the presence of preretinal subhyaloid hemorrhages may imply a poor prognosis, but they may be seen in many other conditions and are not diagnostic. They appear as round "saucerlike" collections of blood that obscure the underlying vessels. Other fundus findings may be signs of chronic hypertension or diabetes, but these are of little help in the acute situation.

Pupils

The size, shape, reactivity, and symmetry of the pupils should be assessed and recorded. Any apparent abnormality of pupil function must be interpreted in the context of the entire clinical history and examination. Abnormalities of pupil function can result from recent or remote eye surgery or trauma, topical or systemic medications or toxins, or other acquired conditions, rather than from disorders of the nervous system.

The size of the pupils is regulated by inputs from both the sympathetic and parasympathetic nervous systems. Pupillary constriction is controlled by parasympathetic fibers that originate from the Edinger-Westphal nucleus located in the midbrain in close association with the ARAS. Failure of the pupils to react to light may indicate a lesion affecting the Edinger-Westphal nucleus, the parasympathetic fibers that travel in association with the third (oculomotor) nerve or blockade of cholinergic neuromuscular junctions in the iris (Fig. 4-4). Dilation of the pupils is controlled by the sympathetic pathway that begins in the hypothalamus and extends through the cervical spinal cord to the upper thoracic cord (T1 level), where the second-order sympathetic axons exit the spinal canal. The fibers ascend in the paraspinal sympathetic chain to the superior cervical ganglion and then travel with the carotid artery to the orbit. Failure of one of the pupils to dilate properly in the presence of dim light (e.g., Horner's syndrome) can indicate a lesion anywhere along this extended sympathetic pathway.

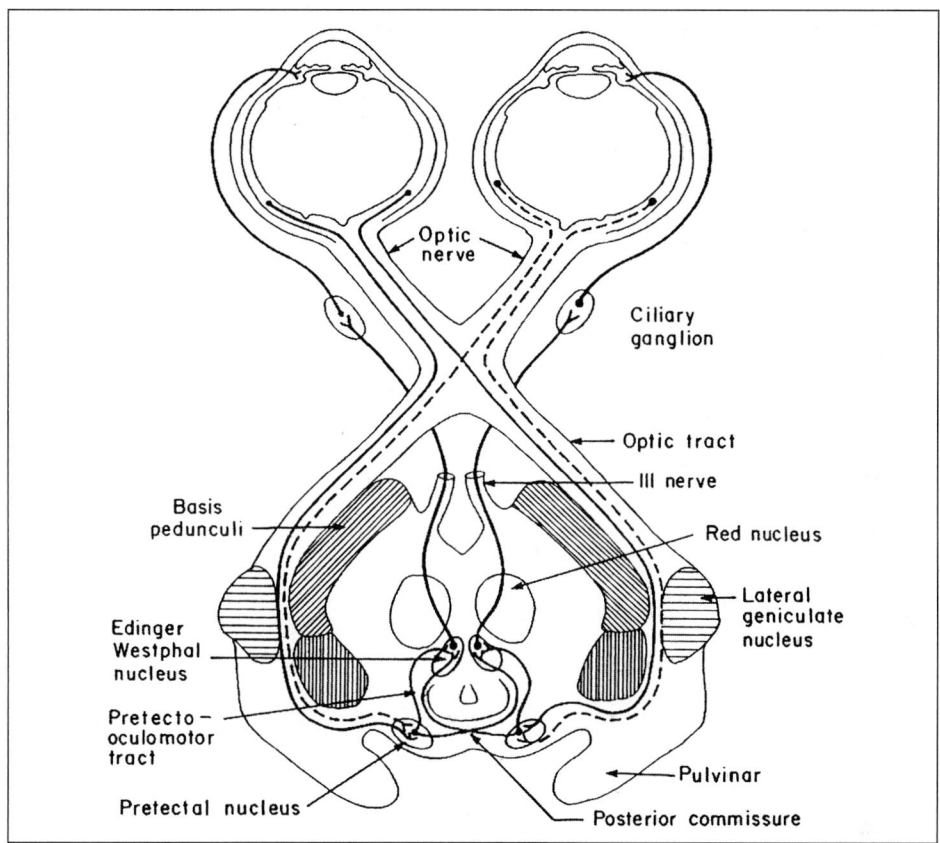

FIGURE 4-4   Diagram of the pupillary light reflex.

The size of the pupils can be affected by a wide variety of drugs and toxins, as well as by structural lesions affecting various parts of the nervous system. Structural lesions of the brain, brainstem, or cranial nerves causing abnormalities of pupil function will virtually always be associated with other abnormalities on neurologic examination, so that abnormalities of pupil size or function without other focal abnormalities on neurologic examination should strongly suggest drug or toxic effects on the pupils. Both intraocular and systemic drugs can affect pupil size. Table 4-1 gives a partial list of drugs and toxins that affect pupil size.

Pupil Reactivity

The pupils will normally constrict abruptly when stimulated with bright light (the light reaction) or when presented with a nearby visual target (accommodation). The light reaction is very resistant to drugs and toxins, although potent topical cycloplegic drugs may completely block the response. Absence of such drugs or failure of both pupils to react to bright light suggests a structural lesion affecting the midbrain tegmentum. Lesions of the cerebral hemispheres will not affect the light reflex. The reflex may be very difficult to see in patients with very small pupils; a magnifying lens (such as a high-plus lens on the

TABLE 4-1

DRUGS AND TOXINS THAT AFFECT PUPIL SIZE
AND FUNCTION

Drugs and Toxins That May Cause Enlarged Pupils
Anticholinergic agents
    Atropine
    Trihexyphenidyl (Artane)
    Benztropine (Cogentin)
    Scopolamine[a]
    Tropicamide[a]
    Cyclopentolate[a]
    Gentamicin[a]
    Jimson weed, nightshade, other plant toxins
    Botulinum toxin
Adrenergic agents
    Epinephrine
    Phenylephrine
    Ephedrine
    Amphetamine, dextroamphetamine
    Cocaine
    Chlorpheniramine[a]

Drugs and Toxins That May Cause Small Pupils
Cholinergic agents
    Pilocarpine[a]
    Methacholine[a]
    Carbachol[a]
    Physostigmine, neostigmine, pyridostigmine[b]
    Organic phosphate esters (insecticides)[c]
Antiadrenergic agents
    Dibenzyline
    Phentolamine
    Tolazoline
    Guanethidine
    Bretylium
    Monoamine oxidase inhibitors
Other agents
    Opiates and synthetic narcotics

[a] Drugs used primarily as topical agents in ophthalmology. Although not causing coma or altered mental status, they may confuse the physical examination.
[b] Used primarily in the treatment of myasthenia gravis.
[c] Rarely encountered in clinical practice; some of these agents have potential for use in terrorist attacks.

ophthalmoscope) should be used to look for any reaction. Any constriction is significant and indicates that the parasympathetic pathway is anatomically intact.

The accommodation reflex cannot be assessed in an unconscious patient. In patients with psychogenic unresponsiveness, sudden presentation of a nearby visual stimulus, such as suddenly holding a mirror in front of the patient, may elicit an accommodation reflex; this indicates intact vision (and preserved consciousness!).

Pupil Symmetry

Drugs or toxins affecting pupil function can be expected to affect both sides equally (unless a topical agent has been used in only one eye). Some asymmetry of the pupils (usually <1 mm) may be seen in normal persons, but such pupils will respond symmetrically to changes in lighting. Asymmetry of the pupil light reflex suggests a structural lesion. When faced with asymmetric pupils, the clinician must first determine which of the pupils is abnormal. Careful observation at different light levels should demonstrate either failure of constriction of the larger pupil, suggesting an oculomotor nerve lesion, or failure of dilation of the smaller pupil, suggesting a Horner's syndrome. If the eyes are open, ptosis on the side of the larger pupil suggests a third nerve lesion; ptosis on the side of the smaller pupil suggests Horner's syndrome. If an oculomotor nerve lesion is present, abnormal eye movements may also be present (see "Eye Movements").

Eye Movements

The control of eye movements is highly complex and depends on the integrated function of multiple areas of the cerebral hemispheres and brainstem. Fortunately, the practical clinical assessment of eye movements, particularly in unconscious patients, is usually quite straightforward.

Lateral movement of each eye is controlled by the ipsilateral sixth (abducens) nucleus via the abducens nerve. Medial, upward, and downward movements of each eye are controlled by the ipsilateral third (oculomotor) nucleus via the oculomotor nerve. [The fourth (trochlear) nucleus and nerve can be ignored in this setting.] The individual cranial nerve nuclei are under the control of supranuclear gaze centers, which serve to ensure that both eyes move together in conjugate fashion. Lateral gaze to each side is controlled by the ipsilateral pontine paramedian reticular formation (PPRF), which is adjacent to the sixth nerve nucleus in the pons; output from the PPRF controls the ipsilateral sixth nerve nucleus and, via the medial longitudinal fasciculus (MLF), the contralateral third nerve nucleus. Thus, activation of the PPRF on one side will induce both eyes to turn to that side (Fig. 4-5). Vertical eye movements are controlled by accessory oculomotor nuclei in the upper midbrain; when activated, these nuclei induce the third nerve nuclei to turn the eyes upward or downward in coordinated fashion. The anatomy is complex, but understanding it is crucial if the physical examination is to yield useful information.

Review of the relevant neuroanatomy will make it clear that lesions at or above the supranuclear gaze centers (the PPRFs and accessory oculomotor nuclei) will cause conjugate disorders of eye movements (both eyes will move together and their movements will be equally impaired). Conversely, a lesion that causes disconjugate eye movements must be located below the level of the gaze centers, i.e., in the brainstem, affecting either the MLF or the cranial nerve nuclei, or outside the central nervous system (CNS), affecting the cranial nerves or the extraocular muscles. A great deal of valuable information can

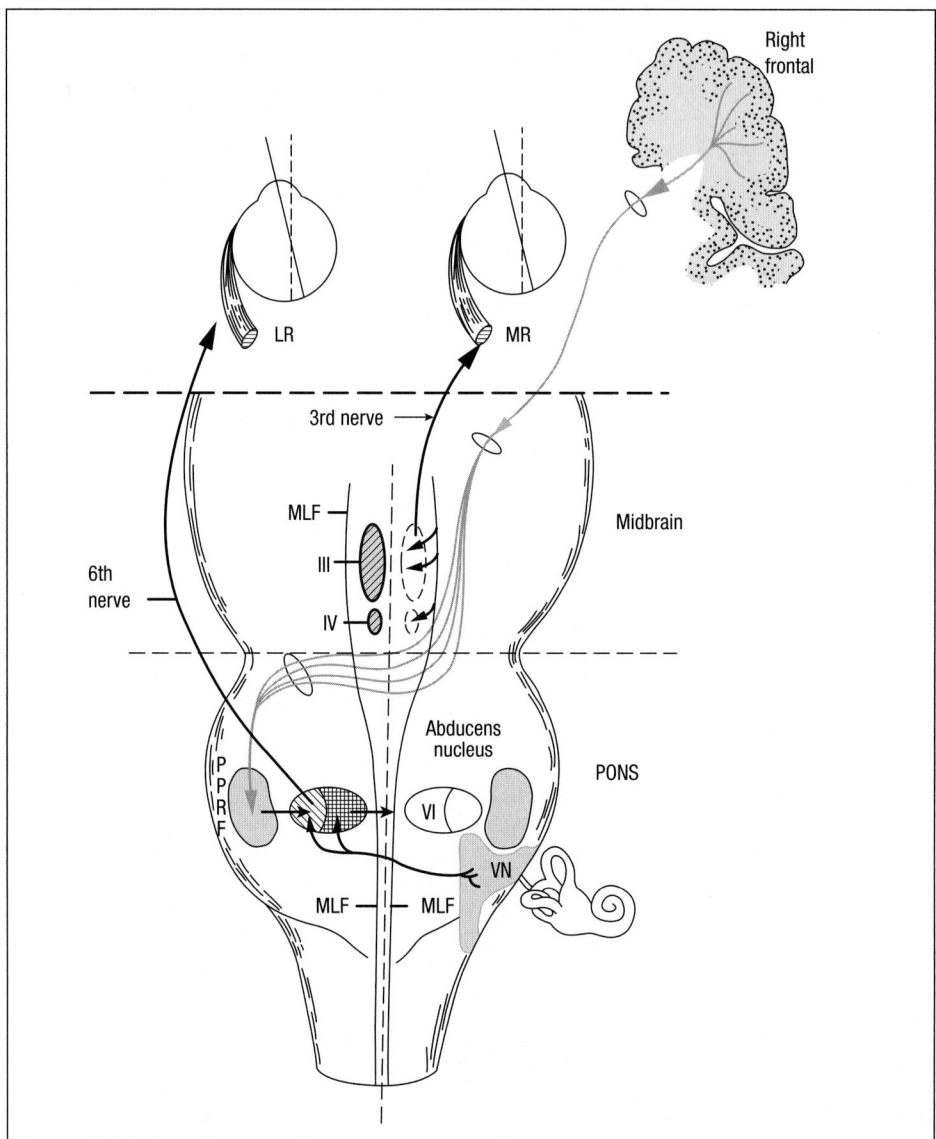

FIGURE 4-5   The supranuclear pathways subserving saccadic horizontal gaze to the left. The pathway originates in the right frontal cortex, descends in the internal capsule, decussates at the level of the rostral pons, and descends to synapse in the left pontine paramedian reticular formation (PPRF). Further connections with the ipsilateral sixth nerve nucleus and contralateral medial longitudinal fasciculus are also indicated. Cranial nerve nuclei III and IV are labeled on the left; the nucleus of VI and vestibular nuclei (VN) are labeled on the right. LR, lateral rectus; MR, medial rectus; MLF, medial longitudinal fasciculus.   (Reproduced with permission from Ropper A, Samuels M. *Adams and Victor's Principles of Neurology*. 9th ed. New York: McGraw-Hill; 2009.)

thus be quickly obtained by observation of voluntary eye movements in conscious patients, and by observation of reflex eye movements in unconscious patients.

Voluntary and pursuit eye movements result when the supranuclear gaze centers are activated by the cerebral cortex. Voluntary movements are initiated in the frontal eye fields; voluntary activation of one of the frontal eye fields results in deviation of the eyes to the opposite side. Focal seizure activity may also induce deviation of the eyes to the contralateral side. Conversely, injury to one of the frontal lobes (such as an acute stroke) may result in deviation of the eyes toward the injured side due to the unopposed output of the intact frontal lobe. This sign is not always present; even when it is present initially, it may resolve within a short time. Pursuit eye movements are controlled by the parieto-occipital areas, but injury to these areas does not produce predictable or reliable localizing signs. Preservation of voluntary or pursuit eye movements implies intact cortical function and consciousness, even in an otherwise unresponsive patient.

Unconscious patients will sometimes exhibit slow roving eye movements. These may be conjugate or disconjugate; disconjugate movements in this setting do not imply a brainstem or cranial nerve lesion as long as both eyes are moving. It should be recalled that these slow roving eye movements cannot be mimicked by a conscious patient.

Reflex eye movements can be elicited by maneuvers designed to activate the supranuclear gaze centers. The oculocephalic (Doll's eye) reflex is elicited by passively moving the patient's head from side to side or forward and backward, and observing any resulting eye movements. The test is contraindicated if there is any suspicion of a cervical spine injury. The patient's eyes are held open and the head is turned briskly first to one side and then to the other. The expected response is conjugate deviation of the eyes to the side opposite the direction of head movement. Similar responses (upward and downward movements of the eyes) can be elicited by passive flexion and extension of the neck. The presence of oculocephalic reflexes implies normal function of the brainstem gaze centers and nuclei; failure of the response suggests brainstem injury. A disconjugate response indicates a focal lesion in the brainstem or cranial nerves. Note that the response cannot be obtained in awake patients (Fig. 4-6).

If the oculocephalic reflex cannot be obtained, or if the test is contraindicated, the oculovestibular (caloric) reflexes can be tested. If performed with ice water (see later), the test is very painful in the awake patient; ice water should only be used to assess brainstem function in patients known to be unconscious. A more gentler version of the test using water only a few degrees below body temperature is used in awake patients to assess vestibular function, usually as part of special testing in persons with balance disorders. It is unnecessary to perform the test in patients with intact oculocephalic reflexes since it is simply a more vigorous test of the same anatomic systems. The test is performed with the patient supine; if possible the head should be elevated about 30 degrees (though this is not strictly necessary). The ear is then irrigated with 50 to 60 mL of ice-cold water via a small catheter. It is preferable (but not strictly necessary) that the ear be clear of impacted cerumen. A normal response in a patient with intact brainstem function is tonic conjugate deviation of the eyes toward the irrigated ear. Absence of any response indicates profound impairment of brainstem function. As with the oculocephalic reflex, a disconjugate response indicates a focal lesion of the brainstem or cranial nerves. Both sides should be tested, with a 5-minute delay between each side (Fig. 4-6 and Tables 4-2 and 4-3). It should be noted that the nystagmus often described with this maneuver (and memorized in the common mnemonic "COWS") occurs only in awake

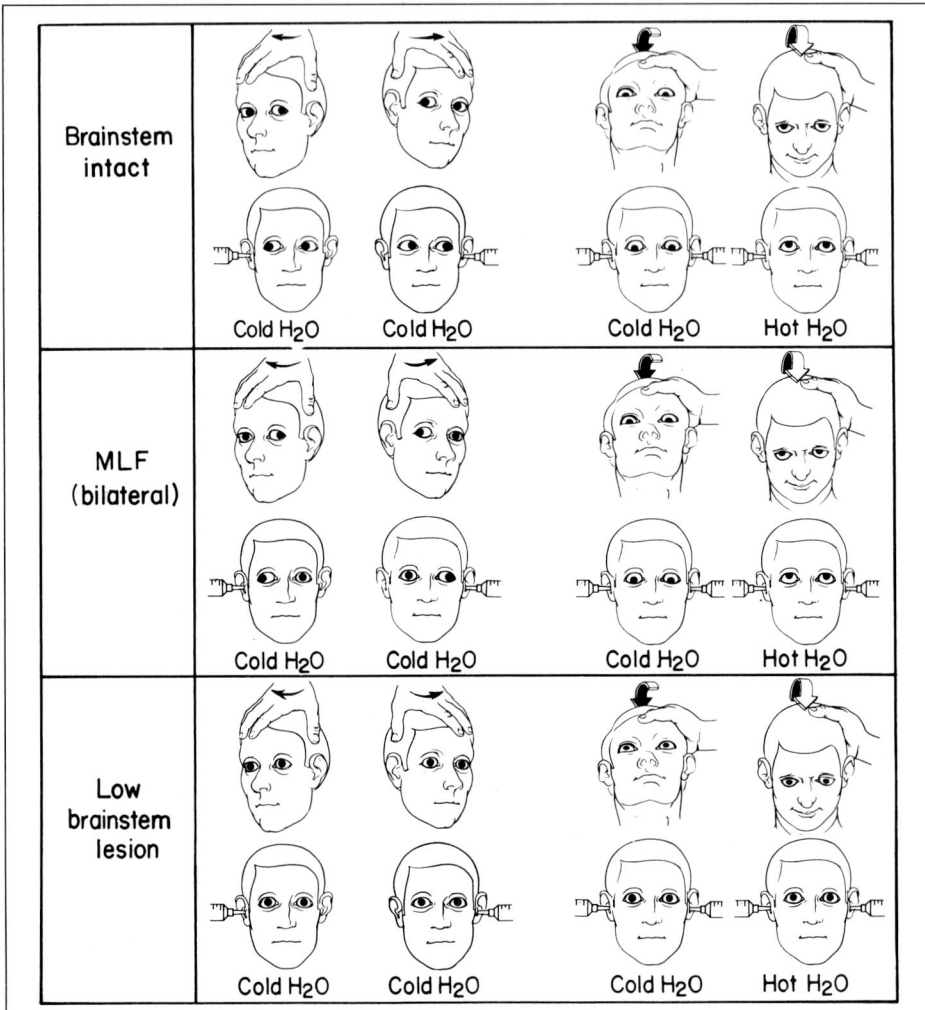

FIGURE 4-6   **Ocular reflexes in unconscious patients.**   (From Plum F, Posner JB. *The Diagnosis of Stupor and Coma.* 3rd ed. Philadelphia: FA Davis; 1982, with permission.)

patients with intact vision; the tonic deviation of the eyes toward the irrigated ear will only occur in unconscious patients. It is important to recognize that failure of these reflexes does not necessarily imply an irreversible process; the reflexes may be abolished by completely reversible profound toxic or metabolic insults (e.g., barbiturate intoxication) or by neuromuscular blockade.

Other Cranial Nerves

Most other tests of cranial nerve function cannot be carried out in unconscious patients. In patients who can be aroused, at least in part, careful examination of facial movements can yield helpful localizing information. Clear, well-articulated speech,

TABLE 4-2
INTERPRETATION OF OCULOCEPHALIC (DOLL'S EYE) REFLEXES[a]

Stimulus	Response	Interpretation
Lateral rotation of head	Eyes remain conjugate, move opposite to head movement	Normal
	No movement either eye with head moved in either direction	Brainstem lesion Bilateral labyrinth dysfunction Drugs/anesthesia
	Eyes move normally with head turned in one direction, no response when head turned in opposite direction	Unilateral lesion in PPRF (lateral gaze center)
	One eye abducts, opposite eye does not adduct	Third nerve lesion Internuclear ophthalmoplegia
Flexion/extension of the head	Eyes remain conjugate, move opposite to head movement	Normal
	No movement either eye with head moved in either direction	Brainstem lesion Bilateral labyrinth dysfunction Drugs/anesthesia
	No upward movement either eye, normal downward movement	Lesions of dorsal midbrain (Parinaud's syndrome)
	Only one eye moves	Third nerve palsy

[a] Drugs that impair vestibular or oculomotor function (anticholinergics, TCAs, neuromuscular blocking agents, and so on) may impair these responses.
Source: Adapted from Berger JR. Clinical approach to stupor and coma. In Bradley WG et al., eds. *Neurology in Clinical Practice.* 2nd ed. Boston: Butterworth-Heinemann; 1996 (with permission).

even if nonsensical, implies normal lower brainstem function. Conversely, the gag reflex yields little useful information and is not a reliable guide to the patient's ability to swallow safely or to protect the airway from aspiration. The presence of the gag and cough reflexes does suggest some preservation of brainstem function but is otherwise of little diagnostic value.

Motor and Sensory Testing

Standard tests of motor function cannot be carried out in unconscious patients; such tests are of limited value even in patients with less severely impaired consciousness since reliable motor testing requires the full cooperation and effort of the patient.

TABLE 4-3

INTERPRETATION OF CALORIC (OCULOVESTIBULAR) TESTING[a]

Stimulus	Response	Interpretation
Cold water in right ear	Nystagmus—slow phase to right, fast phase to left	Normal—brainstem and cortex intact
	No response	Obstructed ear canal, "dead" labyrinth, eighth nerve lesion, brainstem lesion (PPRF)
	Tonic deviation of eyes to right, no nystagmus	Brainstem intact—toxic/metabolic process, structural lesion above brainstem
Cold water in left ear		Responses opposite to above
Warm water in left ear (if no response to cold water in right ear)	Nystagmus—slow phase to right, fast phase to left	Confirms peripheral lesion on right—blocked canal, "dead" labyrinth, eighth nerve lesion—*brainstem and cortex intact*
	Tonic deviation of eyes to right	Confirms peripheral lesion on right (see above)—*brainstem intact*

[a] Drugs that impair vestibular or oculomotor function (anticholinergics, tricyclics, neuromuscular blocking agents, prior use of aminoglycosides) may impair these responses.
Source: Adapted from Berger JR. Clinical approach to stupor and coma. In Bradley WG et al., eds. *Neurology in Clinical Practice.* 2nd ed. Boston: Butterworth-Heinemann; 1996 (with permission).

Patients should be observed carefully for any spontaneous motor activity. Purposeful activity such as rearranging the bedclothes to maintain modesty or to place the limbs in a position of comfort indicates a high level of brain activity, even in an otherwise unresponsive patient. Rhythmic twitching or jerking movements may indicate seizure activity; random twitching and jerking movements (myoclonus) may indicate a diffuse toxic or metabolic brain injury. Movements of the face but not of the body or extremities may indicate a lesion of the cervical spinal cord. Movement of the arms but not the legs may indicate a low cervical or thoracic spinal cord injury. Movement of only one side of the body may indicate hemiplegia.

Movements in response to stimulation should be observed next. Simple withdrawal of a limb from noxious stimulation indicates intact function at spinal cord levels, but movement of two or more extremities when only one is stimulated indicates function at upper brainstem levels. Similarly, decorticate or decerebrate posturing indicates preserved function of the upper brainstem. More complex responses such as purposeful attempts to avoid or remove noxious stimulation indicate higher levels of brain function. Patients with catatonia may have increased muscle tone; muscle rigidity may result from poisoning with neuroleptic drugs (see Chapter 7 for further discussion). Absence of any muscle tone and lack of any response to stimulation suggests a severe brain injury but can be seen as well in patients with cervical spinal cord injuries or with neuromuscular blockade; noxious stimulation above the neck (such as firm pressure on the mastoid processes) should be utilized to be sure there is no response.

Reflexes

Reflex testing is of very limited value in unconscious patients. Asymmetry of reflexes between the two sides or between the upper and lower limbs may have limited localizing value. Similarly, the presence or absence of the Babinski sign is of little help. The Babinski sign is frequently absent in acute lesions of the brain and spinal cord, so absence of the sign is of no diagnostic significance. Presence of the sign indicates only an "upper motor neuron" process—virtually a foregone conclusion in an unconscious patient!

General Physical Examination

The general appearance of the patient should be noted. Cachexia may indicate severe malnutrition or a chronic wasting illness such as AIDS, chronic infection, or cancer.

Head and Neck Region

Signs of trauma, such as hematoma over the mastoid processes (Battle's sign), raccoon eyes, and local tenderness and crepitus, suggest severe neurotrauma and should be sought. Hemorrhage from the nose and ears or discoloration at the base of the skull indicates possible skull fracture. Palpation of the skull may reveal skull fractures or evidence of previous neurosurgical procedures. Palpation of the neck is generally not helpful in the unconscious patient. When in any doubt, it is safer to assume that there may be a cervical spine injury and to take proper precautions until the necessary imaging studies have been obtained. Even without specific signs of trauma to the head and neck region, evidence of significant trauma to the rest of the body should suggest possible trauma to the central nervous system.

Passive flexion of the neck should be attempted; nuchal rigidity should suggest the presence of meningeal irritation from infection or subarachnoid hemorrhage. As usual, this is contraindicated if there is any suspicion of a cervical spine injury.

Skin

Needle tracks suggest IV drug use or recent treatment with intravenous drugs. Cyanosis suggests hypoxemia, polycythemia, or abnormal hemoglobin. Pallor may indicate that the patient has inadequate oxygen-carrying capacity due to blood loss or anemia. A "cherry-red" color of the mucous membranes may indicate carbon monoxide poisoning but this is not reliable. Other skin findings such as multiple abscesses, cellulitis, uremic frost (deposits of white crystalline material on the skin of azotemic patients), or icterus may point to underlying conditions that affect mental status.

Cardiac Examination

Both tachyarrhythmias and bradyarrhythmias can alter mental status because of decreased cardiac output. Paroxysmal arrhythmias, chronic atrial fibrillation, valvular heart disease, or intracardiac shunts may all predispose to embolization and stroke. Infectious endocarditis is also an important risk factor for stroke. Acute myocardial infarction may reduce cardiac output enough to depress consciousness.

Seizures, if present, should be controlled (see Chapter 12).

LABORATORY STUDIES

In general, the use of "routine" laboratory studies is discouraged since such tests rarely yield useful information; it is usually much more efficient to obtain selected tests to answer specific questions. In unconscious patients, however, much of the information (usually obtained through the history and physical examination) is unavailable, and the clinician is often forced to rely on a "shotgun" approach to obtaining laboratory data.

A CBC is appropriate in most patients; severe anemia, marked leukopenia, or leukocytosis should be noted. Marked reduction in the platelet count may indicate sepsis, disseminated intravascular coagulation (DIC), eclampsia (HELLP syndrome), or alcoholism and implies an increased risk of bleeding. Abnormal clotting studies [prothrombin time (PT) and partial thromboplastin time (PTT)] indicate either a coagulopathy or treatment with anticoagulants. Blood glucose should be checked, as either marked hypoglycemia or hyperglycemia can result in coma. Serum electrolytes, osmolality, and BUN should be checked. (Note that elevated BUN, unless acute, is usually not associated with profound alteration of consciousness.) In patients with seizures, assays for commonly used anticonvulsants can be helpful in suggesting a preexisting seizure disorder and assessing the adequacy of treatment.

Arterial blood gases allow assessment of the patient's respiratory status; profound hypoxemia or hypercarbia or severe acidemia or alkalemia may be either the cause or the effect of alterations in mental status. A blood alcohol level may be helpful in excluding alcohol intoxication but is not very helpful in demonstrating that a patient's condition is solely due to alcohol intoxication. Urine drug screens are of little help; these qualitative tests only confirm the presence or absence of a few substances and, even if positive, do not demonstrate that the substance(s) detected is the cause of the patient's symptoms. Once a differential diagnosis is established, further studies may be helpful.

Lumbar puncture can confirm or exclude infectious meningitis or subarachnoid hemorrhage. In unconscious patients, lumbar puncture should be delayed until after a computed tomography (CT) scan of the head has been obtained. If infectious meningitis is suspected, empiric antibiotic treatment should be started immediately and lumbar puncture performed when it is determined to be safe (see "Infection"). Lumbar puncture is essential if subarachnoid hemorrhage is suspected and head CT scan is negative.

Electroencephalography (EEG) is rarely indicated on an emergency basis. However, EEG may be diagnostic when nonconvulsive seizure activity is suspected. This may occur in patients who present with status epilepticus. If patients do not begin to recover after their obvious seizures are controlled, continuing nonconvulsive seizures may be present. Occasional patients who present apparently awake but confused may be having ongoing nonconvulsive seizures. Finally, urgent EEG should be considered in any patient who has required neuromuscular blockade to facilitate management of seizures, to be sure that the seizure activity has actually stopped.

IMAGING STUDIES

As discussed in Chapter 2, there is an increasing array of imaging studies available to the emergency physician and the choice of the best imaging studies depends on the specific questions to be answered. For patients presenting with altered mental status and coma, the most important issue is to exclude an intracranial mass lesion or other structural lesion. For this purpose, CT scanning is usually the procedure of choice. CT images can be obtained very quickly, even in minimally cooperative patients. The entire head can be scanned in less than 15 seconds with most modern scanners. CT imaging is widely available even in locations where other modalities such as MR may not be available on an emergent or urgent basis.

CT will reliably detect most symptomatic epidural and subdural hematomas, intracerebral hemorrhages, cerebellar hemorrhages, abscesses and tumors (if large enough to be the cause of coma), acute hydrocephalus, etc. A CT scan will usually (but not always) detect acute subarachnoid hemorrhage but it is less sensitive in identifying smaller lesions, particularly those in the posterior fossa and brainstem. To assess patients for such lesions, MRI is the procedure of choice. Whenever possible, consultation with a radiologist is the best way to ensure that the most appropriate study is obtained. (See Chapter 2 for full discussion.)

INITIAL MANAGEMENT OF COMA AND ALTERED CONSCIOUSNESS

Appropriate initial management of the patient with altered mental status depends on the severity of the clinical picture, the likely diagnoses, and the patient's clinical course in the ED. Patients with mild confusion, acceptable vital signs, and a stable clinical course may not require acute intervention, allowing the physician time for a relatively "leisurely" assessment prior to initiating any treatment. At the other extreme, the patient in profound coma with signs of brainstem compression needs urgent intervention to try to prevent death and maximize the chance for recovery.

Coma or altered mental status may result from a wide variety of primary or secondary processes affecting the nervous system. Table 4-4 lists some of the more important clinical problems. Much more extensive lists and discussion can be found in the classic text by Posner et al.[8] Fortunately, initial management in the ED can focus on a few clinical syndromes rather than on the wide variety of specific disorders, which may underlie those syndromes. As illustrated in Table 4-4, it is important to distinguish between focal lesions of the CNS and more diffuse lesions as the cause of the abnormal mental status. Focal lesions of the CNS are suggested by any combination of a history of focal symptoms at onset, focal findings on the neurologic examination, and focal abnormalities on imaging studies. Absence of these characteristics suggests a diffuse process.

Empiric Management

In patients with significant alterations of consciousness, intravenous access should be established and blood drawn for laboratory studies (see later). It is common practice to give thiamine 100 mg, glucose 25 to 50 mg, and naloxone 0.8 to 1.6 mg on an empiric basis to virtually all patients with altered mental status. Naloxone may precipitate acute

TABLE 4-4
COMMON CAUSES OF COMA

Focal Lesions
History of focal signs at onset, focal findings on examination, imaging studies
abnormal
  Trauma: epidural or subdural hematomas, intracerebral hemorrhage,
    cerebral or brainstem contusion
  Infection: brain abscess (bacterial, fungal, *Toxoplasma*, etc.), focal
    encephalitis (herpes simplex)
  Stroke: intracerebral hemorrhage, ischemic stroke (large), brainstem stroke,
    or hemorrhage
  Neoplasm: primary or metastatic, especially if large or multiple, or
    associated with significant cerebral edema

Nonfocal (Diffuse) Lesions
No history of focal signs at onset, no focal findings on examination, imaging
studies normal or nondiagnostic
  Trauma: diffuse neuronal injury, increased intracranial pressure, traumatic
    subarachnoid hemorrhage
  Infection: meningitis (especially bacterial), encephalitis
  Vascular: spontaneous subarachnoid hemorrhage, hypertensive
    encephalopathy
  Seizures: convulsive or nonconvulsive, status epilepticus
  Toxic/metabolic disorders:
    Hypoxemia/global ischemia/hypercarbia
    Hypoglycemia/hyperglycemia, ketoacidosis
    Electrolyte disorders
      Hyponatremia/hypernatremia
      Hypercalcemia
    Hepatic failure
    Renal failure
    Thyroid disease: thyroid storm, myxedema coma
    Hyperthermia: heat stroke, neuroleptic malignant syndrome
    Hypothermia: exposure
    Drugs and toxins
      Alcohol intoxication
      Opiates and barbiturates
      Benzodiazepines and other sedatives and anxiolytics
      Antidepressants, phenothiazines, other psychiatric drugs
      Anticonvulsants
      Multiple illicit drugs

narcotic withdrawal, and the physician may suddenly be confronted with a severely agitated or delirious patient, therefore careful titration is recommended. These can be omitted if the available history or initial data (such as a normal or elevated blood glucose level) make it clear that they are unnecessary. Patients potentially at risk for nutritional deficiency (alcoholics or other substance abusers, severely debilitated patients, homeless persons, and others) should be given thiamine when being given glucose.

The next issue to be addressed is management of increased intracranial pressure (ICP). If there are signs of brainstem injury, or if the patient's condition is deteriorating rapidly (deepening coma, worsening focal signs) it is appropriate to begin treatment to lower ICP even before imaging studies are obtained. Patients with coma following head injury and patients with coma following apparent stroke or with other evidence of focal lesions should be assumed to have increased ICP and treated urgently. The fastest way to lower ICP is to correct hypoventilation and possibly to initiate hyperventilation. There is some risk of further compromising cerebral blood flow by abruptly lowering the $PaCO_2$, but it is important to quickly lower the ICP. As discussed in Chapter 10, a target $PaCO_2$ of 30 to 35 mm Hg is recommended, and hyperventilation should be discontinued as soon as possible. A hyperosmolar agent (usually mannitol 0.25–1.0 gm/kg) can be given at the same time; these maneuvers are intended to stabilize the patient until a definitive diagnosis can be made and specific treatment (if any) can be started. Depending on the likely diagnosis, other measures are initiated as discussed in the following sections.[8,10]

Head Trauma

Head trauma can cause coma by several different mechanisms, and more than one mechanism may be important in a given patient. Assessment is complicated by the fact that many head injuries occur in patients with other causes of impaired consciousness, such as drug or alcohol intoxication. Seizures may occur as well, further complicating the situation. Structural lesions resulting from head injury include epidural and subdural hematomas, as well as intracerebral or brainstem hemorrhages and contusions. These lesions may cause coma by increasing ICP, thereby reducing cerebral blood flow; or by compression of the ARAS via herniation syndromes; or by direct injury to the ARAS (as in brainstem hemorrhage). Patients with coma following head injury should be assumed to have increased ICP and be treated as outlined earlier and in Chapter 10. Other measures include neuromuscular blockade and CSF drainage (when available). The initial diagnostic imaging procedure of choice is usually CT scanning since imaging evidence of ICP and most structural lesions likely to cause increased ICP are easily detected by a CT. Neurosurgical consultation should also be obtained.

Another potential consequence of closed head injury is diffuse axonal injury due to shearing forces, as different regions of the brain accelerate and decelerate at different rates or encounter relatively fixed structures such as the free edges of the falx or tentorium. These lesions are often detected with MR imaging (see Chapter 2).

Trauma may also result in diffuse neuronal injury with no identifiable structural lesion. The pathophysiology of this process is complex, but there is marked impairment of cerebral blood flow and increases in the levels of extracellular excitatory amino acids, both of which result in ongoing neuronal injury. These patients develop cerebral edema with a marked rise in ICP, further compromising already tenuous cerebral blood flow. No specific treatment is available and management is controversial; every effort should be made to maintain systemic blood pressure and oxygenation, and neurosurgical consultation should be obtained.

Finally, trauma to major vessels in the neck can cause arterial occlusion or dissection with resultant cerebral infarction.

Stroke

Stroke has been discussed in detail in Chapter 5. Acute ischemic stroke is rarely a cause of coma unless the lesion is in the brainstem. Stroke syndromes that present with a rapid decline in mental status should suggest intracerebral hemorrhage; CT scanning is almost always diagnostic. These patients should be treated empirically for increased ICP until a diagnosis is established. Some patients with acute parenchymal hemorrhage, especially in the cerebellum, may benefit from emergent decompressive surgery, and neurosurgical consultation should be considered. Ischemic stroke may result in secondary cerebral edema with increased intracranial pressure and brain herniation, usually developing over a course of several days; CT scanning is diagnostic for these subacute sequelae of ischemic stroke. Treatment of these patients is expectant and the prognosis is usually bleak.

Other Mass Lesions

Intracranial tumors and abscesses can cause altered mental status and coma, either by increasing ICP or by causing herniation syndromes or both. The onset is rarely abrupt, and the correct diagnosis may well be suggested by the history; imaging studies, especially MR imaging, may be diagnostic. In patients with neoplasms, intravenous corticosteroids (usually dexamethasone) may result in dramatic clinical improvement within 6 to 12 hours. The appropriate dose of dexamethasone remains somewhat uncertain; 10 mg IV is commonly used, but doses up to 100 mg IV have been used by some. Neurosurgical consultation should be obtained.

Infection

Acute bacterial meningitis is virtually always fatal unless treated promptly and aggressively. The classical clinical triad is headache, fever, and nuchal rigidity; mental status changes occur early and patients may present in stupor or coma. Many patients will not present with the classic triad; bacterial meningitis should be considered in any patient who presents with deteriorating mental status and fever. There is usually a history of headache, and nuchal rigidity can often be detected even in comatose patients. Treatment should be initiated as soon as possible after the diagnosis is suspected; it is preferable but not mandatory that a lumbar puncture (LP) be obtained prior to beginning treatment, both to confirm the clinical diagnosis and to obtain CSF for bacteriologic studies. The CSF is characterized by elevated white cells, usually with a marked predominance of polymorphonuclear cells (PMNs), elevated protein, and low glucose. Although it is widely agreed that the risk of herniation following LP in these patients is actually very low, many physicians are reluctant to proceed with LP without antecedent imaging. CT is the examination of choice if imaging is deemed necessary. The emphasis should be on initiating empiric antibiotic therapy quickly with diagnostic studies completed as soon as possible thereafter. CSF cultures may remain positive for several hours following the first dose of antibiotics, and assays for bacterial antigens may yield a specific diagnosis even if cultures are negative. Therapy should be initiated with broad-spectrum antibiotic coverage (including coverage for Listeria) until antibiotic sensitivities are known. Immunosuppressed patients (due to AIDS, chemotherapy, corticosteroids, etc.) may require broader coverage. Dexamethasone, 10 mg IV, can be considered and should be administered shortly prior to or at the time antibiotics are started.[11,12]

Meningitis may be caused by organisms other than bacteria, such as mycobacteria, fungi, spirochetes, and viruses, and by noninfectious processes such as cancer and some drugs. These conditions are loosely grouped under the term aseptic (i.e., nonbacterial) meningitis. They tend to be less acute in onset and less fulminant in their course than bacterial meningitis but ultimately may be no less lethal. They are often characterized by a predominance of lymphocytes in the CSF but this is not reliable, since PMNs may predominate early in the course. These conditions are therefore often difficult or impossible to distinguish reliably from acute bacterial meningitis, especially in the acute setting. In general, it is better to assume that acute meningitis is bacterial until proved otherwise.

Encephalitis is an acute febrile syndrome characterized by fever, headache, and altered mental status. Meningeal signs are common but not always present. Seizures are common and focal neurologic signs may occur as well. The CSF often shows a lymphocytic pleocytosis but PMNs may predominate early in the course. Protein may be normal or slightly elevated and glucose may be normal. The clinical picture is quite nonspecific and may be caused by a wide variety of infectious agents including many viruses, rickettsia (e.g., rocky mountain spotted fever, ehrlichiosis, and others), spirochetes (e.g., Lyme disease), and even protozoa (e.g., *Naegleria*). Likely diagnoses are often suggested by the clinical context. During the summer months, for example, arboviral diseases such as Eastern and Western Equine Encephalitis, West Nile Virus encephalitis, etc., may be present in the community; human infections are often preceded by infections in domestic or wild animals. Specific serologic tests are available for many of these diseases. Treatment and prognosis depend on the specific causative organism.

The most common sporadic viral encephalitis in the United States is caused by *Herpes simplex* type 1 (HSV-1). Early diagnosis is important since specific treatment is available, but is most effective when started early. The illness commonly begins with a prodrome of several days of malaise, irritability, fever and lethargy; patients then develop fever, focal and generalized seizures, focal weakness or hemiplegia, and altered consciousness. CSF findings are nonspecific, with a lymphocytic pleocytosis (sometimes PMNs predominate), mildly elevated protein and normal or slightly low glucose. Red cells are often present. The diagnosis may be supported by MRI evidence of an acute inflammatory lesion, often affecting the temporal lobes and by characteristic EEG abnormalities. Definitive diagnosis is usually by demonstration of HSV-1 DNA in the CSF by the polymerase chain reaction (PCR). Suspected HSV encephalitis should be treated empirically with IV acyclovir 10 mg/kg q8h.

Seizures

Seizure activity may cause altered mental status or coma by several mechanisms. Many seizures, of course, are followed by a postictal period of altered mental status ranging in duration from minutes to hours or even longer. Often the history will suggest the diagnosis; patients will gradually recover without specific treatment, reassuring the physician that the process is benign and self-limited. More difficult to recognize, and less familiar, are situations in which altered mental status or coma are the result of ongoing seizure activity. In patients with prolonged convulsive status epilepticus, the motor manifestations may gradually wane, leaving the patient comatose but without obvious seizure activity. This may occur as well in patients treated for convulsive status; the convulsive movements may stop, giving the physician the illusion that the seizures have been controlled while the brain seizure activity continues unabated. This is a special problem, of course, in the occasional patients who require neuromuscular blocking agents to facilitate the management of their convulsive seizures. In addition, occasional patients are seen with nonconvulsive complex partial or absence seizures. Very careful observation of these patients will often reveal subtle signs of seizure activity such as intermittent or persistent nystagmus, subtle twitching of the mouth, the face, or the extremities, etc. Emergency EEG, if available, will confirm the diagnosis. If the diagnosis is strongly suspected and EEG is not available, empiric treatment for status epilepticus is appropriate (see Chapter 12 for full discussion).

Hypertensive Encephalopathy

Hypertensive encephalopathy (HE) is a fairly unusual condition, more often suspected than confirmed. It occurs as a result of failure of cerebral vascular autoregulation in the face of sustained severe hypertension, usually with mean arterial blood pressure (MAP) greater than 160 mm Hg. The clinical picture is characterized by headache, altered mental status seizures, papilledema, and marked elevation of blood pressure. Confusion and delirium are seen more commonly than frank coma. Focal neurologic signs, if present, are usually mild and transient. Visual field abnormalities are common and may progress to cortical blindness. CT scans may be normal or may reveal extensive, often symmetric, low-density regions in both hemispheres, especially in the parieto-occipital regions. MRI reveals extensive areas of cortical and/or subcortical edema most prominent in the occipital and parietal lobes (Fig. 4-7). HE is a true medical emergency with high mortality if not treated aggressively. The usual treatment is IV nitroprusside to control the blood pressure rapidly, but care must be taken not to lower the blood pressure too far, too fast; in the face of increased ICP, excessive lowering of systemic blood pressure may lead to cerebral ischemia. A safe rule of thumb is to lower the MAP by 25% over the first hour. Other agents such as labetalol and nitroglycerin have also been used with success.

An identical MR appearance can be seen in patients with eclampsia and some toxic/metabolic encephalopathies (see "Toxic and Metabolic Causes of Coma"). The syndrome has acquired several synonyms and has been called the Reversible Posterior Leukoencephalopathy Syndrome (RPLS), the Posterior Reversible Encephalopathy Syndrome (PRES), and Vasoactive Reactive Encephalopathy (VRE). Treatment is directed at the underlying cause, such as lowering the blood pressure in HE, delivering the baby in eclampsia, or reducing the dose or stopping the inciting drug. Despite the dramatic clinical and imaging findings that may be present, the clinical syndrome is almost always completely reversible.

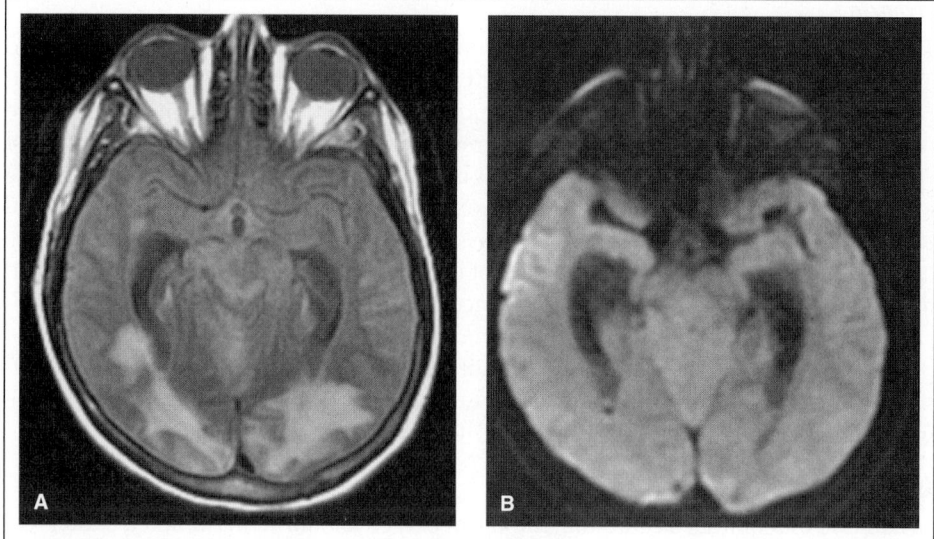

FIGURE 4-7 (A) FLAIR MRI shows extensive bilateral parieto-occipital subcortical vasogenic edema. (B) Diffusion MRI showing lack of abnormality confirms that this is vasogenic edema confirmed by lack of abnormality on the diffusion MR imaging. This patient also demonstrated extensive posterior fossa findings (not shown) which can also be seen in hypertensive encephalopathy.

Toxic and Metabolic Causes of Coma

In most acute care settings, toxic or metabolic disorders are the most common causes of altered mental status. The most common clinical presentations are lethargy and delirium, with stupor and frank coma less frequent. These disorders are generally characterized by absence of focal signs except as noted below and relative preservation of brainstem function. Unfortunately, the clinical syndrome is quite nonspecific and may result from a wide variety of different causes including CNS and systemic infections, metabolic and electrolyte disorders, hypoxemia, decreased CNS perfusion, drugs and toxins, etc. Often, the clinical history offers the best hope for a rapid and accurate diagnosis. A detailed drug history (including both prescribed and nonprescribed drugs and both licit and illicit) is especially helpful. Family members and others should be asked about any other medications or toxins available in the home that may have been ingested by mistake. The "plastic bag test" in which family members are asked to bring in the entire contents of the family medicine chest in a plastic bag may be diagnostic. A complete review of the various toxic/metabolic encephalopathies is beyond the scope of this brief review. Especially in the elderly, acute delirium may complicate virtually any medical condition or may be provoked by a wide variety of drugs and toxins. Accordingly, every effort should be made to obtain a detailed drug history. Regardless of the specific cause, the clinical presentations are quite similar and nonspecific.

As noted earlier, the RPLS syndrome can occur in patients treated with a variety of cytotoxic and immunosuppressive drugs (such as tacrolimus and cyclosporine), and occasionally in patients with no evident predisposing cause. With the increasing use of cytotoxic and immunosuppressive agents in a variety of medical conditions, this syndrome may become more frequent in the future.[13]

Hypoxia

The brain is dependent on a continuing supply of oxygen and metabolic substrates to maintain its intense metabolic activity and even a very brief interruption leads to impaired consciousness or coma. Cerebral hypoxia most commonly results from perfusion failure (see "Disorders of the Cerebral Hemispheres") but may also result from impairment of ventilation, or impairment of pulmonary gas exchange from pulmonary embolism, severe pneumonia, acute respiratory distress syndrome, or pulmonary edema. Another potential cause is reduced blood–oxygen carrying capacity, as in carbon monoxide (CO) poisoning or methemoglobinemia. CO poisoning is not uncommon; the diagnosis is often suggested by the history. A clinical clue is the presence of hypoxemia without cyanosis; the well-known cherry-red color of the mucous membranes is uncommon and not reliable. The prognosis depends on the severity and duration of hypoxia, but may be favorable if perfusion is maintained during the period of hypoxemia. There is no effective treatment for the brain disorder per se in hypoxia; treatment should be directed at the underlying disorder.

Ischemia

In addition to requiring a continuing supply of oxygen and nutrients as noted earlier, the brain requires continuous perfusion to remove the toxic byproducts of its metabolism. Cerebral ischemia delivers a double insult, both depriving the brain of oxygen and substrates and allowing the toxic by-products of anaerobic metabolism to accumulate rapidly. With complete cessation of cerebral perfusion, permanent neuronal injury may occur within minutes.

Global cerebral ischemia most often results from pump failure (cardiogenic shock, cardiac arrest, etc.) but may also develop as a consequence of profound systemic hypotension of whatever cause. The mainstay of treatment is to restore adequate brain perfusion as quickly as possible. Several recent trials suggest that prognosis is improved in patients treated with mild induced hypothermia to 33°C to 34°C for 12 to 24 hours, at least in patients whose initial rhythm was ventricular fibrillation (VF).[14,15] The utility of this approach in patients with other arrest rhythms such as PEA or asystole is unknown, but induced hypothermia may be considered in these patients as well. There is no other specific care for the brain lesion. Depending on the clinical circumstances, several days of observation may be needed to reliably estimate the prognosis in these patients and to make decisions about further treatment.[16]

Hypoglycemia and Hyperglycemia

Profound hypoglycemia is a fairly common cause of altered mental status in the acute care setting. This may be due to inadequate food intake in patients taking insulin or oral hypoglycemic agents or overdose of these medications. The treatment is rapid replacement of glucose (with thiamine, as indicated). Hyperglycemia, with or without ketoacidosis, is also an important cause of coma. It must be remembered that either hypoglycemia or hyperglycemia may cause seizures (including focal seizures) and focal neurologic deficits mimicking stroke. The appropriate treatment is to normalize the blood sugar; anticonvulsants and stroke-treatment protocols are ineffective and not indicated.

Electrolyte Abnormalities

Severe hyponatremia may cause altered mental status or coma. Symptoms usually do not occur unless the serum sodium is <125 mEq/L; seizures and coma usually do not occur unless the serum sodium is <115 mEq/L. The severity of the clinical syndrome depends both on the sodium level and on the rate of decrease of the sodium; even profound hyponatremia may be well tolerated if developed over a long period of time. The treatment of severe hyponatremia remains somewhat controversial, since too rapid corrections can have severe consequences, including osmotic demyelination (central pontine myelinolysis). In general, the more acute the hyponatremia, the more rapidly replacement can proceed. Hypernatremia is less commonly encountered and is most often the consequence of dehydration. It may be encountered in patients receiving parenteral feedings, especially if they are also receiving diuretics. It should be considered in chronically debilitated patients, especially the very elderly, with altered mental status. The treatment is rehydration; this should be undertaken with care to avoid the risk of water intoxication. Hypercalcemia is an occasional cause of obtundation and coma, particularly in patients with cancer.

Hepatic and Renal Failure

Either hepatic or renal failure may produce a clinical syndrome characterized by progressive obtundation, asterixis and/or myoclonus, and eventual coma. This clinical syndrome is nonspecific and similar to that seen in a wide variety of other toxic/metabolic encephalopathies. The diagnosis in each case will be based on clinical suspicion and appropriate laboratory studies. It should be remembered that these clinical syndromes are often reversible, so that aggressive evaluation and treatment should be pursued.

Alcohol Intoxication

Ethyl alcohol is the most common intoxicant encountered in the acute care setting. The effects of alcohol are usually transient and no treatment is required. It is essential that the physician not assume that the presence of alcohol, even at high levels, is necessarily the only cause of a given patient's altered mental status. Any of the other causes of altered mental status or coma, including potentially lethal conditions such as intracranial mass lesions, meningitis, and others, may well be present but overlooked in the apparently intoxicated patient. Accordingly, each patient needs careful assessment. Other alcohols such as methanol or ethylene glycol are occasionally used as intoxicants as well. Their presence should be suspected in an apparently intoxicated patient with a significant osmolal gap and negative ethanol level.

Drugs

An enormous number of drugs may cause obtundation and coma, usually, but not necessarily, when taken in overdose. Prescription drugs, over-the-counter drugs, and recreational drugs all may be responsible. Common urine drug screens are qualitative and indicate only that a patient has used a drug recently; such screens do not indicate that any given drug is the cause of the patient's clinical symptoms. Specific quantitative assays are available for some agents and may be very helpful. Opiates are common offenders; the diagnosis is established by the prompt response to intravenous naloxone. The physician should recall that the duration of action of the offending drug may exceed that of naloxone and that repeated doses of naloxone may be needed. Barbiturates are also a common cause, but no diagnostic or therapeutic antidote is available. It should be recalled that barbiturates per se have no permanent adverse effects on the brain and that even profoundly depressed patients may make a full recovery. Benzodiazepines rarely cause coma by themselves but may potentiate other intoxicants; flumazenil will reverse benzodiazepine effects but may provoke acute withdrawal with agitation, delirium, and seizures.

Anticholinergic drugs such as atropine, trihexyphenidyl, and benztropine, as well as agents such as tricyclic antidepressants (e.g., amitriptyline) often cause a severe agitated delirium; patients present with dilated pupils, tachycardia, and hot, dry, flushed skin—a syndrome summarized by the phrase, "mad as a hatter, red as a beet, dry as a bone." Treatment with physostigmine may result in dramatic, albeit transient, improvement. With any drug-induced or metabolic encephalopathy, specific treatment depends on the specific cause. Supportive measures include keeping the patient in a quiet and comfortable space; a family member or other person may help to keep the patient calm. Pain should be controlled. Pharmacologic treatment should be avoided if possible. When needed, antipsychotic drugs such as haloperidol and others are probably the drugs of choice. Benzodiazepines are also widely used, but there is not much data regarding their effectiveness in this setting.[5]

SUMMARY

The patient with severely altered mental status or coma is a true medical emergency with a high likelihood of death or permanent disability. The physician's immediate actions should be as follows:

1. Assess the patient's vital signs and stabilize if necessary.
2. Determine whether the underlying disorder is structural or diffuse.
3. Initiate emergency treatment.
4. Determine the specific diagnosis.
5. Arrange appropriate consultation and continuing treatment.

The initial emphasis should always be on the rapid identification and management of potentially treatable conditions. It is much less critical if the diagnosis of a self-limited or untreatable condition is missed.

REFERENCES

1. Kanich WS, Brady WJ, Huff SJ. Altered mental status in the emergency department: most efficient diagnostic tools and most frequent causes. *Ann Emerg Med.* 2001;37:547.
2. Rummans TA, Evans JM, Krahn LE, et al. Delirium in elderly patients: evaluation and management. *Mayo Clin Proc.* 1995;70:989.
3. Hustey FM, Meldon SW. The prevalence and documentation of impaired mental status in elderly emergency department patients. *Ann Emerg Med.* 2002;39:248.
4. Sanders AB. Missed delirium in older emergency department patients: a quality-of-care problem. *Ann Emerg Med.* 2002;39:338.
5. American Psychiatric Association Workgroup on Delirium. Practice guideline for the treatment of patients with delirium. *Am J Psychiatry.* 1999;156(suppl):1-20.
6. Johnson MH. Assessing confused patients. *J Neurol Neurosurg Psychiatry.* 2001;71(suppl I):i7.
7. Cartlidge N. States related to or confused with coma. *J Neurol Neurosurg Psychiatry.* 2001; 71(suppl I):i18.

8. Posner JB, Saper CB, Schiff ND, Plum F. *Plum and Posner's Diagnosis of Stupor and Coma.* 4th ed. New York: Oxford University Press; 2007.

9. Sapira JD. An internist looks at the fundus oculi. *Dis Mon.* 1984;30(14):1-64.

10. Chesnut RM. Guidelines for the management of severe head injury: what we know and what we think we know. *J Trauma.* 1997;42(suppl):S19.

11. Roos KL, Tyler KL. Meningitis, encephalitis, brain abscess, and empyema. In: Fauci AS, Braunwald E, Kasper DL, et al. *Harrison's Principles of Internal Medicine.* 17th ed. New York: McGraw Hill Medical; 2008;2621-2641.

12. Tunkel AR, Scheld WM. Bacterial infections of the central nervous system. In: Hall JB, Schmidt GA, Wood LDH, eds. *Principles of Critical Care.* 3rd ed. chap 52. New York: McGraw Hill; 2005 http://accessmedicine.com/content.aspx?aID=2291393.

13. Lee VH, Wijdicks EF, Manno EM, Rabinstein AA. Clinical spectrum of reversible posterior leukoencephalopathy syndrome. *Arch Neurol.* 2008;65(2):205.

14. Dine CJ, Abella BS. Therapeutic hypothermia for neuroprotection. *Emerg Med Clin North Am.* 2009;27:137-139.

15. Bernard S. Hypothermia after cardiac arrest: expanding the therapeutic scope. *Crit Care Med.* 2009;37(suppl 7):S227-S233.

16. Young GB. Neurologic prognosis after cardiac arrest. *N Engl J Med.* 2009;361:605-611.

5

ACUTE FOCAL NEUROLOGIC DEFICITS

Patients with acute focal neurologic deficits are frequently seen in the acute care setting and can pose difficult challenges to the clinical skills of physicians. It is not uncommon for such patients to be assigned a tentative but virtually meaningless diagnosis such as "rule out stroke." A vague or incorrect diagnosis may effectively limit the search for the correct diagnosis and potentially deprive the patient of some effective treatment, or may expose him or her to the potential hazards of an unneeded treatment. Especially for patients with suspected stroke, this problem has become more serious with the advent of thrombolytic therapy, which may offer significant benefit, but which carries significant risk as well.

An acute neurologic deficit will be defined as one that develops over 24 hours or less. In fact, many such deficits evolve much more rapidly, often over a period of only a few minutes. A focal deficit implies injury or dysfunction in a localized area of the nervous system. The focal nature of the neurologic deficit may not always be immediately apparent. A patient who appears confused or disoriented at first glance, suggesting a diffuse brain disorder, may be found on careful evaluation to actually have dysphasia, a disorder of language function caused by a discrete focal lesion of the brain. Conversely, a patient who complains of weakness in the lower extremities, suggesting a focal disorder, may be found to actually have generalized weakness and decreased reflexes, suggesting a more diffuse process. As always, the correct diagnosis depends on careful clinical assessment.

CLINICAL ASSESSMENT

The process of clinical diagnosis depends first on a clear understanding of what is to be diagnosed. Accordingly, the importance of a clear and adequate history cannot be overemphasized. Failure to obtain an adequate history can result in expensive, invasive, potentially hazardous, and ultimately useless investigation of symptoms never actually experienced by the patient; at the same time, necessary and appropriate studies may be omitted. Even with patients who are confused, disoriented, or unconscious (signs usually suggesting a diffuse process), a proper history, obtained from family or other witnesses, may suggest a focal onset to the clinical syndrome.

The most important goal of getting the history is to obtain as accurate and detailed description as possible of the specific symptoms experienced by the patient. When obtainable, a good history will often suggest the correct diagnosis, or at least sharply limit the number of reasonable possible diagnoses. For example, pain in the left shoulder and left arm may be due to a cervical radiculopathy, a brachial plexus lesion, a torn rotator cuff, or coronary artery disease (among other possibilities); an adequate history will often distinguish among these. Similarly, a complaint of "dizziness" may actually refer to vertigo, dysequilibrium, impending syncope, or lightheadedness. Each of these symptoms implies a different differential diagnosis, and investigation of any one of them will probably not help in the diagnosis of any of the others. It is especially helpful to ask about any specific functional impairment as this will often give the physician a much better insight into the patient's complaints than a simple recitation of symptoms. Once the character of the patient's symptoms is clearly understood, the usual questions concerning onset, progression, associated symptoms, etc., should be pursued.

The next step in the clinical assessment is the neurologic examination. This is discussed in detail in Chapter 3 and only a few comments will be added here. The examination should serve to:

1. Clarify the exact nature of the clinical symptoms. For example, is a "weak" leg truly weak, or is it actually numb, clumsy, or stiff? Does a patient with slurred speech actually have dysphasia or dysarthria?
2. Identify additional clinical findings not reported by the patient. For example, is a weak leg reported by the patient accompanied by slight weakness of the face and arm on the same side?
3. Suggest the anatomic basis for the symptom. For example, leg weakness accompanied by increased reflexes and an upgoing toe suggests an upper motor neuron lesion, while muscle atrophy and decreased reflexes suggest a lower motor neuron lesion, and thus a completely different differential diagnosis.

In many cases, a fairly comprehensive neurologic examination will be needed, but a "complete" examination is rarely needed even if it were possible. The examination should be carefully planned so as to avoid missing crucial information. It is better to be too detailed than to be too superficial. It is particularly important to "examine the complaint," that is, to observe the patient attempting to perform the specific activity that is problematic. A patient with a gait disorder, for example, should be observed while trying to walk and cannot be fully examined while lying supine on a gurney.

At the conclusion of the initial clinical assessment, the physician should be prepared to give tentative answers to three questions:

1. Are the patient's symptoms probably due to a focal lesion in the nervous system?
2. Where is the lesion?
3. What is (are) the likely cause(s) of the lesion?

Note that the likely location of the lesion must be determined before a differential diagnosis can be suggested. The ability to localize the lesion depends primarily on the

TABLE 5-1 —————————————————————————————

CLUES TO CLINICAL LOCALIZATION

Brain Lesions

Language disorders (aphasias)[a]
Agnosias and apraxias[b]
Visual field defects (affecting both eyes)[c]
Motor deficits, sensory deficits involving the face, arm, and leg on the same side
  of the body (the side opposite the lesion)
Alterations of consciousness, perception, or behavior
"Cortical" sensory impairment—astereognosis, impaired graphesthesia, etc.

Brainstem Lesions

Cranial nerve abnormalities[d]
Alternating hemiplegia—weakness of cranial nerve function on one side and of
  the body on the opposite side

Spinal Cord Lesions

Sensory or motor "levels"
Mixed "upper motor neuron" and "lower motor neuron" signs
Sensory dissociation (impaired pain/temperature sensation on one side of the
  body, impaired vibration/position sense on the opposite side)
Sensory/motor dissociation (impaired pain/temperature sensation on one side of
  the body, impaired motor function on the opposite side)
Early impairment of bladder, bowel, or sexual function

Peripheral Nerve/Root Lesions

Motor impairment, sensory impairment, or both confined to the distribution of a
  single peripheral nerve or nerve root
Pain confined to the distribution of a single peripheral nerve or nerve root

---

[a] Aphasia implies a lesion in the dominant (usually the left) hemisphere. The many subtypes of aphasias discussed in textbooks are rarely seen in pure form in clinical practice and are of little localizing value in the emergency setting.

[b] These are most often recognized in patients with right parietal lesions (in whom language function is preserved).

[c] Vision deficits confined to only one eye are caused by lesions anterior to the optic chiasm on the affected side, not by lesions of the brain.

[d] Cranial nerve lesions due to brainstem lesions will virtually always be associated with clinical signs affecting other parts of the nervous system (e.g., long tract signs).

physician's skill in performing the neurologic examination and interpreting the findings. The more sophisticated the physician's clinical skills, the more accurate the anatomic diagnosis and the shorter the differential diagnosis is likely to be. A brief list of some common clues to localization is given in Table 5-1. Once a differential diagnosis is established, the necessary laboratory and imaging studies can be obtained to confirm the correct diagnosis and to exclude the others. An imaging study of the wrong part of the body (e.g., a CT scan of the head in a patient who has a spinal cord problem) is unlikely to contribute much to diagnostic clarity.

Acute focal neurologic deficits may be due to a wide variety of entities. The most likely causes in a particular patient are determined by the part of the nervous system affected, the time course, and the clinical context. The most common causes of lesions in various parts of the nervous system are discussed as follows.

ACUTE FOCAL LESIONS OF THE BRAIN AND BRAINSTEM

The most common causes of acute focal lesions affecting the brain and brainstem are listed in Table 5-2.

Stroke

The most common cause of an acute focal lesion affecting the brain, the brainstem, or the cerebellum is stroke. A stroke is defined as an acute focal loss of brain function caused by a disruption of brain blood flow. Depending on their mechanism, strokes are classified as either ischemic or hemorrhagic; most strokes (approximately 85%) are ischemic. The term *stroke* is not ordinarily applied to the more global ischemic injury resulting from profound hypotension, cardiac arrest, etc. Subarachnoid hemorrhage, in which

TABLE 5-2

ETIOLOGIES OF ACUTE FOCAL LESIONS OF THE BRAIN AND BRAINSTEM

Vascular disorders
Stroke (ischemic or hemorrhagic)
Transient ischemic attack (TIA)
Migraine
Venous thrombosis

Infectious disorders
Brain abscess (bacterial, fungal, protozoan, etc.)
Encephalitis (especially herpes simplex)

Mass lesions
Neoplasms (primary and metastatic)
Epidural/subdural hematomas/empyemas

Metabolic disorders
Hypoglycemia/hyperglycemia

Seizures
Focal seizures
Postictal (Todd's) paralysis

Inflammatory/granulomatous disorders
Multiple sclerosis
Sarcoidosis
Cerebral vasculitis (with or without systemic vasculitis)

bleeding occurs into the subarachnoid space, often from a ruptured aneurysm or other vascular lesion, is not included in this definition of stroke.

Ischemic stroke occurs as a result of partial or complete occlusion of a vessel supplying blood to the brain. Depending on the adequacy of any collateral circulation, the cerebral blood flow (CBF) to the affected region of the brain is reduced. Reduction of CBF below 50% of normal (i.e., to approximately 20 mL blood/100 g brain tissue/min) results in neuronal dysfunction and the appearance of neurologic deficits. Reduction of CBF below 25% of normal causes metabolic failure and initiates a cascade of events leading to cell death. The current view is that an ischemic stroke is characterized by an *ischemic core*, in which CBF is markedly reduced or absent, and in which permanent neuronal injury occurs within minutes. The core is surrounded by an *ischemic penumbra*, a zone of less severe reduction of CBF in which permanent neuronal injury may be delayed for several hours. The size of the infarcted zone (the core) relative to the size of the ischemic zone (the penumbra) depends on multiple factors such as the size of the occluded vessel, the abruptness of the occlusion, and the state of the collateral circulation. The goal of acute stroke therapy is to enhance the prospects for survival of this potentially salvageable penumbra tissue, either by restoring adequate perfusion to ischemic tissue before permanent damage occurs or by enhancing the ability of brain tissue to withstand ischemic stress.[1] To date, efforts in stroke treatment have been focused on restoring perfusion (explained later) because despite multiple attempts, no effective neuroprotective agents have yet been identified.

Hemorrhagic stroke occurs as a result of leakage of blood from a damaged vessel into the surrounding brain; local tissue damage may occur as a result of the physical disruption of brain parenchyma, displacement or distortion of nearby structures (mass effect), and toxic effects of extravasated blood. In addition, hemorrhages may cause more diffuse effects from raised intracranial pressure and mass effects. In some cases, an initial ischemic infarction can be complicated by *hemorrhagic transformation*, in which there is secondary hemorrhage into the infarcted tissue.

It is important to recall that both ischemic and hemorrhagic strokes occur as the final result of some underlying process; effective management requires recognition and treatment not only of the stroke syndrome but of the underlying cause as well. Table 5-3 lists some potential causes for stroke. Clearly, many of these diagnoses will require more extensive evaluation than would be carried out in the acute care setting.

Clinical Evaluation

In many cases, the clinical diagnosis of stroke is straightforward. The abrupt onset of symptoms consistent with an acute focal brain injury is virtually diagnostic. Often the clinical picture will suggest a lesion in a specific vascular territory, such as the middle cerebral artery or one of its branches, the vertebrobasilar system, and other locations. Strokes in the territory of the middle cerebral arteries typically present with weakness of the contralateral face and arm, often with a contralateral visual field deficit, and with less severe weakness of the leg. With left hemisphere lesions, aphasia is often present as well. Dense weakness of the face, arm, and leg on the same side, and with sparing of visual fields and language, suggest a lesion in the deep white matter of the brain, such as the internal capsule. Lesions in the anterior cerebral artery territory commonly cause weakness of the contralateral leg with relative sparing of the arm and face, generally without visual field deficits. Lesions of the posterior cerebral arteries cause contralateral visual

TABLE 5-3 ————————————————————————————

CAUSES OF STROKE[a]

A. Ischemic stroke

Vascular disorders
Atheromatous disease (extracranial or intracranial)
Small-vessel vasculopathy (diabetes, hypertension, lupus, etc.)
Primary vascular disease (fibromuscular dysplasia, congenital stenosis or atresia, moya moya, etc.)
Arterial dissection (spontaneous or traumatic)
Infectious/inflammatory disease (meningitis, granulomatous angiitis, etc.)

Cardiac disorders
Atrial fibrillation
Myocardial infarction
Valvular heart disease, endocarditis
Cardiomyopathies
Intracardiac shunts (patent foramen ovale, atrial septal defects, etc.)
Atrial myxoma

Hematologic disorders
Sickle cell disease
Hyperviscosity syndromes
Hypercoaguable states (pregnancy, oral contraceptives, coagulopathies)

B. Hemorrhagic stroke
Small vessel vasculopathy (hypertension, diabetes, amyloid angiopathy, etc.)
Vascular anomalies (arteriovenous malformation, hemangiomas, etc)
Intracranial aneurysms (including mycotic aneurysms)
Coagulation disorders (primary and iatrogenic)

---

[a] This list is not intended to be exhaustive, but rather to give the reader some sense of the wide range of different disorders that may present with stroke.

field deficits, usually with minimal motor deficits. Strokes in the brainstem may cause a variety of cranial nerve signs, especially diplopia, vertigo, and dysequilibrium, together with unilateral or bilateral motor deficits. Most patients with stroke present with one of a small number of common and easily recognized syndromes.

The time of onset of the symptoms should be accurately determined, if possible. This is especially critical if the patient is to be considered a possible candidate for thrombolytic therapy (see later). The manner of onset and subsequent evolution of the symptoms may suggest the likely mechanism of the stroke. Abrupt onset, with the clinical deficit reaching its maximum extent within minutes, suggests embolic occlusion of a vessel, the embolus having originated either in a larger more proximal vessel or in the heart. Multiple lesions in different arterial distributions also suggest embolism from a central source such as the heart. A stuttering course suggests progressive occlusion of an extra- or intracranial vessel, or recurrent embolism from a nearby vessel such as the common carotid artery at its bifurcation or the internal carotid artery. A history of premonitory transient ischemic attacks (TIAs) suggests atheromatous disease of the ipsilateral internal carotid artery. The presence of severe headache at onset, abrupt loss of consciousness, or steady progression of a neurologic deficit should suggest intracerebral hemorrhage.

The clinical context may also suggest the likely mechanism of the stroke. The presence of atrial fibrillation, a history of cardiac valve disease (or replacement), or evidence of recent myocardial infarction should all suggest possible cardiogenic embolism. Strokes in younger patients are often cryptogenic, but may suggest inflammatory vasculopathy, a cardiac lesion, arterial dissection, or (rarely) a coagulopathy.

In the initial evaluation of patients with suspected stroke, a structured rating scale such as the National Institutes of Health Stroke Scale (NIHSS) can be very useful to record the neurologic deficits and grade the severity of the stroke (Table 5-4). The initial Stroke Scale Score provides a convenient baseline against which one can measure progression or resolution of stroke symptoms. The NIHSS is based on a structured neurologic examination and yields scores between 0 and 42; scores over 20 are generally considered to indicate "severe" stroke. However, it is important to remember that even a "low" score, such as in a patient with an isolated aphasia (NIHSS score 2 or 3) may be associated with a devastating and life-altering event.

Differential Diagnosis

Even in patients with seemingly "obvious" stroke, it is important to recall that there is ample opportunity for diagnostic error, and error rates as high as 25% in the clinical diagnosis of stroke have been reported.[2–4] The potential differential diagnoses include virtually every cause of an acute focal deficit. The conditions most commonly mistaken for stroke in one series of 411 patients are listed in Table 5-5. Even though many of these conditions may cause symptoms that appear to be acute, the neurologic deficits more commonly develop over hours or days or longer. Careful questioning may be necessary to extract a reliable history from anxious patients and families, many of whom will have already made their own diagnosis of stroke before coming to the emergency department.

Imaging Studies

Computed tomography (CT) remains the imaging procedure of choice for most patients with suspected acute stroke (see Chapter 2). CT scans can be performed very quickly and without concern for possible implanted metal, pacemakers, infusion pumps, and other devices. Critically ill or unstable patients can be more easily monitored and managed in the CT environment than in the MR suite. In addition, adequate images can usually be obtained even in minimally cooperative patients. Contrast administration is usually not necessary but should be considered after the noncontrast examination if there is concern about lesions other than stroke, such as neoplasms or infection. CT is virtually 100% sensitive in detecting intracranial blood and is highly sensitive for intracranial mass effect from whatever cause, conditions that must be excluded before patients can be considered for thrombolytic therapy (see later). It is true that CT is not very sensitive for acute ischemic lesions with approximately 30% detectable at 3 hours and 60% at 24 hours. In patients with large ischemic lesions, subtle changes may be evident within hours but are not reliably present. Even apparently "positive" scans must be interpreted with caution, because a lesion detected on the scan may not be the lesion responsible for the patient's acute symptoms.

Magnetic resonance imaging (MRI) is considerably more sensitive than CT in detecting acute ischemic lesions.[5] Although modern MRI systems can obtain images

TABLE 5-4

THE NIH STROKE SCALE

Examination Item	Response	Points
1a. Level of consciousness	Alert	0
	Drowsy	1
	Stuporous	2
	Comatose	3
1b. Level of consciousness	Both correct	0
Ask patient age and	One correct	1
current month	Both incorrect	2
1c. Level of consciousness	Both correct	0
Ask patient to close eyes	One correct	1
Ask patient to make a fist	Both incorrect	2
2. Best gaze	Normal	0
	Partial gaze palsy	1
	Forced deviation of eyes	2
3. Visual fields	Normal	0
	Partial hemianopia	1
	Complete hemianopia	2
	Bilateral hemianopia (cortical blindness)	3
4. Facial weakness	Normal	0
	Minor weakness	1
	Partial weakness	2
	Complete paralysis	3
5–8. Motor function	No drift	0
(test all four limbs)	Drift present	1
	Some effort against gravity	2
	No effort against gravity	3
	No movement	4
	Not testable	9
9. Limb ataxia	Absent	0
(Score if *present*—	Present in one limb	1
cannot be scored in a	Present in two limbs	2
plegic limb or if patient		
unable to perform)		
10. Sensory (pinprick)	Normal	0
	Partial loss	1
	Complete loss	2
11. Best language	No aphasia	0
	Mild/moderate aphasia	1
	Severe aphasia	2
	Mute	3

TABLE 5-4

THE NIH STROKE SCALE (*Continued*)

Examination Item	Response	Points
12. Dysarthria	Normal articulation	0
	Mild/moderate dysarthria	1
	Unintelligible	2
	Untestable	X
13. Neglect/inattention	None	0
	Partial neglect	1
	Complete neglect	2
Total		0–42

The NIH Stroke Scale—Instructions[a]

1a. The examiner must choose a response even if full evaluation is prevented by obstacles such as an ET tube, language barrier, or bandages—note that the level of arousal, not the content of consciousness, is being evaluated.

1b. Score only the first answer to each question—not partial credit for "close" answers. Do not repeat the questions or "coach" the patient. Aphasic or stuporous patients are scored "2." Patients who cannot speak because of physical barriers (e.g., an ET tube) are scored "1."

1c. Test the nonparetic hand. Another suitable one-step command may be used if the hands cannot be tested. Score only the first response. If the patient does not respond to command, the requested movement can be demonstrated by the examiner.

2. Only horizontal movements are tested. Voluntary, pursuit, or oculocephalic reflex movements can be tested, but not caloric responses.

3. Fields can be tested using confrontation, finger counting, or visual threat. Note that visual *fields* are being tested, not vision in each eye; this can be done even in a patient with monocular blindness. Patients who are blind (from any cause) are scored "3."

4. Ask or use pantomime to encourage the patient to show teeth and to close the eyes. Score grimace to noxious stimulus in the patient who cannot respond.

5 & 6. The limb is placed in the appropriate position—arm extended 90 degrees (patient sitting) or 45 degrees (patient supine); the leg is placed at 30 degrees elevation (patient supine). Each limb is tested separately. Score drift if the arm drifts downward before 10 seconds or the leg drifts downward before 5 seconds.

7. Use standard finger-nose-finger and heel-shin maneuvers. Ataxia is scored only if out of proportion to weakness—ataxia is not scored if the patient cannot understand or if the tested limb is plegic. Score 9 only for amputation or joint fusion.

(*continued*)

TABLE 5-4

THE NIH STROKE SCALE (*Continued*)

8. Use pinprick or other noxious stimulus. Only sensory loss attributable to stroke can be scored (e.g., do not score sensory loss secondary to peripheral neuropathy).
9. Be sure to distinguish true aphasia from dysarthria (#10). Patients in coma are scored as "3."
10. If aphasia is present, any spontaneous speech is scored. Patients who are mute are scored "2." Score "3" only if speech is physically impossible (e.g., intubated patient).
11. Neglect is scored only if clearly present. Note that neglect may not be testable in patients with severe sensory loss; such patients are scored as normal on this item.

[a] This is only a brief summary of the instructions. Use of the scale should be demonstrated by an experienced user or by instructional video to obtain maximum reliability and reproducible results.
[b] Scores of "9" (untestable items) are not included in the final score.

within minutes, the usefulness of MRI is limited by technical considerations. MRI cannot be performed on patients with implanted pacemakers or similar devices, or on patients with ferromagnetic metals in the body. Although technically possible, MRI is more difficult in patients who require mechanical ventilation. In addition, MRI requires that the patient remain very still throughout the examination, and may be impossible in confused, aphasic, or agitated patients. Finally, effective MRI requires the immediate availability of equipment and staff, as well as physicians experienced in the interpretation of the images. Despite these limitations, the use of MRI in acute stroke patients is likely to become more widespread, especially as new and more powerful techniques are developed that may directly affect acute treatment decisions. Diffusion- and perfusion-

TABLE 5-5

CONDITIONS THAT MIMICKED STROKE IN 411 PATIENTS

Condition	Frequency (%)
Seizure	13 (16.7)
Systemic infection	13 (16.7)
Brain tumor	12 (15.4)
Toxic/metabolic	10 (12.8)
Positional vertigo	5 (6.4)
Cardiac	4 (5.1)
Syncope	4 (5.1)
Other	17 (4.1)

Other conditions included trauma, subdural hematoma, herpes encephalitis, transient global amnesia, dementia, demyelinating disease, cervical spine fracture, myasthenia gravis, parkinsonism, hypertensive encephalopathy, and conversion disorder.
Source: From Libman RB et al. Conditions that mimic stroke in the emergency department. *Arch Neurol* 1995;52:1119-1122. (with permission)

weighted imaging (see Chapter 2) may allow accurate delineation of the core and penumbra regions of acute strokes and in the near future may permit rapid identification of patients more or less likely to benefit from thrombolytic therapy. MR angiography (MRA) can provide rapid noninvasive imaging of vascular occlusions and may help select patients who are candidates for intra-arterial thrombolytic therapy. MR technology is developing rapidly, and regular consultation with radiologists should be obtained so that stroke patients can receive the benefits of the most effective available imaging studies. At present, these approaches are still evolving, and their ultimate usefulness in the acute setting is uncertain.[6] The reader is referred to Chapter 2 for additional discussion of imaging options in acute stroke patients.

Atheromatous disease of the extracranial and intracranial carotid and vertebrobasilar arterial systems are important causes of stroke. Other vascular disorders such as vascular dissection, fibromuscular dysplasia, congenital vascular anomalies, or vasculitis may be important in some patients. Vascular imaging studies may provide important information regarding the cause of a stroke or TIA (see later) and may help suggest appropriate treatment to reduce the risk of recurrent stroke. At this time, however, these studies are of little help in guiding the initial management of the patient with a completed stroke. Available techniques for vascular imaging include ultrasound (extracranial and transcranial), MR angiography, CT angiography, and contrast angiography, among others. The advantages and limitations of these studies are reviewed in Chapter 2. Local availability, expertise, and experience will guide the choice of the most appropriate studies until more definitive comparison data become available.

Laboratory Studies

The diagnosis of stroke depends largely on the clinical assessment and imaging studies, but laboratory studies may help to elucidate the likely cause of the stroke and may be helpful in guiding therapy. The most recent American Heart Association Guideline (2007) suggests basic data to be obtained in all patients with suspected stroke should include:

- an electrocardiogram (ECG)
- complete blood count (CBC) with platelet count
- coagulation studies; PT/INR and PTT
- electrolytes, renal function studies
- blood glucose
- markers for cardiac ischemia
- oxygen saturation

Other laboratory studies, including chest x-ray, arterial blood gases, pregnancy tests, liver function studies, lumbar puncture, and EEG, should be ordered as indicated. Lumbar puncture is indicated in patients with suspected subarachnoid hemorrhage when the CT scan is negative or in patients with suspected meningeal disease (such as infection, tumor infiltration, etc.). EEG may be helpful if nonconvulsive seizure activity is suspected.[7]

Acute Stroke Management

Thrombolytic Therapy

For much of medical history, treatment of patients with acute stroke has consisted largely of supportive care and there has been no direct intervention to reduce the severity of stroke and improve clinical outcomes. Recognition that many strokes were due to arterial occlusions by blood clots, and that many apparent strokes included regions of potentially salvageable brain tissue (the ischemic penumbra) suggested that urgent recanalization of occluded vessels might offer significant clinical benefit. Anticoagulants have proved ineffective and their use is associated with increased risk of hemorrhagic transformation of the ischemic stroke. Direct lysis of the offending clot with a thrombolytic agent also seemed to be a reasonable approach. Initial trials with a variety of thrombolytic agents demonstrated no benefit and were associated with unacceptable rates of intracerebral hemorrhage and increased mortality.

In 1995, the rt-PA Stroke Study Group of the National Institute of Neurologic Disorders and Stroke (NINDS) published a randomized clinical trial (RCT) of recombinant tissue plasminogen activator (rt-PA) inpatients with acute stroke. They reported that intravenous rt-PA given within 3 hours of stroke symptom onset resulted in improvement in patient outcome.[8] The benefits were modest, with an absolute increase of 11% to 13% in the proportion of treated patients with normal or near-normal neurologic function at 3 months compared with placebo-treated controls (the relative benefit was 24%–35%). This benefit did come at a substantial price, as 6.4% of treated patients had symptomatic intracerebral hemorrhage compared to only 0.6% in the placebo group. Despite the increased risk of intracerebral hemorrhage in the treated group, overall mortality was the same in the two groups. Although the NINDS trial has been challenged on methodological grounds (see Ref. 9 for a brief review), it remains to date the only RCT using rt-PA within the 3-hour "window." Other trials, reported at around the same time,[10,11] also demonstrated an increased risk of hemorrhage but did not confirm any clinical benefit. These trials were different in several respects; most importantly, they used a 6-hour "window" rather than the 3 hours in the NINDS trial.

Based in a large part on the results of the NINDS trial, the FDA approved rt-PA for treatment of patients with acute ischemic stroke within 3 hours of symptom onset and the American Heart Association/American Stroke Association recommended treatment with intravenous rt-PA for selected patients within 3 hours of stroke onset.[7,12]

Despite this and other similar recommendations, use of rt-PA in clinical practice has remained quite limited, and only a very small proportion of patients with acute ischemic stroke (less than 2%) actually receive thrombolytic treatment. The most important reasons for this include:

1. Most patients do not arrive in the emergency department or other treatment facility sufficiently soon after the onset of their symptoms to allow for a complete evaluation and initiation of treatment within 3 hours of symptom onset. Many strokes (approximately 25%) occur during sleep so that the time of symptom onset is uncertain,[13] Even when patients are awake, when their stroke symptoms begin, they often delay seeking treatment for many hours.

   Even when patients do arrive in a timely fashion, it may be difficult or impossible to complete the evaluation sufficiently and quickly. Although well-designed stroke protocols can speed the process,[14] some requirements, such as the need for urgent performance/interpretation of imaging studies, may be beyond the capabilities of some treatment facilities.

2. The NINDS protocol, used as the basis for current treatment guidelines, includes many contraindications to thrombolytic treatment (see Table 5-6).

TABLE 5-6

INCLUSION/EXCLUSION CRITERIA FOR THROMBOLYTIC THERAPY

Inclusion criteria
1. Ischemic stroke with a measurable defect on NIHSS[a]
2. Clearly defined time of onset within 3 hours of start of treatment[b]
3. Age >18 years

Exclusion criteria
1. Evidence of ICH on pretreatment CT scan[c]
2. Clinical presentation consistent with subarachnoid hemorrhage, even if CT scan is negative
3. Known arteriovenous malformation or aneurysm
4. Prior intracranial hemorrhage
5. Active internal bleeding
6. Known bleeding diathesis including, but not limited to:
   platelet count <100,000/mm^3
   prothrombin time >15 sec; international normalized ratio >1.7, or current use of oral anticoagulants
   use of heparin within 48 hr and prolonged partial thromboplastin time
7. Systolic blood pressure >185 mmHg, or diastolic blood pressure >110 mmHg (repeated measurements at the time treatment is to begin); aggressive measures should not be used to reduce blood pressure to these limits
8. Intracranial surgery, serious head trauma, stroke within past 3 months
9. Major surgery with past 14 days
10. Pregnancy
11. Post–myocardial infarction myocarditis

Warnings
1. Rapid improvement of neurologic signs
2. Mild stroke or isolated neurologic deficits[d]
3. Gastrointestinal or genitourinary bleeding within past 21 days
4. Recent lumbar puncture
5. Recent arterial puncture at noncompressible site
6. Blood glucose <50 or >400 mg/dL
7. Seizure at stroke onset

[a] NIHSS, National Institutes of Health Stroke Scale—see Table 5-4 and text.

[b] Note that time interval is from symptom onset to time of treatment (not time of presentation). Time of onset is the last time at which the patient was known to be normal. For patients in whom stroke onset was not observed or in whom stroke occurs during sleep, this will often preclude treatment.

[c] The scan must be interpreted by a physician with demonstrated expertise in the interpretation of brain CT. See text for discussion.

[d] Some isolated deficits (e.g., aphasia) may be devastating even without a high NIHSS score, and treatment may well be appropriate.

3. Many physicians remain concerned about the balance between the apparently modest benefits of rt-PA and the significant risks, especially the risk of intracerebral bleeding. In addition, the diagnosis of stroke is often uncertain, with error rates as high as 25% as noted earlier. Physicians are appropriately reluctant to expose patients to the risks of thrombolytic therapy for diagnoses other than acute ischemic stroke.

There have been several attempts to increase the proportion of patients able to receive thrombolytic therapy. One approach has been to expand the treatment "window" beyond three hours. In the United States, the ATLANTIS trial, an RTC to assess the efficacy of rt-PA from 3 to 5 hours after stroke onset, found no evidence of benefit, but did find a 6.7% risk of hemorrhage, comparable to the NINDS trial.[15] A more recent European study (ECASS III) of patients treated between 3 and 4.5 hours after stroke onset did demonstrate benefit for thrombolytic therapy. The risk of symptomatic hemorrhage was between 1.9% and 7.9% depending on the definition used.[16] Not surprisingly, these apparently conflicting results have generated a lively debate (see Refs. 17 and 18 for examples). Nonetheless, based on the results of ECASS III, The American Heart Association / American Stroke Association has recommend that rt-PA be administered to eligible patients within the 3 to 4.5 hour time window[18a]. At least one commentator has suggested that this recommendation is "premature"[18b, 18c, 18d] and rt-PA is not currently approved by the FDA for this indication. It seems clear that there remains considerable uncertainty about the appropriate use of thrombolytic therapy, and further clinical trial data are needed.[19]

Another potential approach to increasing the number of patients treated with rt-PA is to relax some of the exclusion criteria used in the NINDS trial. One recent observational study has suggested that rt-PA may be reasonably safe and effective in patients who wake up with stroke.[13] Others have suggested that the outcome for patients with apparently mild or improving symptoms may not be as good as has been assumed and that more aggressive treatment should be considered for some of these patients. The NINDS trial did not specify any definition of "mild" symptoms and did not specify any stroke score below which treatment should be withheld. As noted earlier, even a "low" stroke score may imply a serious and disabling neurologic injury.[20,21] These proposals also need to be assessed by RCTs before being adopted into clinical practice.

At this time, intravenous thrombolysis with rt-PA remains the only direct treatment with potential benefit to patients with acute ischemic stroke. However, the applicability of the results of RCTs, conducted in specialized stroke centers, to community clinical practice remains an important source of concern for many physicians. One early observational study of 3948 patients managed in 29 community hospitals found that symptomatic intracerebral hemorrhages occurred in 15.7% of treated patients (twice the rate in the NINDS trial), and inhospital mortality was also higher in treated patients. In addition, protocol violations occurred in 50% of treated patients.[22] By contrast, the European SITS–MOST study evaluated 6483 patients treated in 285 centers. Of these centers, 50% were said to have little previous experience in stroke thrombolysis. The rate of symptomatic hemorrhage was 7.3% in treated patients (compared with 8.3% of pooled treated patients from previous RCTs), and a 3-month mortality was 11.3% (compared with 17.3% in pooled treated patients from previous RCTs).[23] These data suggest that rt-PA can be used with reasonable safety in a community setting. It appears appropriate for treatment facilities using rt-PA to regularly review and assess their results.

Based on current information, the following recommendations seem reasonable:

1. rt-PA should be used only in patients with acute ischemic stroke and only in patients in whom intracerebral hemorrhage has been excluded. Reference has already been made to the potentially high rates of diagnostic error in patients with suspected stroke. Accordingly, all such patients should be evaluated by physicians with adequate experience and expertise in neurologic diagnosis and diagnostic image interpretation. Appropriate consultation should be obtained when needed.

2. rt-PA should be considered only for patients who meet the inclusion and exclusion criteria used in the NINDS trial, and the trial protocol should be followed. Based on current data, there is no reason to "push the envelope" by using rt-PA in patients outside the 3-hour "window," in patients in whom the diagnosis of stroke is uncertain, or in patients for whom there is uncertainty about the time of stroke onset. A well-defined written protocol should be available to guide treatment.

3. If rt-PA is utilized, every effort should be made to initiate treatment as quickly as possible. Current view is that the "time is brain"; although no RCT data bear directly on the point, it seems likely that any delay in treatment will decrease any potential benefit and may increase the risk of complications.

4. rt-PA should be used only in settings where there are adequate staff and facilities for close observation and immediate management of patients with bleeding complications (intracranial or elsewhere).

5. rt-PA should be used only with the fully informed consent of the patient or other appropriate decision makers.

6. Centers using rt-PA should periodically assess their experience and outcomes.

Ongoing and future clinical trials using advanced imaging technology may improve our ability to better identify patients likely to benefit from thrombolysis or more likely to suffer complications. Several trials have also suggested that intra-arterial rt-PA may be an option for patients who are not candidates for intravenous treatment or even for patients who have failed intravenous treatment. This approach requires advanced imaging capability and a qualified interventional radiologist, and it is currently under investigation.

Anticoagulant Therapy

Anticoagulation with heparin, and more recently with low-molecular-weight heparins, has been widely used in the management of patients with acute ischemic stroke for many years. Despite this extensive clinical experience and multiple clinical trials, there are as yet no data to suggest that acute anticoagulation with heparin or similar agents offers any benefit in the management of acute stroke. Even in patients with progressing strokes or with presumed cardioembolic stroke, groups in whom anticoagulation has been most commonly advocated and used, there is little evidence of any benefit. There is an increased risk of intracerebral bleeding in stroke patients treated with anticoagulants. The current American Heart Association guideline does not recommend the use of heparin or similar agents in the management of acute ischemic stroke, regardless of the presumed mechanism of the stroke.[8] Long-term anticoagulation does reduce the risk of recurrent stroke in patients with presumed cardiogenic embolism, and low-dose treatment with heparin or similar agents is recommended to reduce the risk of venous thromboembolism in patients with impaired mobility.

Antiplatelet Therapy

Currently available data suggest that aspirin produces a small but definite net reduction in the risk of early recurrent stroke in patients with acute stroke. The optimum dose of aspirin remains unclear, but the current American Heart Association guideline recommends an initial dose of 325 mg. Aspirin should be withheld for 24 hours in patients treated with rt-PA. There are no data available regarding the efficacy of other antiplatelet agents (ticlopidine, clopidogrel, dipyridamole, glycoprotein IIb/IIIa inhibitors) in patients with acute stroke and their use is not currently recommended.[8]

Supportive Care

Hypertension is common in patients with acute stroke. In most cases, immediate treatment is unnecessary because blood pressure often declines spontaneously over time, and lowering blood pressure acutely may be contraindicated. The normal autoregulation of cerebral blood flow is thought to fail in the region of the ischemic penumbra; thus blood flow in this zone of relative ischemia may be further reduced when blood pressure falls, potentially enlarging the zone of infarction. In fact, some degree of hypertension may actually be beneficial in patients with acute stroke. There are no data at this time to suggest a specific blood pressure which requires urgent intervention.[24] Current American Heart Association guidelines suggest cautious treatment if the systolic pressure exceeds 220 mm Hg or if the mean arterial pressure exceeds 130 mm Hg. Patients with evidence of acute end-organ damage or other risk from acute hypertension such as acute myocardial infarction, congestive heart failure, or aortic dissection should be treated as necessary for these conditions.

If thrombolytic therapy is being considered, current guidelines suggest that the blood pressure not exceed 185/110 mm Hg at the time of treatment (Table 5-6). The guidelines are based on those utilized in the NINDS trial and are not supported by experimental evidence. If blood pressure exceeds the recommended level, one or two small doses of IV labetalol (10–20 mg) may be given to reduce blood pressure to this level. If this is ineffective, the patient should not be treated with rt-PA. The NINDS and similar protocols also suggest, again without any experimental evidence, that a marked increase in blood pressure following rt-PA administration should be treated aggressively to maintain blood pressure no higher than 185/110 mm Hg. It must be emphasized that there are no reliable experimental data to guide physicians in this situation; this is another area in which well-designed RCTs would be of great benefit.[8]

Diabetes and hyperglycemia have been associated with worsened outcome in acute stroke. It is not clear whether the hyperglycemia actually causes the worse outcome, possibly by facilitating continued anaerobic metabolism in areas of relative brain ischemia, or whether the elevated blood sugar is a stress reaction in patients with more severe stroke. Treatment with insulin may be appropriate to achieve normal glucose levels, but no clinical trials are available that bear directly on this point.[25,26]

Hyperthermia is also associated with worse outcome in patients with stroke. Even mild elevations in temperature are associated with a measurable deleterious effect. Accordingly, antipyretics should be used when temperature is elevated; of course, the cause of the elevated temperature should be sought and treated.[8]

Seizures occur in approximately 5% of patients with stroke. When present, seizures should be treated in the usual fashion; there is general agreement that prophylactic treatment with anticonvulsants is not indicated.

Increased intracranial pressure resulting from brain edema is not usually a problem in the early stages of acute stroke; when present, the swelling and associated mass effect is usually maximum 3 to 5 days after the stroke. Patients with large infarcts and early areas (<12 hours) of hypodensity on CT scans may be at increased risk. Management is difficult. Corticosteroids are not helpful; hyperventilation, mannitol, or CSF drainage ventriculostomy may be beneficial. Some patients may benefit from decompressive surgery such as hemicraniectomy, but indications, timing, and outcomes remain unclear. Neurosurgical consultation should be sought. In patients with large cerebellar strokes, early swelling may cause progressive brainstem compression during the acute phase. In these cases, early neurosurgical intervention may be lifesaving and may result in a good outcome.[8]

General Medical Care

Common secondary medical problems in stroke patients include aspiration pneumonia, urinary tract infection, and deep venous thrombosis (DVT) with pulmonary embolism. Although the continuing care of stroke patients is often not the responsibility of the acute care physician, some appropriate care can be initiated in the acute care setting. Patients should be kept NPO until there is no doubt about their swallowing function; in case of any doubt, a formal swallowing study should be obtained. Indwelling bladder catheters are usually unnecessary and should be used only when clearly required, rather than for the convenience of physicians and nursing staff. Appropriate prophylaxis for DVT should be initiated, but all anticoagulants should be withheld for 24 hours in patients treated with thrombolytic agents.

Intracerebral Hemorrhage

Approximately 15% of acute strokes are due to intracerebral hemorrhage (ICH) rather than ischemia. ICH often cannot be reliably distinguished from ischemic infarction on clinical grounds, but severe headache or vomiting or sudden loss of consciousness at the onset of a stroke, or rapid decline in consciousness soon after the onset of a stroke should suggest possible ICH. Continuing progression of a neurologic deficit over several hours, especially with a decline in mental status, also suggests ICH. The deterioration in mental status may be due to mass effect from the extravasated blood, increased intracranial pressure, or intraventricular or subarachnoid extension of the hemorrhage. The diagnosis is usually confirmed by a CT scan; in experienced hands, CT is virtually 100% sensitive for ICH, although small or subtle hemorrhages can be overlooked. Lumbar puncture is not indicated.

The most common cause of ICH is degenerative disease of small blood vessels associated with chronic hypertension; the second most common cause is cerebral amyloid angiopathy. In addition, ICH is well recognized as a complication of anticoagulant and antiplatelet therapy, and the frequency of ICH due to these causes appears to be increasing. Other potential causes include vascular disorders such as vascular malformations or aneurysms (congenital or mycotic), hemorrhage into tumors (primary or metastatic), and trauma. Rarer causes include vasculitis, moyamoya disease, and others.

Until recently, management of patients with ICH has been largely supportive, as outlined for patients with acute ischemic stroke. There has been increasing interest in more aggressive management and reason to hope that more effective management may soon be available,[27] but so far few reliable experimental data are available to guide treatment. Management of hypertension in patients with acute ICH remains controversial; the patients often have chronic hypertension and frequently develop severe reactive hypertension. Although it seems intuitively obvious that lowering the blood pressure would reduce the risk of further bleeding, patients with ICH often have increased intracranial pressure, and reducing the systemic pressure may lower the cerebral perfusion pressure, compromising cerebral blood flow and worsening the neurologic injury. Current guidelines suggest that the mean arterial pressure (MAP) be kept below 130 mm Hg. For patients with marked elevations in blood pressure (systolic pressure >230 mm Hg or diastolic pressure >140 mm Hg), intravenous nitroprusside should be used. For patients with systolic pressures between 180 and 230 mm Hg or diastolic pressures between 105 and 140 mm Hg, labetalol or similar agents can be used.[28,29] Several trials of more aggressive blood pressure management are under way and may provide better evidence to support treatment decisions.[30] As in patients with ischemic stroke, hypotension should be avoided and treated if necessary.

There is similar uncertainty about the optimal management of patients with ICH associated with anticoagulant (usually warfarin) therapy. It is generally agreed that the coagulopathy should be corrected as quickly as possible, but there is no general agreement on how best to do this. Options include administration of vitamin K, fresh frozen plasma, prothrombin complex concentrate, and recombinant Factor VIIa, either singly or in various combinations. No RCTs are available yet to demonstrate the clinical benefit of these agents or to compare their effectiveness.[31]

Neurosurgical intervention may also be beneficial in selected patients with cerebral hemorrhage, especially those with initially less severe deficits who show signs of progressive deterioration, but there are few data to guide patient selection or to determine the best surgical treatment. At this point, there is little reason to expect much benefit from surgery in patients with massive hemorrhages or in those who are moribund at presentation. Special mention should be made of patients with acute cerebellar hemorrhage, in whom neurosurgical intervention may be lifesaving and may result in good outcome.[28] The clinical picture of cerebellar hemorrhage is characterized by the abrupt onset of headache, dizziness, and ataxia, as well as vomiting. Brainstem signs are often present, and the diagnosis is confirmed by CT scanning.

Transient Ischemic Attack

The classic definition of a transient ischemic attack (TIA) has been "a temporary and focal episode of neurologic dysfunction of presumed vascular origin, typically lasting from 2 to 15 minutes, but occasionally as long as 24 hours, which clears without any residual symptoms."[32] It has since become evident from imaging studies that many patients with symptoms lasting <24 hours have nonetheless had a stroke, and a change in the definition of TIA has been recommended to "a brief episode of neurologic dysfunction caused by a focal disturbance of brain or retinal ischemia, with clinical symptoms typically lasting less than one hour, and without evidence of infarction."[33] The critical clinical point is that most TIA are very brief, commonly lasting only a few minutes, and thus many will have resolved by the time the patient comes to medical attention. Therefore, the diagnosis must often be based entirely on the history. The onset of the attack is usually abrupt, with symptoms developing over only a few seconds or minutes. A detailed account of the attack should be obtained to establish that the symptoms were consistent with a focal lesion of the brain or brainstem. An especially subtle form of TIA, often ignored by patients, is *amaurosis fugax*, an episode of transient monocular blindness caused by acute retinal ischemia. Patients typically describe a "shade" coming down over one eye with temporary loss of vision; the other eye is unaffected. Normal vision is restored after a few minutes. As with virtually all TIAs, the episode is painless and its significance often unrecognized. In general, nonfocal symptoms such as syncope or light-headedness are not due to TIA. Similarly, symptoms such as vertigo, dysarthria, double vision, etc., occurring in isolation are not usually due to TIA.[34]

TIA should be regarded as a medical emergency, as it is well established that patients with TIA are at substantially increased risk for subsequent strokes. The risk of stroke is approximately 5% within the first 7 days, and 10% to 15% within 90 days.[35] Estimation of the actual risk is difficult because the rate of error in diagnosing TIA is as high as 50% to 60% in some studies.[36,37] The stroke risk in patients with true TIA may well be higher; one study estimates the risk of subsequent stroke in patients with "true" TIA (that is, with a confirmed diagnosis) at up to 24% within 90 days.[38] These risks are similar to those associated with a "minor" stroke, and it seems appropriate to regard TIA as a stroke from which the patient was fortunate enough to make a full recovery. In addition, most recent studies of stroke risk following TIA and prior stroke include patients on various antiplatelet and other regimens, so that the true stroke risk in untreated patients is presumably higher.

Despite these risks, the majority of patients with TIA will have a benign course, and it would be very helpful to have some method to identify those patients most at risk of imminent stroke and therefore most in need of urgent assessment and intervention. Rothwell et al. proposed a clinical score ("ABCD") to stratify the risk of subsequent stroke and this was later modified by Johnston et al. ("ABCD2") to better predict the risk of stroke with 48 hours of TIA.[37,39] The ABCD2 score is determined by the following table.

Age >60 years	1 point
Blood pressure >140/90 mm Hg	1 point
Clinical features	
Unilateral weakness	2 points
Speech disturbance without weakness	1 point
Duration	
>60 minutes	2 points
10–59 minutes	1 point
Diabetes	1 point

Scores from 0 to 3 were associated with a 48-hour stroke risk of 1%; scores of 4 to 5 predicted a stroke risk of 4.1%, and scores of 6 to 7 predicted a risk of 8.1%. In part, the predictive value of the ABCD score may derive from increased accuracy in diagnosing "true" TIA.[39] Subsequent studies have suggested that the predictive value of the ABCD2 score can be further enhanced if MRI evidence of new ischemic lesions (using diffusion-weighted images) and likely TIA etiology (large-vessel atherosclerosis and atrial fibrillation) are considered as well.[40,41]

Given the substantial risk of early stroke, patients with TIA require urgent assessment to identify any potentially remediable causes for stroke and to initiate treatment. At a minimum, patients should have a blood glucose level, electrolytes, CBC with platelet count, urinalysis, PT/INR, PTT, ECG, and cardiac monitoring. A CT of the brain should be obtained; in view of recent data cited earlier regarding risk stratification, MR imaging should be obtained if available. Vascular imaging (carotid ultrasound, CT angiography, or MR angiography) may also be obtained on an urgent basis (see Chapter 2). Additional studies (e.g., echocardiography) should be obtained if the initial workup does not reveal a likely cause for the TIA. As with other stroke patients, the best results will likely be obtained when a well-defined protocol or clinical pathway is established to guide the assessment.[42,43] Clearly, most of the workup can be accomplished in the ED or on an outpatient basis; there is little evident benefit to admitting most of these patients to the hospital unless admission would significantly facilitate the workup. It has been suggested that "high risk" patients (e.g., with ABCD2 scores of 6–7) should be admitted so that immediate rt-PA treatment will be available in the event of an acute stroke, but there are no outcomes data directly supporting such an approach at this time.[36]

Treatment depends to some extent on the presumed cause of the TIA. Where a specific treatable cause for TIA is identified, specific treatment is indicated. For patients with high-grade (>70%) stenosis in an accessible neck vessel, carotid endarterectomy is often the procedure of choice. The relative roles of open endarterectomy and percutaneous endovascular surgery are not yet clear. Patients with carotid stenosis between 50% and 69% may benefit from endarterectomy, but the benefits are less clear and careful patient selection is necessary. For patients with stenosis less than 50%, surgery appears not to be superior to medical management. For patients with atrial fibrillation or presumed cardiogenic emboli, long-term anticoagulation is beneficial; but anticoagulation is not recommended in patients with noncardioembolic stroke. For most patients with TIA and stroke, antiplatelet therapy is recommended. Aspirin 50 to 325 mg/d, clopidogrel, and aspirin plus extended-release dipyridamole are all acceptable options. The most recent American Heart Association/American Stroke Association guidelines favor the use of a combination product containing aspirin 25 mg and sustained-release dipyridamole 200 mg (Aggrenox) twice daily as initial therapy.[44] Hackam et al. suggest that a combined regimen of dietary modification, exercise, aspirin, a statin, and an antihypertensive agent could reduce relative stroke risk by as much as 80%.[45] Clearly, some of these interventions are not initiated or implemented in the ED, and the patient should be referred to the primary physician.

Migraine

The diagnosis and management of migraine are discussed in Chapter 8. Focal neurologic symptoms are quite common in patients with migraine. Most common are the familiar visual auras, which may include central or peripheral scotomas, visual field loss, or even complete blindness. Although both eyes are usually involved, unilateral visual loss (amaurosis fugax) may occur and be mistaken for a TIA.[46] Other focal neurologic symptoms may include aphasia or speech arrest, motor weakness or paralysis (even hemiplegia), or sensory symptoms. The attacks may or may not be associated with headaches.

Recognition of this syndrome and distinction from TIA requires a careful history. A history of previous similar attacks, some associated with typical migraine headaches, may be diagnostic. In general, migraine symptoms evolve gradually over a period of 5 to 10 minutes or more; patients may describe numbness or weakness beginning in one hand, gradually spreading up the arm, and then spreading to the face, the trunk, or elsewhere. When present, this history is virtually diagnostic and quite distinct from the more abrupt onset of symptoms characteristic of TIA and stroke. In some cases, of course, the story will not be so clear. There is no laboratory or imaging study that will permit a clear distinction between migraines and TIA; when in doubt, it is reasonable to pursue the workup for TIA.

Cerebral Vein Thrombosis

Thrombosis of the cortical veins and/or dural venous sinuses is much less common than arterial occlusive disease. The diagnosis is often difficult but is suggested by a somewhat slower evolution of clinical symptoms and frequently by the presence of bilateral signs. Signs of increased intracranial pressure (especially depressed level of consciousness, vomiting, and papilledema) are often present, and seizures are often prominent. CT or MRI scanning may reveal extensive bilateral cortical and subcortical hemorrhagic infarction, but the findings may be quite subtle. The diagnosis can be confirmed with MR venography.

Cerebral vein thrombosis occurs most often in the setting of an underlying coagulopathy such as pregnancy (or recent delivery), systemic cancer, sickle cell disease, or primary coagulopathy, including mutations in the factor V Leiden gene.[34] Because of the frequent association with primary coagulopathy, extensive medical evaluation may be needed in these patients. Other conditions associated with cerebral venous thrombosis include severe dehydration and local or systemic infection.

There are few controlled trials to guide treatment. Based on the little data available, current clinical guidelines from the American Heart Association/American Stroke Association recommend anticoagulation with heparin or low-molecular-weight heparin.[34]

Other Disorders

The clinical picture in patients with brain abscess is nonspecific, and may be indistinguishable from that in patients with other intracranial masses, with headache, seizures, and focal signs. Signs of increased intracranial pressure may be present as well. As in patients with tumors, the onset of clinical symptoms is usually subacute rather than abrupt. The diagnosis is often suggested by CT or MRI with evidence of a mass lesion, often enhancing following contrast administration. These lesions may be difficult to distinguish from neoplasms, although the correct diagnosis is sometimes suggested by the clinical context. Brain abscess should be considered in patients with evidence of systemic infection, patients with sinus or mastoid infections, patients with suspected endocarditis, congenital or valvular heart disease, patients using IV drugs, patients with CSF leaks, and patients with a history of recent head trauma or a neurosurgical procedure. Biopsy may be needed to confirm the diagnosis and to identify the causative organism. Brain abscesses can be caused by a wide variety of bacterial infections, both aerobic and anaerobic, and polymicrobial infections are common. In immunocompromised hosts (especially patients with AIDS), fungal infections or protozoan infections (e.g., toxoplasmosis) should also be considered. Although many brain abscesses are caused by hematogenous spread of infection, fever and signs of systemic infection may be absent.

Definitive treatment ultimately depends on the size and location of the lesion(s), the stage of development of the lesion (early "cerebritis" or a well-developed mature abscess with a thick capsule), and identification of the causative organism. Neurosurgery may be needed for both diagnosis and treatment, and early consultation is appropriate. Depending on the clinical urgency of the situation, treatment may be delayed until a definitive diagnosis is established or empiric antibiotic treatment can be started, based on the most likely clinical diagnoses. For patients with probable bacterial infection from sinus infection or cardiac sources, a third-generation cephalosporin (e.g., ceftriaxone 2 g IV q12h) and metronidazole 30 mg/kg/d (divided into four doses) is appropriate. For patients with head trauma or neurosurgery, coverage for staphylococci should be given. For patients with AIDS, coverage for toxoplasmosis should be considered. Early consultation with a specialist in infectious diseases should be sought.

The clinical syndrome of acute encephalitis is characterized by fever, headache, altered mental status, and sometimes focal neurologic signs. The most common cause of acute encephalitis is *Herpes simplex* virus (HSV), but a wide variety of other viruses, as well as bacterial and other infections, can produce a similar picture. Treatment with acyclovir or other antiviral agents may be beneficial in HSV encephalitis (see Chapter 4).

Intracranial tumors are occasionally present with the apparent onset of acute focal neurologic deficits; in many of these cases, a careful history will reveal a more subacute or chronic course. However, symptoms are occasionally abrupt in onset. Potential mechanisms include sudden hemorrhage into a previously "silent" tumor, the onset of seizure activity, or disruption of local blood supply by the tumor. Either primary or metastatic tumors may present in this way.

Brain metastases may be suspected in patients with a prior history of systemic cancer, but either primary or metastatic tumors may present with no antecedent history. The diagnosis is often first suggested by the appearance of a mass lesion on CT or MR scanning, although low-grade primary brain tumors may be subtle on CT scans. MRI with enhancement is usually the imaging procedure of choice, but does not have to be done urgently once CT has ruled out significant intracranial mass effect. Emergency treatment is usually not required unless there is substantial mass effect or impending herniation, in which case intravenous corticosteroids (e.g., dexamethasone 10 mg initially, then 4 mg q6h) may be beneficial. Patients with marked decrease in their level of consciousness should be managed as outlined in Chapter 4. Prophylactic anticonvulsants are not necessary.

Epidural hematomas are generally due to arterial bleeding secondary to head trauma with an associated skull fracture. The classic clinical picture is that of a patient with a head injury who acutely loses consciousness and then recovers, at least in part (the so-called "lucid interval"), before beginning progressive deterioration. In many patients, the temporary improvement in consciousness does not occur. Focal signs such as worsening hemiparesis are common, and may be followed by signs of progressive herniation. The diagnosis is usually evident on CT scanning. The treatment is neurosurgical intervention. Subdural hematomas may be clinically much more subtle. They result from venous bleeding and may evolve over a prolonged period (days to weeks to months) as a result of small recurrent hemorrhages. There is often, but not always, a history of head trauma, sometimes seemingly trivial. Diagnosis is by CT scan. As with epidural hematomas, neurosurgical consultation should be obtained.

Hypoglycemia and hyperglycemia are typically present with altered mental status, as discussed in Chapter 4. However, either condition may cause focal signs; these usually resolve promptly with treatment. If focal signs persist following normalization of blood glucose, alternative causes should be sought.

Focal motor seizures ordinarily cause no diagnostic difficulty when observed by the physician. However, sensory seizures, unaccompanied by any abnormal movements, may occur as well and may be very difficult to recognize. Simple focal seizures (either motor or sensory) are not associated with any alteration of consciousness. Focal seizures imply the presence of an underlying focal brain lesion and focal seizures of new onset should prompt a thorough evaluation. This can usually be done on a nonurgent or elective basis. Focal seizures (with or without secondary generalization) may result in focal weakness (Todd's paralysis) that persists after the seizure has resolved. This can cause diagnostic confusion in a patient who comes for medical attention after an unwitnessed seizure; the clinical picture is of altered mental status with focal weakness, with a large differential diagnosis. Usually the correct diagnosis will be suggested by rapid improvement, but Todd's paralysis may occasionally last a day or more, particularly after frequent or prolonged seizures. The presence of a Todd's paralysis implies a focal onset to the seizure, even if the seizure appeared clinically to be generalized at onset (see Chapter 12).

Multiple sclerosis (MS) may present with acute focal neurologic deficits. In one classic study, nearly 20% of patients presented with acute deficits of abrupt onset.[47] In such cases, the clinical picture may be difficult to distinguish from acute stroke. CT scans may be normal or may reveal one or more low-density lesions, often periventricular. MRI scanning is far more sensitive and specific for demyelinating lesions but may also be nondiagnostic in new-onset cases. The subsequent workup of patients with suspected MS may include evoked potential studies and lumbar puncture, none of which need to be accomplished in the acute care setting.

In patients with established MS, acute intercurrent illnesses such as urinary tract infections or other infections, marked temperature elevations from other causes (even a hot bath!) may exacerbate pre-existing MS deficits and cause the rapid development of focal neurologic deficits. These episodes do not represent an exacerbation of the underlying MS, and the focal deficits may improve quickly with treatment of the acute illness. Of course, a history of MS does not exclude other causes of acute focal weakness. Patients with MS can therefore present a major diagnostic and therapeutic challenge to the acute care physician.

Acute Focal Lesions of the Spinal Cord

The clinical anatomy of the spinal cord is reviewed in Chapter 10; only a few brief points will be discussed here. The spinal cord extends from the foramen magnum to approximately the level of the L1 vertebra. There is therefore essentially no spinal cord in the lumbar spinal canal and imaging studies of the lumbosacral spine are not indicated in patients with suspected spinal cord lesions! There are 31 pairs of spinal nerves, numbered according to the vertebral levels at which they exit the spinal canal via the neural foramina. These same numbers are also used to designate the spinal cord levels at which each pair of nerves originates. As the spinal cord is shorter than the vertebral column, the spinal levels and the vertebral levels do not match. It is important to remember this fact when planning and interpreting clinical findings and imaging studies of the spine and spinal cord in patients with suspected spinal cord lesions (Table 5-7 and Fig. 5-1).

Several anatomic features make the spinal cord highly susceptible to injury from compression by mass lesions within the spinal canal. The cord is tightly confined within the spinal canal, with little room for displacement by a mass lesion. In addition, the major blood supply to the spinal cord (the anterior spinal artery) depends on a small number of

TABLE 5-7

SPINAL CORD LEVELS AND VERTEBRAL LEVELS

Spinal Cord Level	Vertebral Level
C1	C1
T1	C7–C8
T6	T4
T12	T9–T10
L1–L5	T10–T12
S1–S5	T12–L1

feeding vessels derived from segmental branches from the aorta, with the result that much of the cord depends on a somewhat tenuous blood supply. Compression or occlusion of these vessels can result in infarction of the spinal cord. The spinal cord may also be injured by intrinsic processes. Table 5-8 lists some of the more common lesions that may affect the spinal cord. It is imperative that extrinsic compression of the spinal cord be recognized as quickly as possible, as emergency treatment may lead to dramatic improvement. Conversely, delay in treatment can quickly lead to irreversible injury to the spinal cord.

Clinical Assessment

The most common cause of acute lesions of the spinal cord is trauma; the possibility of spinal cord injury should be considered in all injured patients and appropriate steps taken to evaluate and treat such injuries (see Chapter 10). Nontraumatic extrinsic and intrinsic lesions of the spinal cord are less common and are more easily overlooked; recognition of a spinal cord lesion may require a high index of suspicion and a high degree of skill in the performance and interpretation of the neurologic examination. The neurologic examination is reviewed in Chapter 3; clinical findings that indicate a spinal cord lesion are summarized in Table 5-1 and are also discussed later in this chapter. It is important to remember that symptoms involving the face and head (e.g., facial weakness or numbness) are not caused by spinal cord lesions.

A sensory level, with impairment of sensation below a specific spinal level on the trunk or neck, is diagnostic of a spinal cord lesion; the anatomic organization of the nervous system is such that a true sensory level will not result from lesions elsewhere in the nervous system. It is important to recall that the patient may be completely unaware of the sensory impairment, which can therefore be overlooked unless specifically sought by the examiner. Sensory levels may be very difficult to recognize in the extremities and may be difficult to distinguish from the distal sensory impairment seen in patients with peripheral nerve lesions.

A motor level is usually characterized by weakness in the lower extremities more than in the upper extremities. This finding is less clearly diagnostic than a true sensory level, but a spinal cord lesion should be suspected especially if there is severe weakness in the lower extremities with normal strength in the upper extremities. Careful examination can sometimes reveal weakness in the lower abdominal or trunk muscles more than the upper muscles, suggesting a lesion in the lower thoracic spinal cord, but this is frequently very subtle and difficult to detect.

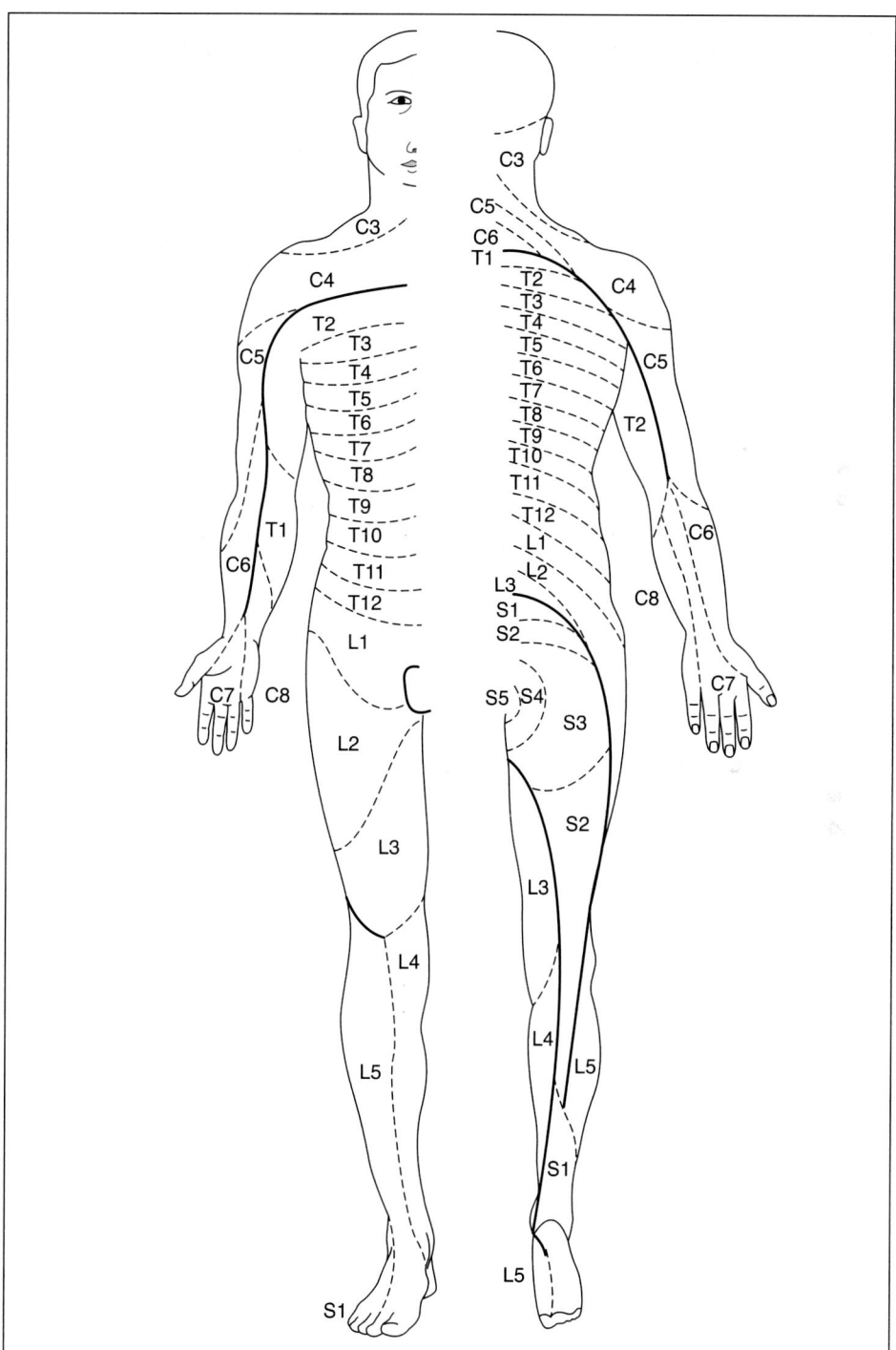

FIGURE 5-1   The sensory dermatomes.

TABLE 5-8

ETIOLOGIES OF SPINAL CORD LESIONS

Extrinsic (compressive) lesions
Spondyloarthropathy
Disc protrusion/herniation[a]
Neoplasms (primary/metastatic)[a]
Epidural abscess[a]/hematoma[a]
Trauma[a]

Intrinsic lesions
Vascular (spinal cord infarction)[a]
Neoplasms (primary/metastatic)
Inflammatory/granulomatous
   Multiple sclerosis[a]
   Transverse myelitis[a] (idiopathic or postinfectious)
   Vasculitis

[a] Lesions most likely to present with acute spinal cord dysfunction. See text for details.

Sensory dissociation is characterized by impairment of pain and temperature sensation on one side of the body and impairment of position and vibration sense on the opposite side; this finding can only result from a spinal cord lesion and implies a lesion affecting one side of the spinal cord but sparing the other side.

Sensory–motor dissociation means impairment of motor function on one side of the body and impairment of pain and temperature sensation on the opposite side; as with sensory dissociation (explained earlier), this too can only result from a spinal cord lesion.

Additional symptoms that should suggest a spinal cord lesion include early involvement of bladder function, bowel function, or sexual function. The presence of neck pain or back pain in association with weakness of the lower extremities or impaired bowel, bladder, or sexual function, also strongly suggests a spinal cord or cauda equina lesion. Finally, the combination of both "lower motor neuron" and "upper motor neuron" signs should suggest a spinal cord disorder.

If a spinal cord lesion is suspected, additional clinical history may suggest the etiology. The patient should be asked about recent trauma. A history of localized pain in the neck or back, especially in association with percussion tenderness, suggests a lesion of the spine or meninges. A history of prior cancer, even if remote, should suggest metastatic disease. A history of systemic infection, or of unexplained fever, especially if associated with back pain, should suggest a spinal or epidural abscess. A history of HIV infection suggests opportunistic infection or abscess, or HIV myelopathy. Chest pain or abdominal pain in association with signs of spinal cord injury may be due to thoracic or abdominal aortic aneurysm or dissection.

Once a spinal cord lesion is suspected, it is essential to try to determine whether the lesion is extrinsic or intrinsic to the spinal cord. Although various clinical clues have been used to make this distinction (e.g., the presence or absence of "sacral sparing"), these are not sufficiently reliable, and an urgent imaging study is indicated to determine if the patient has a structural lesion affecting the spinal cord.

Spinal Cord Imaging

MRI with contrast administration is the study of choice for patients with suspected intrinsic or extrinsic lesions of the spinal cord. In patients with trauma, only the region of the trauma needs to be scanned, and no contrast needs to be administered. In patients with suspected spinal cord compression from neoplasm or infection, the entire spinal cord should be scanned. In patients with suspected intrinsic lesions of the cord, consultation with a radiologist and careful consideration of the clinical question to be answered will help to select the most appropriate study. MRI provides detailed images of the spinal cord, the subarachnoid space, and the surrounding structures. These images distinguish the extrinsic cord lesions from the intrinsic ones and often indicate the specific diagnosis. Even in patients with x-ray evidence of an acute spinal lesion (e.g., collapse of a vertebral body), an MRI will indicate the extent of injury to the spinal cord. Accordingly, emergency MRI, if available, should be obtained in virtually all patients with acute spinal cord syndromes. If emergency MRI is not immediately available, contrast myelography followed by CT imaging, should be performed. Myelography followed by CT scanning will not miss the structural lesions detected by MR imaging, but it is a more invasive study. Plain radiographs, or CT without intrathecal contrast, are rarely, if ever, adequate. If neither MRI nor myelography is immediately available, arrangements should be made for emergency transfer of the patient with a suspected acute spinal cord lesion to an appropriate facility. Diagnostic imaging should be accomplished as soon as it is feasible.

As noted previously, clinical assessment is needed to ensure that the appropriate region of the spine is scanned; even exquisitely detailed images of the thoracic spinal cord are of no diagnostic value in a patient with a cervical spinal cord lesion. Consultation with a radiologist may help to ensure that the appropriate regions are scanned and the appropriate imaging sequences are obtained.

Extrinsic Compression of the Spinal Cord

As noted earlier, the spinal cord is subject to extrinsic compression from any mass lesion within the spinal canal; potential causes include primary and metastatic tumors, abscesses, bony overgrowth from degenerative disease of the spine, epidural bleeding, deformities of the spine due to vertebral collapse, extruded intervertebral disc material, etc. In most cases, the likely culprits will be suggested by the clinical context. It is important that the physician maintain a high index of suspicion for spinal cord compression as prompt decompression may prevent permanent disabling injury.

Epidural metastasis from systemic cancer is not an uncommon cause of extrinsic compression of the spinal cord. The most common mechanism is metastases to one or more vertebral bodies with direct extension of tumor into the epidural space. Less common mechanisms include extension of extraspinal tumors through the intervertebral foramina or (rarely) direct metastasis to epidural fat. Especially in the case of vertebral metastasis, pain is a common early symptom, occurring in over 90% of patients. Unlike most mechanical back pains, the pain is typically not relieved by rest or changes in position and may actually become worse when the patient lies down. The diagnosis of vertebral metastasis should be suspected in any patient with systemic cancer and worsening back pain, but it should also be considered in patients with a similar pattern of steadily worsening pain even without known cancer. Spinal canal metastasis with cord compression is not rare as the initial manifestation of systemic cancer. The initial neurologic symptoms may be mild and subtle, with clumsy gait, vague numbness or tingling, or mild weakness or heaviness of the legs. Bladder, bowel, or sexual dysfunctions occur later, and the patient should be questioned carefully about these symptoms. Once neurologic symptoms develop, progression may be very rapid, and diagnosis and treatment are urgent. It is a rule of thumb that patients who lose their ability to walk will never regain it. As noted previously, once the diagnosis is suspected, emergency MRI scanning is mandatory.

Emergency treatment usually consists of high-dose corticosteroids (e.g., dexamethasone 100 mg IV immediately, then 25 mg IV q6h), followed by emergent radiation therapy.[48] Surgery is generally reserved for those patients in whom the diagnosis is unclear, in whom there is evidence of spinal instability, or who have undergone prior radiation of the affected area.

Epidural abscess is an unusual but important potential cause of spinal cord compression. The abscess may develop as a result of direct extension from osteomyelitis of a vertebral body or from direct seeding of the epidural space from the blood. Important predisposing causes include diabetes mellitus, immunodeficiency syndromes (including AIDS), and systemic sepsis. The clinical symptoms generally include severe and progressive pain, similar to that seen in patients with metastatic disease. Fever and malaise are common. Neurologic symptoms, once present, may evolve rapidly; as with metastatic disease, treatment should begin as soon as possible after diagnosis. The diagnosis is most often made by MRI. Treatment is with antibiotics and surgical drainage; surgery serves to decompress the spinal cord and to obtain positive identification of the causative organism (most often *Staphylococcus aureus*).

Herniation of an intervertebral disc is an occasional cause of acute spinal cord compression, most often as a result of trauma (see Chapter 10). Degenerative disease of the spine can also cause spinal cord compression, as a result of either disc disease or spondylosis or both. This is most often a chronic process, and a good history will usually indicate the presence of chronic, slowly evolving symptoms. If the process is long-standing, emergency treatment is not usually required, and an appropriate referral should be made.

Unusual causes of spinal cord compression include epidural hematomas which occur most often as a result of trauma but which can occasionally occur following lumbar puncture, especially in patients with coagulopathies. Diagnosis usually depends on imaging studies obtained in a patient with a clinically suspected spinal cord lesion.

Intrinsic Lesions of the Spinal Cord

Acute lesions of the spinal cord without evidence of extrinsic compression can result from a wide variety of causes including spinal cord infarctions, immune-mediated inflammatory disorders, and acute viral infections. In addition, many are idiopathic.[49] Establishing a definitive diagnosis often requires an extensive assessment not usually undertaken in the ED, and the emergency treatment options are very limited in any case.

Infarction of the spinal cord (spinal cord stroke) occurs as a result of occlusion of the anterior spinal artery or of one of the segmental arteries that supply blood to the cord. The most common cause is occlusion of segmental arteries by aortic dissection or as a result of surgery on the aorta. Other potential causes include systemic vasculitides, coagulopathies, decompression sickness (the bends), and cocaine use; occasional cases are seen with no evident cause. The clinical syndrome is characterized by the abrupt onset of paralysis (including sphincter paralysis) below the level of the lesion. There is commonly a sensory level to pain and temperature sensation below the level of the lesion, but there is often relative sparing of posterior column sensory functions such as vibration sense, light touch sensation, and joint position sense. The clinical findings are typically bilateral and symmetric. The infarction is usually seen on MRI scanning of the spine within hours of the injury. Unfortunately, there is no effective treatment.

Immune-mediated inflammatory lesions of the cord can occur in a wide variety of disorders including connective tissue diseases, following viral illnesses, etc. The most common specific cause is multiple sclerosis, and an acute transverse myelitis may be the initial clinical manifestation of MS. Clinically, transverse myelitis is characterized by bilateral weakness and sensory loss below the level of the lesion, often quite severe. Fifty percent of patients develop complete paralysis of their lower extremities and virtually all have autonomic symptoms such as impaired bladder and bowel function. Unlike in spinal cord infarction, there is no sparing of posterior column sensory functions. The onset of symptoms is acute or subacute, over a period of several days or longer. MRI scans are frequently, but not invariably, abnormal. Acute treatment usually consists of intravenous corticosteroids such as methylprednisolone 1000 mg IV qd $\times$ 3 to 5 days.[50] As described earlier, patients with MS may also experience acute deterioration in their clinical symptoms as a result of fever or other systemic illness (e.g., urinary tract or respiratory infections). These symptoms need not indicate any activity of their underlying MS and will improve rapidly when the secondary disease is treated. Therefore, in patients with known MS who present with sudden worsening of their symptoms, a careful evaluation is needed to exclude some other disorder. Treatment is directed toward the secondary disorder, and corticosteroids are not required.

ACUTE FOCAL LESIONS OF THE PERIPHERAL NERVES

Acute focal lesions of peripheral nerves are fairly common and they may cause diagnostic difficulty in the acute care setting. Many peripheral nerve lesions are due to obvious trauma such as lacerations, penetrating injuries, or fractures, and ordinarily present no diagnostic difficulty. Acute nontraumatic lesions of peripheral nerves may be less easily recognized for several reasons. First, many acute care physicians who are presented with a patient with an acute focal neurologic deficit, may be predisposed to consider potentially life-threatening or serious central nervous system lesions such as stroke, and may overlook clinical clues suggesting a peripheral lesion. Second, nontraumatic lesions are often incomplete and result in clinical syndromes that are partial or incomplete rather than "classic." Finally, some symptoms of peripheral nerve lesions, such as pain, paresthesias, or sensory loss, are entirely subjective and difficult to define accurately.

In the following discussion, the term peripheral nerve will include cranial nerves III through XII, the motor and sensory spinal roots, the brachial and lumbosacral plexuses, and the peripheral nerves. Potential causes of focal lesions of peripheral nerves are listed in Table 5-9.

TABLE 5-9

ETIOLOGIES OF ACUTE FOCAL LESIONS
OF PERIPHERAL NERVES

Extrinsic lesions
Direct trauma (blunt trauma, lacerations, avulsions, etc.)
Mass lesions (neoplasms, spondyloarthropathy, disc protrusion/herniation)
Pressure palsies

Intrinsic lesions
Vascular (diabetes, vasculitis, etc.)
Inflammatory
Idiopathic

Clinical Assessment

As in the case of spinal cord lesions, recognition of peripheral nerve disorders depends on the clinical acumen of the examining physician. The task for the physician is to recognize that a patient's clinical symptoms indicate a lesion of a specific peripheral root or nerve rather than a more central lesion. This requires a detailed knowledge of the clinical anatomy of the peripheral nervous system. There are hundreds of peripheral nerves, and it is virtually impossible for physicians to recall all of the relevant anatomic and clinical details (Table 5-10 and Fig. 5-2). Fortunately, there are several excellent references available that summarize the anatomy and the necessary techniques for an effective clinical examination.[51,52] Access to one of these or similar references should be a part of the basic armamentarium of every physician who confronts patients with neurologic symptoms. With such a reference, and with the willingness to consider the possibility of peripheral nerve disorders, accurate diagnosis is usually straightforward. For example, the syndrome of severe pain in the posterolateral aspect of the lower extremity, weakness of plantar flexion of the foot, and loss of the ankle reflex suggest a lesion of the S1 nerve root. If weakness of dorsiflexion of the foot were also present, the lesion would more likely affect the sciatic nerve; this is because the clinical findings would not be compatible with a single root lesion (S1 does not innervate the anterior tibial muscles) but would be consistent with a sciatic nerve lesion. Similarly, weakness of the wrist and finger extensor muscles in the forearm, without weakness of other muscles, suggests a radial nerve lesion; a brain or spinal cord lesion would not cause symptoms limited to the distribution of a single peripheral nerve.

Laboratory and Imaging Studies

Laboratory studies are usually of little value, especially in the acute care setting. Electromyography (EMG) and nerve conduction velocity (NCV) studies are often helpful in characterizing and confirming the localization of peripheral nerve lesions but are usually not done in the acute care setting. Often, EMG and NCV abnormalities are not evident until 2 to 3 weeks or more after an acute injury, so that such studies are unhelpful even if performed.

TABLE 5-10 PRINCIPAL MUSCLES AND THEIR NERVE SUPPLY

Action Tested	Roots	Nerves	Muscles
Cranial			
Closure of eyes, pursing of lips, exposure of teeth	Cranial 7	Facial	Orbicularis oculi Orbicularis oris
Elevation of eyelids, movement of eyes	Cranial 3, 4, 6	Oculomotor, trochlear, abducens	Levator palpebrae, extraocular
Closing and opening of jaw	Cranial 5	Motor trigeminal	Masseters Pterygoids
Protrusion of tongue	Cranial 12	Hypoglossal	Lingual
Phonation and swallowing	Cranial 9, 10	Glossopharyngeal, vagus	Palatal, laryngeal, and pharyngeal
Elevation of shoulders, anteroflexion and turning of head	Cranial 11 and upper cervical	Spinal accesory	Trapezius, steromastoid
Brachial			
Adduction of extended arm	**C5**, C6	Brachial plexus	Pectoralis major
Fixation of scapula	C5, C6, C7	Brachial plexus	Serratus anterior
Initiation of abduction of arm	**C5**, C6	Brachial plexus	Supraspinatus
External rotation of flexed arm	**C5**, C6	Brachial plexus	Infraspinatus
Abduction and elevation of arm up to 90°	**C5**, C6	Axillary nerve	Deltoid
Flexion of supinated forearm	C5, C6	Musculocutaneous	Biceps, brachialis
Extension of forearm	C6, **C7**, C8	Radial	Triceps
Extension (radial) of wrist	C6	Radial	Extensor carpi radialis longus
Flexion of semipronated arm	C5, **C6**	Radial	Brachioradialis
Adduction of flexed arm	C6, **C7**, C8	Brachial plexus	Latissimus dorsi

(continued)

TABLE 5-10 — PRINCIPAL MUSCLES AND THEIR NERVE SUPPLY (*Continued*)

Action Tested	Roots	Nerves	Muscles
Supination of forearm	C6, C7	Posterior interosseous	Supinator
Extension of proximal phalanges	**C7**, C8	Posterior interosseous	Extensor digitorum
Extension of wrist (ulnar side)	**C7**, C8	Posterior interosseous	Extensor carpi ulnaris
Extension of proximal phalanx of index finger	**C7**, C8	Posterior interosseous	Extensor indicis
Abduction of thumb	**C7**, C8	Posterior interosseous	Abductor pollicis longus and brevis
Extension of thumb	**C7**, C8	Posterior interosseous	Extensor pollicis longus and brevis
Pronation of forearm	C6, C7	Median nerve	Pronator teres
Radial flexion of wrist	C6, C7	Median nerve	Flexor carpi radialis
Flexion of middle phalanges	C7, **C8**, T1	Median nerve	Flexor digitorum superficialis
Flexion of proximal phalanx of thumb	C8, *T1*	Median nerve	Flexor pollicis brevis
Opposition of thumb against fifth finger	C8, *T1*	Median nerve	Opponens pollicis
Extension of middle phalanges of index and middle fingers	C8, *T1*	Median nerve	First, second lumbricals
Flexion of terminal phalanx of thumb	**C8**, T1	Anterior interosseous nerve	Flexor pollicis longus
Flexion of terminal phalanx of second and third fingers	C8, T1	Anterior interosseous nerve	Flexor digitorum profundus
Flexion of distal phalanges of ring and little fingers	C7, **C8**	Ulnar	Flexor digitorum profundus
Adducation and opposition and fifth finger	C8, *T1*	Ulnar	Hypothenar

Extension of middle phalanges of ring and little fingers	Ulnar	C8, *T1*	Third, fourth lumbrical
Adduction of thumb against second finger	Ulnar	C8, *T1*	Adductor pollicis
Flexion of proximal phalanx of thumb	Ulnar	*C8*, T1	Flexor pollicis brevis
Abduction and adduction of fingers	Ulnar	C8, *T1*	Interossei
Crural			
Hip flexion from semiflexed position	Femoral	*L1, L2*, L3	Iliopsoas
Hip flexion from externally rotated position	Femoral	L2, L3	Sartorius
Extension of knee	Femoral	L2, *L3, L4*	Quadriceps femoris
Adduction of thigh	Obturator	*L2, L3*, L4	Adductor longus, magnus, brevis
Abduction and int. rotation of thigh	Superior gluteal	*L4, L5*, S1	Gluteus medius
Extension of thigh	Inferior gluteal	*L5, S1*, S2	Gluteus maximus
Flexion of knee	Sciatic	L5, *S1*, S2	Biceps femoris Semitendinosus Semimembranosus
Dorsiflexion of foot (medial)	Peroneal (deep)	*L4*, L5	Anterior tibial
Dorsiflexion of toes (proximal and distal phalanges)	Peroneal (deep)	*L5*, S1	Extensor digitorum longus and brevis

(continued)

TABLE 5-10 —— PRINCIPAL MUSCLES AND THEIR NERVE SUPPLY *(Continued)*

Action Tested	Roots	Nerves	Muscles
Dorsiflexion of great toe	*L5*, S1	Peroneal (deep)	Extensor hallucis longus
Eversion of foot	L5, S1	Peroneal (superficial)	Peroneus longus and brevis
Plantar flexion of foot	*S1*, S2	Tibial	Gastrocnemius, soleus
Inversion of foot	L4, *L5*	Tibial	Tibialis posterior
Flexion of toes (distal phalanges)	L5, *S1*, *S2*	Tibial	Flexor digitorum longus
Flexion of toes (middle phalanges)	*S1*, *S2*	Tibial	Flexor digitorum brevis
Flexion of great toe (proximal phalanx)	S1, S2	Tibial	Flexor hallucis brevis
Flexion of great toe (distal phalanx)	L5, *S1*, *S2*	Tibial	Flexor hallucis longus
Contraction of anal sphincter	S2, S3, S4	Pudendal	Perineal muscles

Source: From Victor M, Ropper AH. *Adams and Victor's Principles of Neurology.* 7th ed. New York: McGraw-Hill; 2001:1468-1469. (with permission)

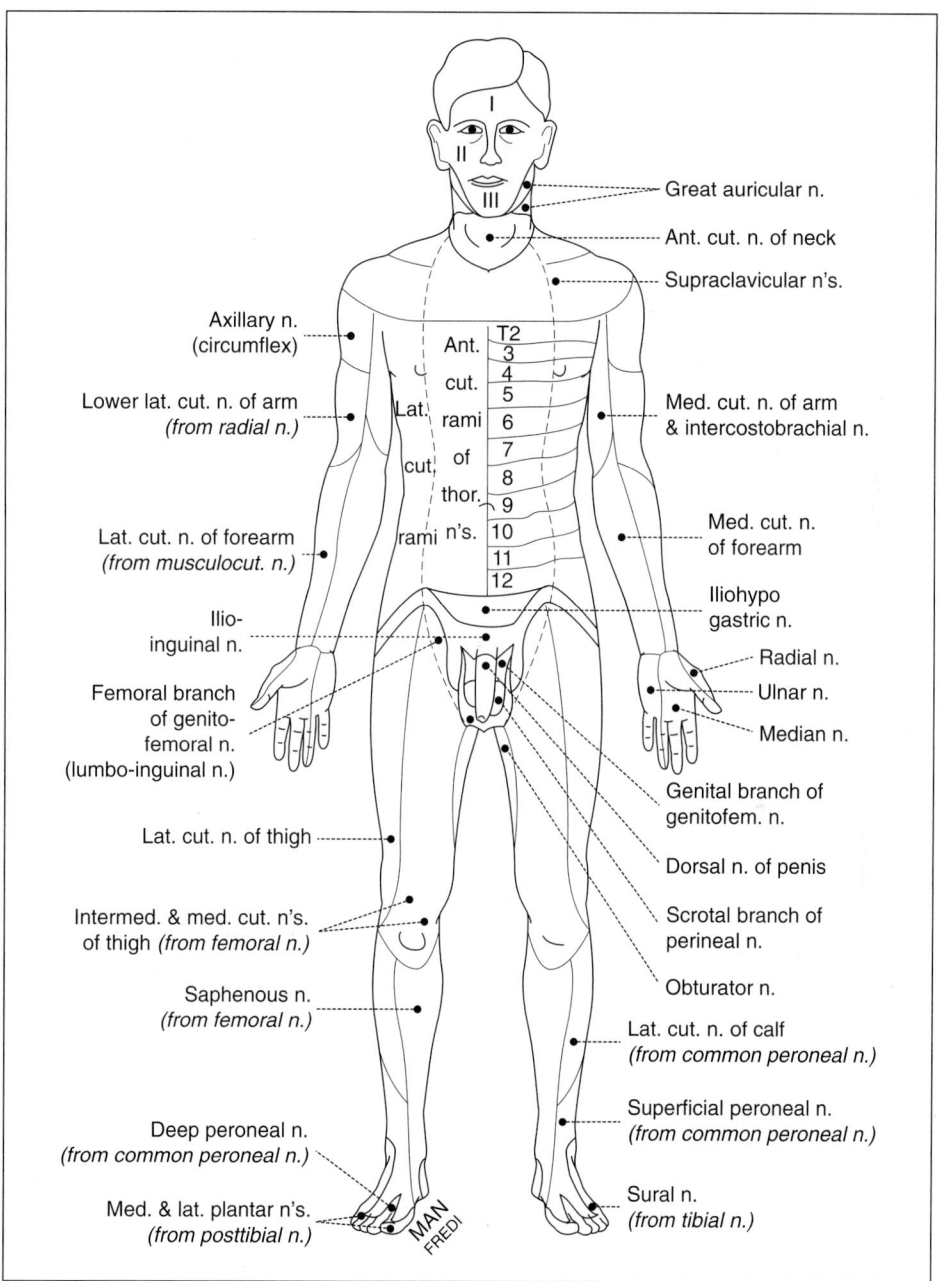

FIGURE 5-2 Cutaneous fields of the peripheral nerves. (*continued*)

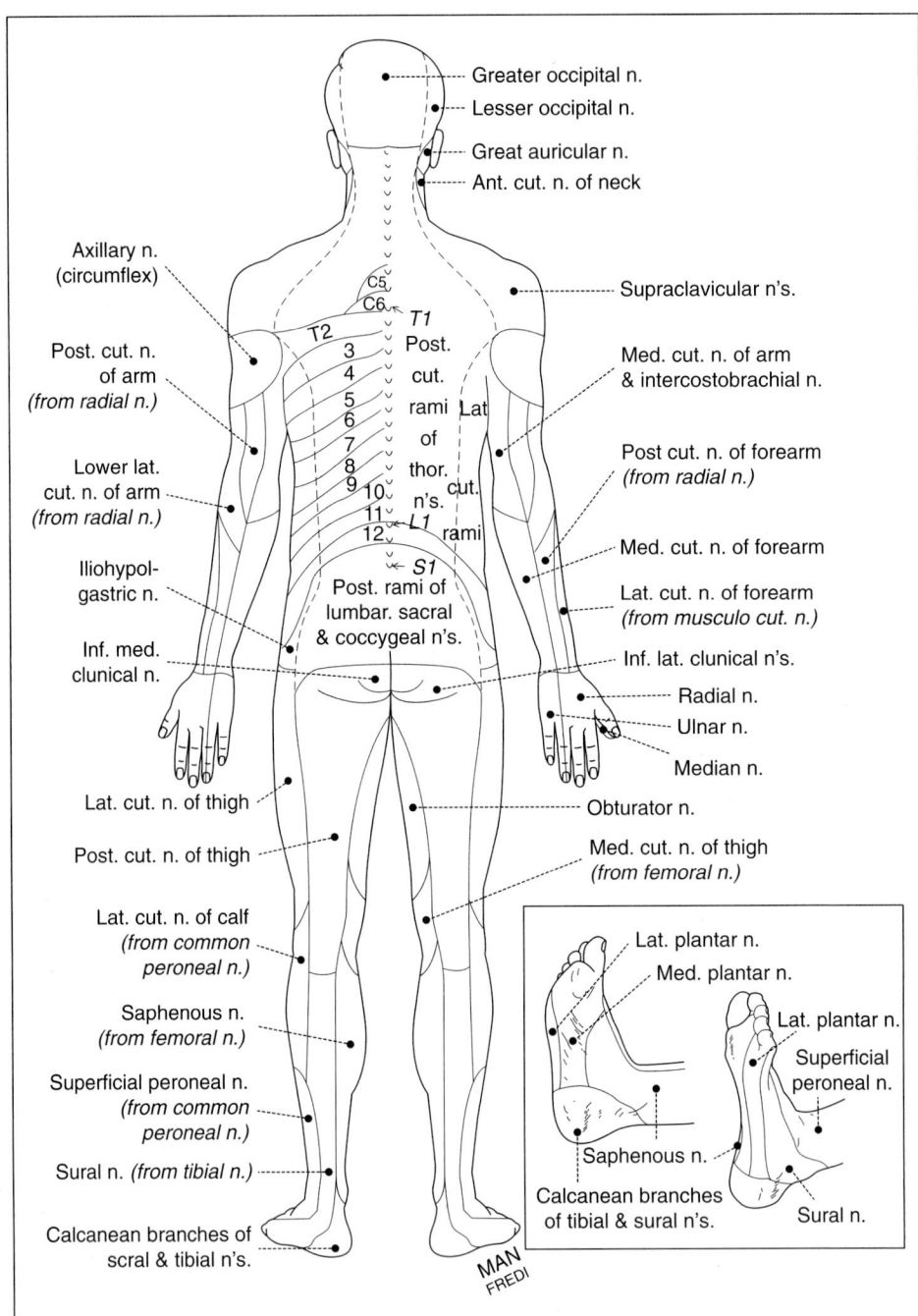

FIGURE 5-2   (*Continued*)

MRI has revolutionized the diagnostic evaluation of peripheral nerve injuries due to structural lesions, but it is usually of little help in other cases. Effective use of MRI requires that an accurate "anatomic" diagnosis be made so that the appropriate body region can be imaged. As a practical matter, MRI is rarely needed in the acute care setting to evaluate peripheral nerve lesions.

Cranial Nerve Lesions

Trigeminal neuralgia is characterized by severe pain in the distribution of one or more divisions of the trigeminal nerve (most often the mandibular and maxillary divisions). The pain is typically very intense and occurs in brief paroxysms, each lasting only a few seconds; the pain usually has a burning, stabbing, or searing quality. The stabs of pain may be isolated or occur in bursts. Bursts of pain may be associated with involuntary twitches or jerks of the face, hence the synonym *tic douloureux*. Attacks are often stimulated by touching trigger zones on the face or in the mouth, by chewing or eating, or even by a breath of wind; patients will often walk about with a hand held over the face (but not touching the face) to ward off any contact. The physical examination is normal, and there are no associated neurologic symptoms or findings. The syndrome may occur without warning in a previously healthy patient and thus provoke a visit to the emergency department. It is important to distinguish this condition from more slowly evolving persistent pain or sensory loss in the face, which suggest infiltration or compression of the trigeminal nerve by tumor, infection, connective tissue disease, dental disease, or other causes. This syndrome is usually called trigeminal neuropathy, and diagnosis may require a very detailed workup that would not be undertaken on an emergency basis.

For patients with classic trigeminal neuralgia, emergency imaging studies are not required. Pain medication is usually of little benefit. Many patients respond promptly to anticonvulsant medications, and carbamazepine is commonly used with success. Long-term management is complicated, and patients should be referred to a neurologist.

Facial nerve palsy is characterized by acute weakness or paralysis of the muscles on one side of the face. Typically, in lesions of the facial nerve, the upper and lower portions of the ipsilateral face are affected equally; in "central" lesions (e.g., stroke), the lower portion of the contralateral face is affected while the upper portion is spared. This well-known clinical pearl is not entirely reliable; some patients with acute hemispheric strokes will have weakness affecting both the upper and the lower face, and some patients with more distal lesions of the facial nerve, for example in the parotid gland, may have selective weakness of the lower face. A more reliable approach is to examine the patient carefully for evidence of any other neurologic deficit; if the only deficit is weakness of the face, a peripheral lesion is likely. Weakness of an arm or leg on the ipsilateral side suggests a contralateral hemisphere lesion; ipsilateral abducens palsy or gaze palsy or a contralateral hemiparesis indicates an ipsilateral brainstem (pons) lesion. As the weakness of the facial muscles makes it difficult or impossible to close the eye on the affected side, many patients complain of "blurred vision" on the affected side, but careful examination shows no actual visual impairment. Some patients with facial nerve palsy may experience hyperacusis on the affected side; some will complain of an abnormal sense of taste, but the actual loss of taste sensation is difficult to demonstrate.

The most common cause of facial nerve palsy is Bell's palsy; by definition this is idiopathic, although recent data suggest that a significant proportion of these cases may be due to infection by HSV. A similar clinical picture with the added features of pain in the ear and a vesicular eruption in the external ear canal is caused by herpes zoster (the Ramsay Hunt syndrome). In typical Bell's palsy, the onset is acute, and weakness develops over a few hours to a day or two, occasionally longer. The onset of weakness may be preceded by a few days or hours of temporal headache or pain behind the ear. If the weakness develops more slowly, over a period of weeks or longer, infiltration or compression of the nerve should be suspected. In general, in cases of isolated facial weakness, diagnostic study is not an emergency and can be undertaken on an elective basis if the diagnosis is uncertain.

Treatment of Bell's palsy remains somewhat controversial. Fortunately, most patients (70%–80%) make a full spontaneous recovery over several weeks to months. Corticosteroids (prednisone 40 to 60 mg/d for 5 to 10 days), if started early, may shorten the course and improve outcome and should be given if there are no contraindications. The role of antiviral agents (acyclovir and others) is less clear and they are not generally recommended.[53,54] It is important to remember to protect the patient's eye on the affected side; because the patients may be unable to close the eye, they are at risk of excessive drying of the eye, and its damage from foreign bodies and infection. Depending on the severity of the weakness, treatment may range from liberal use of eyedrops or ointments to patching or taping the eye shut, or even to tarsorrhaphy. Patients should be instructed to seek medical attention without delay if they develop pain or other problems in the eye.

Isolated lesions of other cranial nerves may occur as well. Lesions of the oculomotor (III), trochlear (IV), and abducens (VI) nerves cause diplopia; oculomotor lesions may also cause ptosis and pupil abnormalities. Careful physical examination is needed to decide which nerve is affected and to look for any evidence of brainstem involvement. These are discussed in Chapter 9. Isolated mononeuropathies of the lower cranial nerves are much less common.

Spinal Root Lesions

The most common symptom of lesions affecting single spinal roots is pain in the dermatome of the affected root. Sensory loss is highly variable or may be absent entirely in patients with single-root lesions. Reflexes are typically reduced or absent in the affected root distribution. Weakness, if present, is confined to muscles innervated by the affected root; complete paralysis does not occur because individual muscles are innervated by nerve fibers from several roots (Table 5-10). The most common cause of an acute root lesion is herniation of an intervertebral disc; the cervical and lumbosacral roots are most often affected. The patient can often recall some specific activity, trauma, or other cause that provoked the symptoms. Other structural lesions such as osteophytes, tumors, and others can also cause root lesions, more often with a subacute or chronic course.

The clinical diagnosis of an acute root lesion ordinarily presents no difficulty. A careful examination is necessary to assess for any evidence of spinal cord involvement. In the usual case of an isolated single root lesion, urgent imaging studies are not required. Initial treatment usually consists of aspirin, NSAIDs, and sometimes muscle relaxants. In patients with severe pain, a short course of corticosteroid therapy may be beneficial (e.g., prednisone 1 mg/kg/d for 5–7 days followed by a tapering dose over the next 5–7 days). Narcotic analgesics may be needed if the pain is very severe.

There are three situations in which urgent imaging (MRI) and neurosurgical referral may be needed. First is the patient with marked weakness of the affected muscles. Second is the patient with signs and symptoms suggesting spinal cord compression. Third is the patient with pain in the perineum or pain and sensory loss in a "saddle" distribution involving the perineum and medial thighs. These findings suggest possible compression of the cauda equina in the lumbar spinal canal; bladder and bowel function may be compromised as well. Urgent surgical treatment may be needed to minimize the extent of permanent injury.

Brachial and Lumbosacral Plexus Lesions

Plexus lesions should be suspected when symptoms are not confined to the distribution of a single nerve or nerve root, but instead indicate injury to several anatomically related nerves. The anatomy of the brachial and lumbosacral plexuses is quite complex, and a detailed analysis of these lesions requires careful examination.[50,51] Fortunately, a detailed assessment is not required in the acute care setting and these patients can be referred for elective evaluation.

Acute lesions of the brachial plexus are often due to trauma. Violent stretching or twisting of the neck, shoulder, or upper arm are obvious potential causes. Less immediate obvious causes are compression injuries from shoulder straps. An idiopathic (possibly inflammatory or immune-mediated) brachial plexopathy (Parsonage-Turner syndrome) is also well described. It is usually characterized by severe pain in the shoulder and upper arm; weakness of the arm muscles, sensory loss, and impaired reflexes involving several different nerve distributions are also seen. Acute treatment consists of pain management and rest; steroids are often prescribed but are of unknown benefit.

Acute lesions of the lumbosacral plexus can result from pelvic fractures. Other potential causes of particular interest in the acute care setting include a leaking abdominal aortic aneurysm or retroperitoneal hemorrhage, especially in patients on anticoagulant therapy. Infiltration of the plexus by cancer or compression from retroperitoneal or psoas muscle abscess also occur but generally have a subacute or chronic course.

Peripheral Mononeuropathy

Isolated acute lesions can affect virtually every peripheral nerve, each resulting in a characteristic clinical syndrome. As noted previously, recognition of these syndromes depends on the skill of the examining physician; because of the bewildering variety of these syndromes, liberal use should be made of appropriate tables and references. A few of these syndromes are so common that they should be easily recognized by acute care physicians. In the upper extremity, common syndromes include those of the median, ulnar, and radial nerves. In the lower extremity, the common syndromes are those of the lateral femoral cutaneous nerve and the femoral, sciatic, and peroneal nerves. It is important to recall that the clinical syndromes are frequently incomplete; it is generally best to base the diagnosis on those findings that are present rather than on those that are absent. For example, weakness of the extensor muscles of the wrist and fingers should suggest radial nerve palsy even in the absence of the typical sensory findings.

As noted previously, many peripheral nerve injuries are caused by obvious trauma. However, the peripheral nerve injury itself may not be obvious, especially in the face of pain, or limited motion, caused by the primary injury. The acute care physician should always consider the possibility of peripheral nerve injury in trauma patients and should carry out any needed examination. A less obvious cause of peripheral nerve injury is pressure palsy, resulting from sustained compression of a nerve, often against a bony surface. There is usually no obvious trauma, and the patient may be unaware of the cause of the injury. There are several quite common pressure palsies in the acute care setting.

Radial nerve palsy results from compression of the radial nerve against the medial surface of the humerus in the upper arm. This can result when an arm is allowed to hang over the back of a chair or over the side of a bed for an extended period ("Saturday night palsy"), or when a heavy object, such as a companion's head, is allowed to rest on the inside of the upper arm ("honeymooner's palsy"). The nerve is occasionally injured in the axilla in patients using crutches. A more restricted radial palsy, characterized by pain and numbness on the back of the hand, but without weakness, can result from compression of the superficial sensory branches of the nerve from handcuffs.

Median and *ulnar nerve* palsies can also result from compression of the nerves in the axilla, at the elbow, or at the wrist. The median nerve can be injured at the wrist (carpal tunnel syndrome) by a variety of mechanisms. Although usually chronic, these are occasionally seen as an acute problem in pregnant women or following forceful hyperextension of the wrist (as in motor vehicle accidents).

Sciatic nerve palsies can result from local pressure on the sciatic nerve from prolonged sitting in a fixed position, particularly in patients who drive long distances; a large billfold in a hip pocket may be the culprit. The sciatic nerve may also be injured when a leg is allowed to hang over the edge of the bed for a prolonged period, as when a patient falls asleep while intoxicated.

Peroneal nerve palsy results from compression of the peroneal nerve where it passes under the head of the fibula. This can occur when patients sit for long periods with one leg crossed over the other, or in bedridden patients who are unable to move their legs. The nerve is sometimes injured when the legs are placed in stirrups to maintain the lithotomy position during obstetrical delivery, gynecologic examinations, etc.

Femoral nerve palsy can result from compression of the femoral nerve at the inguinal ligament; this can result from hematomas following arterial puncture or from forceful flexion of the hips during childbirth or gynecologic procedures. Compression of the femoral nerve within the abdomen by an enlarged uterus is an occasional complication of pregnancy. The femoral nerve can also be injured with retroperitoneal bleeding.

Lateral femoral cutaneous nerve injury causes pain and paresthesias in the anterolateral thigh (*meralgia paresthetica*). This is a pure sensory nerve and there are no motor symptoms. The cause is usually obscure, but the nerve is occasionally injured by pressure from the enlarged abdomen in pregnant patients or grossly obese patients or occasionally by tight undergarments.

Finally, isolated peripheral nerve palsies may occur for a number of other reasons. Some of these, especially in patients with diabetes or other microangiopathic diseases, are thought to result from nerve infarction; others are probably immune-mediated. In some cases, no explanation can be found.

In most cases of isolated peripheral nerve palsies, no urgent treatment is necessary or available. Fortunately, the prognosis is usually good unless the nerve is transected. It is important to be able to reassure the patient that he or she has not had a stroke or other neurologic catastrophe.

Mononeuritis multiplex is a rare clinical syndrome in which two or more isolated peripheral nerves are affected nearly simultaneously. This is most often the result of microvascular infarction of nerves and may be seen in polyarteritis nodosa or other vasculitides, or in diabetes. Other potential causes include multifocal motor neuropathy (an autoimmune-mediated disorder), sarcoidosis, and others.

SUMMARY

Patients with acute focal weakness are frequently seen in the acute care setting. The crucial step in the evaluation of these patients is localization of the anatomic lesion causing the clinical symptoms. A useful technique is for the physician to consider, in each case, about whether the symptoms could have been caused by a lesion in the brain, the brainstem, the spinal cord, the peripheral nerves, or the muscles. The clinical history and neurologic examination are the sources for the necessary information. Accurate localization of the lesion and the clinical course should suggest a differential diagnosis; the differential diagnosis should then suggest the appropriate laboratory and imaging studies. There are relatively few causes of acute focal weakness that may require emergency management; often the task of the acute care physician should be to determine that the patient does not require emergency intervention.

The most common emergency condition is acute stroke. It is becoming clear that thrombolytic therapy should be considered in patients who present with acute stroke, but there is still considerable controversy about the most appropriate use of this therapy, with some physicians more convinced by the accumulated observational data and the limited RCT data than others. It is to be hoped that developments in diagnostic imaging will serve to better define a population of patients most likely to benefit from this approach. The pathophysiology of stroke implies that the effectiveness of any treatment will depend in large measure on the rapid identification of appropriate patients. It seems likely that the choice of therapy will vary depending on the probable mechanism of the stroke, placing a high premium on rapid clinical assessment. Close attention should be paid to supportive measures ensuring oxygenation and perfusion.

A second category of patients who may benefit from urgent intervention are those with acute brainstem lesions. Although such conditions are less likely to respond to specific treatment, these patients are at substantial risk from respiratory failure and aspiration, and protection of the airway and support of ventilation should be considered.

The final category of patients who require emergency treatment are those with spinal cord syndromes, especially spinal cord compression from mass lesions. Urgent decompression may reduce or prevent permanent damage to the spinal cord.

REFERENCES

1. Hakim AM. Ischemic penumbra: the therapeutic window. *Neurology*. 1998;51:544-546.
2. Kothari RU et al. Emergency physicians: accuracy in diagnosis of stroke. *Stroke*. 1995;26: 2238-2241.
3. Libman RB et al. Conditions that mimic stroke in the emergency department. *Arch Neurol*. 1995;52:1119-1122.

4. Moeller JJ, Kurniawan J, Gubitz GJ, et al. Diagnostic accuracy of neurological problems in the emergency department. *Can J Neurol Sci*. 2008;35:335-341.

5. Chalela JA, Kidwell CS, Nentwich LM, et al. Magnetic resonance imaging and computed tomography in emergency assessment of patients with suspected acute stroke; a prospective comparison. *Lancet*. 2007;369:293-298.

6. Kane I, Sandercock P, Wardlaw J. Magnetic resonance perfusion diffusion mismatch and thrombolysis in acute ischemic stroke; a systematic review of the evidence to date. *J Neurol Neurosurg Psychiatry*. 2007;78(5):485-491.

7. Adams HP, del Zoppo G, Alberts, MJ, et al. Guidelines for the early management of adults with acute ischemic stroke: a guideline from the American Heart Association/American Stroke Association Stoke Council, Clinical Cardiology Council, Cardiovascular Radiology and Intervention Council, and the Atherosclerotic Peripheral Vascular Disease and Quality of Care Outcomes in Research Interdisciplinary Working Groups. *Stroke*. 2007;38: 1655-1711.

8. The National Institute of Neurological Disorders and Stroke rt-PA Stroke Study Group. Tissue plasminogen activator for acute ischemic stroke. *N Engl J Med*. 1995;333:1581-1587.

9. Jenkins PO, Turner MR, Jenkins PF. What is the place of thrombolysis in acute stroke? A review of the literature and a current perspective. *Clin Med*. 2008;8(3):253-258.

10. Hacke W, Kaste M, Fieschi C, et al. Intravenous thrombolysis with recombinant tissue plasminogen activator for acute hemispheric stroke. The European Cooperative Acute Stroke Study (ECASS). *JAMA*. 1995;274:1017-1025.

11. Hacke W, Kaste M, Fieschi C, et al. Randomised double-blind placebo-controlled trial of thrombolytic therapy with intravenous alteplase in acute ischaemic stroke (ECASS II). Second European-Australasian Stroke Study Investigators. *Lancet*. 1998;352:1245-1251.

12. Adams HP et al. Guidelines for thrombolytic therapy for acute stroke: a supplement to the guidelines for the management of patients with acute ischemic stroke. A statement for healthcare professionals from a special writing group of the Stroke Council, American Heart Association. *Circulation*. 1996;94:1167-1174.

13. Barreto AD, Martin-Schild S, Hallevi H, et al. Thrombolytic therapy for patients who wake-up with stroke. *Stroke*. 2009;40(3):827-832.

14. Gorelick AR, Gorelick PB, Sloan EP. Emergency department evaluation and management of stroke: acute assessment, stroke teams, and care pathways. *Neurol Clin*. 2008;26(4): 923-942.

15. Clark WM, Wissman S, Albers GW, et al. Recombinant tissue-type plasminogen activator (Alteplase) for ischemic stroke 3 to 5 hours after symptom onset. The ATLANTIS Study: a randomized controlled trial. *JAMA*. 1999;282:2019-2026.

16. Hacke W, Kaste M, Bluhmki E, et al. Thrombolysis with Alteplase 3 to 4.5 hours after acute ischemic stroke. *N Engl J Med*. 2008;359(13):1317-1329.

17. Lyden P. Thrombolytic therapy for acute stroke—not a moment to lose [editorial]. *N Engl J Med*. 2008;359(13):1393-1394.

18. Clark WM, Madden KP. Keep the three hour TPA window: the lost study of Atlantis [letter]. *J Stroke Cerebrovasc Dis*. 2009;18(1):78-79.

18a. del Zoppo GJ, Saver JL, Jauch EC, et al. Expansion of the time window for treatment of acute ischemic stroke with intravenous tissue plasminogen activator: a science advisory from the American Heart Association/American Stroke Association. *Stroke*. 2009;40:2945-2948.

18b. Alper BS, Brown CB. Expanding recombinant tissue plasminogen activator time window is premature. *Stroke*. 2009;40:e632.

18c. Asimos AW. Guidelines for extending the tissue plasminogen activator window for ischemic stroke. *Stroke*. 2009;40:e633.

18d. del Zoppo GJ, Saver JL, Jauch EC, et al. Response to letters by Asimos and by Alper and Brown. *Stroke*. 2009;40:e634-e635.

19. Albers GW, Amarenco P, Easton JD, et al. Antithrombotic and thrombolytic therapy for ischemic stroke: American College of Chest Physicians Evidence-Based Clinical Practice Guidelines (8th Edition). *Chest*. 2008;133(suppl 6):630S-669S.

20. Smith EE, Abdullah AR, Petkovska I, et al. Poor outcomes in patients who do not receive intravenous plasminogen activator because of mild or improving ischemic stroke. *Stroke*. 2005;36;2497-2499.

21. Köhrmann M, Nowe T, Huttner HB, et al. Safety and outcome after thrombolysis in stroke patients with mild symptoms. *Cerebrovasc Dis*. 2009;27:160-166.

22. Katzan IL et al. Use of tissue-type plasminogen activator for acute ischemic stroke: the Cleveland area experience. *JAMA*. 2000;283:1151-1158.

23. Wahlgren N, Ahmed N, Davalos A, et al. Thrombolysis with alteplase for acute ischemic stroke in the safe implementation of thrombolysis in stroke monitoring study (SITS-MOST): an observational study. *Lancet*. 2007;369:275-282.

24. Powers WJ. Acute hypertension after stroke: the scientific basis for treatment decisions. *Neurology*. 1993;43:461-467.

25. Quinn TJ, Lees KR. Hyperglycaemia in acute stroke-to treat or not to treat. *Cerebrovasc Dis*. 2009;27(suppl 1):148-155.

26. Gray CS, Hildreth AJ, Sandercock PA, et al. Glucose-potassium-insulin infusions in the management of post-stroke hyperglycaemia: the UK Glucose Insulin is Stroke Trial (GIST-UK). *Lancet Neurol*. 2007;6:397-406.

27. Grotta JC. Intracerebral hemorrhage: effective therapy at last? *Int J Stroke*. 2006;1:30-31.

28. Broderick JP et al. Guidelines for the management of spontaneous intracerebral hemorrhage: a statement for healthcare professionals from a special writing group of the Stroke Council, American Heart Association. *Stroke*. 1999;30:905-915.

29. Rincon F, Mayer SA. Current treatment options for intracerebral hemorrhage. *Curr Treat Options. Cardiovasc Med*. 2008;10(3):229-240.

30. Testai FD, Aiyagari V. Acute hemorrhagic stroke pathophysiology and medical interventions: blood pressure control, management of anticoagulant-associated brain hemorrhage and general management principles. *Neurol Clin*. 2008;26:963-985.

31. Aguilar MI, Hart RG, Kase CS, et al. Treatment of warfarin-associated intracerebral hemorrhage: literature review and expert opinion. *Mayo Clin Proc*. 2007;82(1):82-92.

32. Committee on Cerebrovascular Diseases. Classification and outline of cerebrovascular diseases II. *Stroke*. 1975;6:564-616.

33. Sacco RL, Adams R, Albers G, et al. Guidelines for prevention of stroke in patients with ischemic stroke or transient ischemic attack: a statement for healthcare professionals from the American Heart Association/American Stroke Association Council on Stroke. *Stroke*. 2006;37:577-617.

34. Lewandowski CA, Rao CP, Silver B. Transient ischemic attack: definitions and clinical presentations. *Ann Emerg Med*. 2008;52(2):S7-S16.

35. Giles MF, Rothwell PM. Transient ischemic attack: clinical relevance, risk prediction and urgency of secondary prevention. *Curr Opin Neurol*. 2009;22(1):46-53.

36. Prabhakaran S, Silver AJ, Warrior L, et al. Misdiagnosis of transient ischemic attacks in the emergency room. *Cerebrovasc Dis*. 2008;26(6):630-635.

37. Rothwell PM, Giles MF, Flossman E, et al. A simple score (ABCD) to identify individuals at high early risk of stroke after transient ischemic attack. *Lancet*. 2005;366:29-36.

38. Josephson SA, Sidney S, Pham TN, et al. Higher ABCD2 score predicts patients most likely to have true transient ischemic attack. *Stroke*. 2008;39(11):3096-3098.

39. Johnston SC, Rothwell PM, Nguyen-Huynh MN, et al. Validation and refinement of scores to predict very early stroke risk after transient ischemic attack. *Lancet*. 2007;369:283-292.

40. Coutts SB, Eliasziw M, Hill MD, et al. An improved scoring system for identifying patients at high early risk of stroke and functional impairment after an acute transient ischemic attack or minor stroke. *Int J Stroke*. 2008;3(1):3-10.

41. Calvet D, Touzé E, Oppenheim C. DWI lesions and TIA etiology improve the prediction of stroke after TIA. *Stroke*. 2009;40(1):187-192.

42. Jagoda A, Chan YF. Transient ischemic attack overview: defining the challenges for improving outcomes. *Ann Emerg Med*. 2008;52(2):S3-S6.

43. Messé SR, Jauch EC. Transient ischemic attack: diagnostic evaluation. *Ann Emerg Med*. 2008;54(2):S17-S26.

44. Adams RJ, Albers G, Alberts, MJ, et al. Update to the AHA/ASA recommendations for the prevention of stroke in patients with stroke and transient ischemic attack. *Stroke*. 2008;39: 1647-1652.

45. Hackam DG, Spence JD. Combining multiple approaches for the secondary prevention of vascular events after stroke; a quantitative modeling study. *Stroke*. 2007;38:1881-1885.

46. Harbison J, Palmer K, Ochs A. Migraine amaurosis fugax? Investigate [abstract]. *Stroke*. 1987;18:225.

47. McAlpine D, Lumsden CE, Acheson ED. *Multiple Sclerosis: A Reappraisal*. 2nd ed. Edinburgh, UK: Churchill Livingstone; 1972.

48. Mundy Stephanie B, Manzullo Ellen. Oncologic emergencies. In: Kantarjian HM, Wolff RA, Koller CA, eds. *MD Anderson Manual of Medical Oncology*. chap 39. http://www.accessmedicine. com/content.aspx?aID=2800143.

49. Bruna J, Martinez-Yélamos S, Rubio F, Arbizu T. Idiopathic acute transverse myelitis: a clinical study and prognostic markers in 45 cases. *Mult Scler*. 2006;12:169-173.

50. Greenberg BM, Thomas KP, Krishnan C, et al. Idiopathic transverse myelitis: corticosteroids, plasma exchange, or cyclophosphamide. *Neurology*. 2007;68:1614-1617.

51. Guarantors of Brain. *Aids to the Examination of the Peripheral Nervous System*. 2nd ed. London: Baillière-Tindall; 1986.

52. Devinsky O, Feldmann E. *Examination of the Cranial and Peripheral Nerves*. New York: Churchill Livingstone; 1988.

53. Madhok V, Falk G, Fahey T, Sullivan FM. Prescribe prednisolone alone for Bell's palsy diagnosed within 72 hours of symptom onset. *BMJ*. 2009;338:b255.

54. Sullivan FM, Swan IRC, Donnan PT, et al. Early treatment with prednisolone or acyclovir in Bell's palsy. *N Engl J Med*. 2007;357(16):1598-1607.

6

ACUTE
GENERALIZED
WEAKNESS

Much of the central and peripheral nervous system is dedicated to the initiation and control of voluntary movement. As a result, abnormal function in virtually any part of the nervous system may result in weakness of voluntary muscles. Chapter 5 reviewed the evaluation and management of patients with acute focal weakness; this chapter reviews the evaluation and management of patients with more diffuse or generalized weakness. Many of the disorders causing generalized weakness are chronic or even lifelong; this discussion focuses on those disorders that develop over a few hours or days rather than over periods of weeks or longer.

Strictly speaking, the term *weakness* means loss of muscle power or strength. However, the word is often used by patients to denote a variety of different symptoms in addition to actual loss of strength. The term *weakness* is sometimes used to describe such symptoms as malaise, fatigue, or lassitude, conditions characterized more by a disinclination to move than by actual loss of strength. Patients with movement disorders, discussed in Chapter 7, such as Parkinson's disease, often describe themselves as weak even though their actual muscle power may be normal. Patients with pain may also describe themselves as weak owing to their inability to move around as they wish. A careful history is therefore often necessary to distinguish patients with actual weakness from those with other symptoms. If true weakness is present, the next step is to try to localize the responsible lesion(s) within the nervous system. As with focal lesions, the location of the lesion will suggest the most likely diagnostic possibilities.

CLINICAL ASSESSMENT

History

The first and most important step in clinical diagnosis is to be as clear as possible about exactly what symptoms are to be diagnosed. The differential diagnosis of true generalized weakness of acute onset is fairly limited, whereas the differential diagnosis of the multiple symptoms that may masquerade as weakness is enormous. The best clinical clue to the presence of true muscle weakness is loss or impairment of function. It is often helpful to ask patients to describe their symptoms without using the term "weakness" or to ask them to describe any specific activities that are limited or prohibited by their weakness. For example, a patient who is unable to climb stairs is more likely to have true weakness than the patient who feels tired or exhausted after climbing stairs. Similarly, a patient who cannot get up from a chair is more likely to have true weakness than one who gets up slowly and with difficulty. A patient unable to lift her arms over her head is more likely to have true weakness than one who feels exhausted after carrying out her usual daily activities. If true weakness seems likely, the physician should try to determine which muscles are affected and to what extent.

Once the basic nature of the patient's complaints is clear, the usual questions should be asked regarding the onset, progression, and severity of the symptoms. Patients commonly date the onset of symptoms from the time they first became aware of them; what seems to the patient to be acute weakness may actually have been slowly evolving over months or even years. Careful questioning may reveal subtle changes in function that began well before the patient became aware of the weakness. It is crucial to determine whether the weakness is constant or variable, provoked by activity, or relieved by rest. The patient should be questioned carefully about any recent or chronic illnesses and recent or chronic use of drugs, prescribed or otherwise, including alcohol. Drugs of particular importance include diuretics, thyroid replacement, corticosteroids, and lipid-lowering agents such as the statins. A prior history of similar symptoms should be sought. The presence or absence of bladder or bowel dysfunction, sexual dysfunction, pain, paresthesia, sensory loss, or muscle cramps and spasms should be determined. A family history of similar symptoms should be sought.

Physical Examination

A fairly comprehensive neurologic examination is usually necessary in these patients. A "focused" neurologic examination carries a risk of missing essential information. When in doubt, it is usually better to be overinclusive rather than underinclusive. The neurologic examination is discussed in Chapter 3, and only a few points will be reviewed here. The goals of the neurologic examination, as always, are to

1. clarify the exact nature of the clinical symptoms. Does the patient have true loss of strength, or are his/her symptoms due to pain, lethargy, etc.?
2. identify symptoms not identified by the patient. For example, is weakness of the legs accompanied by mild but less evident weakness in the arms? Is the weakness accompanied by sensory loss not recognized by the patient?
3. clarify the anatomic basis for the symptoms. For example, is weakness accompanied by altered reflexes or an up going toe, or by muscle atrophy and fasciculations?

On physical examination, strength is commonly graded on a numerical scale where:

O = no trace of movement
1 = a trace of motion, but insufficient to move an extremity
2 = movement of the extremity in the horizontal plane, but not against gravity
3 = movement of an extremity against gravity, but not against additional resistance
4 = movement of an extremity against resistance, but with less than full strength
5 = normal strength

Although useful as a way of recording clinical findings, use of such scales can create the impression that assessment of muscle strength is "objective" and easily quantified. In fact, assessment of muscle strength is quite subjective and is dependent on the skill and insight of the physician. Reliable assessment of strength requires that the patient exert a maximum effort, thus patients' apparent strength can be greatly affected by their willingness and ability to cooperate with the examiner. It may be difficult or impossible to assess strength reliably in an individual with severe pain or who is unwilling to make a maximum effort. Patients with severe anxiety or depression may not be motivated to make a full effort. Although true malingering is uncommon, patients with subjective weakness may try to "help" the examiner by exaggerating the extent of their weakness.

A substantial disparity between the strength of the examiner and the patient may also cause confusion. It is not uncommon for elderly patients to have their strength graded as "4/5," indicating a degree of true weakness, when in fact their only problem is that they were examined by younger (and presumably stronger) physicians. Similarly, a small or slight examiner may be unable to detect even significant weakness in a much stronger patient. Accordingly, assessment of strength ultimately requires a subjective judgment by the physician that an individual patient is as strong, or less strong, than expected. When in doubt, it is better simply to acknowledge that strength cannot be adequately assessed than to "guess" that the patient is or is not weak.

An excellent way to assess strength is to observe the patient attempting to perform the specific activities that are affected by the reported weakness. Thus, watching a patient get up from a chair and walk may be much more revealing than direct manual muscle testing. Careful observation of a patient's spontaneous activity during the interview and when his or her attention is distracted can yield important information.

If weakness is present, its distribution should be determined. Are all four limbs affected? Are axial muscles (especially the neck and back) affected? Does the weakness primarily affect proximal or distal muscles of the extremities? Is there involvement of muscles innervated by the cranial nerves, such as the extraocular muscles, the eyelids, or the face? Is there any involvement of speech or swallowing? A careful search should be made for any sign of an underlying focal disorder. Weakness affecting only the legs and sparing the arms may suggest a lesion of the thoracic spinal cord, while weakness affecting all four extremities but completely sparing the face may indicate a lesion of the upper cervical spinal cord. Involvement of muscles innervated by the cranial nerves, especially if asymmetric, may indicate a brainstem lesion. A sensory "level" indicates a spinal cord lesion. The presence of hyperactive reflexes or a Babinski sign indicates a central (brain or spinal cord) lesion, but recall that complete areflexia may also be seen in patients with acute lesions of the spinal cord (see Chapters 5 and 10 for further discussion).

A general physical examination should be performed. Special attention should be directed to any signs of chronic systemic illness, occult neoplasms, chronic infection, or endocrine dysfunction such as hyperthyroidism or hypothyroidism or Cushing's disease or syndrome.

DIFFERENTIAL DIAGNOSIS

As noted earlier, acute generalized weakness can result from disorders affecting virtually any part of the nervous system. The differential diagnosis and diagnostic strategy depend on the likely location of the lesion. For example, generalized weakness resulting from a diffuse brain disorder is likely to be associated with abnormalities of consciousness, behavior, memory, judgment, etc., and the primary focus of the evaluation will be the altered mental status, discussed in Chapter 4. Similarly, focal disorders of the brainstem and spinal cord will virtually always be associated with localizing signs; their evaluation is discussed in Chapter 5.

In the acute care setting, the most important causes of acute generalized weakness without localizing signs are disorders affecting the peripheral nerves, the neuromuscular junction, and the muscles themselves. Clinical features that help to distinguish among these are listed in Table 6-1. Inspection of the table reveals that the clinical features of these disorders are variable and overlap to a considerable extent, so a reliable diagnosis cannot often be based on one or two features but rather will depend on the entire clinical picture.

Peripheral nerve disorders may involve isolated nerves, as discussed in Chapter 5; disorders that affect the peripheral nerves in a more diffuse or generalized fashion, such as the Guillain-Barré syndrome, are termed polyneuropathies. These conditions may primarily affect either the myelin sheath (demyelinating polyneuropathies) or the axons themselves (axonal polyneuropathies) or both. Depending on the particular population of nerve fibers affected, the primary symptoms may be motor weakness, sensory loss, paresthesia, pain, or any combination of these.

Demyelinating neuropathies are commonly not painful, and patients may complain of "numbness" of the affected extremities. Reflexes are diminished or lost early in the course, even before weakness is clinically evident. Sensory loss, when detectable, involves

TABLE 6-1

GENERALIZED WEAKNESS: PERIPHERAL LOCALIZATION

Clinical Sign	Neuropathy	N-M Junction	Myopathy
Weakness (pattern)	Distal > proximal	Variable	Proximal > distal
Weakness (severity)	Constant, progressive	Variable	Constant, progressive
Sensory loss	Distal > proximal	Absent	Absent
Pain	Variable, distal	Absent	Usually absent
Muscle atrophy	Variable, often early	Absent	Variable, usually late
Reflexes	Decreased or absent	Normal	Normal or slightly decreased
Fasciculations	Sometimes	Absent	Absent
CSF protein	Normal or increased	Normal	Normal
CK level (serum)	Normal	Normal	Increased
Edrophonium test	No response	May respond	No response

vibration sense, position sense, and light touch sense with relative preservation of pain and temperature sensation. Axonal disorders, on the other hand, are commonly painful; the pain often has a tingling or burning quality. Reflexes are often preserved until the neuropathy is more advanced and weakness is evident. Pain and temperature sensation are affected early.

Because longer nerve fibers are commonly affected first, peripheral neuropathy symptoms often begin distally and spread proximally. In more chronic conditions, there may be atrophy of distal muscles, and fasciculations may be seen. Reflexes are often markedly diminished or absent, even in muscles not obviously weak or otherwise affected. Muscle enzymes (e.g., creatine kinase [CK]) may be normal or elevated.

Neuromuscular junction disorders, such as myasthenia gravis, are characterized by variable weakness that may be relieved by rest. The weakness is frequently asymmetric and often does not respect anatomic boundaries. Cranial nerve muscles and spinal nerve muscles are often affected together. Sensory symptoms and pain are absent. Reflexes are generally preserved unless the weakness is severe. Muscle enzymes are usually normal.

Muscle disorders are characterized by fairly symmetric weakness affecting proximal more than distal muscles; axial muscles are often affected as well. Although muscle pain and tenderness are sometimes present, sensory symptoms are absent. Reflexes are generally preserved unless weakness is severe. Muscle enzymes may be normal or markedly elevated.

By the time a patient's illness has progressed to the point of severe generalized weakness, these clinical patterns may be obscured. However, a careful history can often reveal how the symptoms began and progressed and thus suggest the likely location of the disorder.

Peripheral Nerve Disorders

Many of the more common disorders that affect the peripheral nervous system, such as the polyneuropathies associated with diabetes and other metabolic disorders, drug toxicity, genetic disorders, and others are chronic conditions. These patients present when their symptoms cause increased functional impairment or when they seek treatment for pain, weakness, gait disorders, or other symptoms. In most such cases, a brief history will reveal that the neuropathy is long-standing, and the focus of care will be relief of the acute symptoms rather than diagnosis and management of the underlying disorder. There are a few important conditions in which peripheral nerve disorders cause acute or subacute weakness and which require urgent evaluation and treatment (Table 6-2).

The *Guillain–Barré syndrome* (GBS) is known by a variety of eponyms, most derived by stringing together the various names of the many authors who have described components of the clinical syndrome during the past century. GBS is an autoimmune-mediated disorder in which the immune response to an infectious agent is misdirected against peripheral nerve antigens structurally similar to antigens presented by the infection. Approximately 70% of cases develop a few weeks after apparent infectious illness (often mild), but many cases develop without any evident prodrome. Some 20% to 30% of cases are associated with infections with *Campylobacter jejuni*, but other cases have been associated with multiple infectious agents including CMV, HIV, and mycoplasma among others. The most common form of the disorder is a demyelinating disorder of peripheral nerves, often designated *acute inflammatory demyelinating polyradiculoneuropathy* (AIDP), but axonal forms and mixed axonal/demyelinating forms are known as well.

TABLE 6-2

ACUTE PERIPHERAL NERVE DISORDERS

I. Acute motor paralysis[a]
  A. Guillain-Barré syndrome
  B. Diphtheritic polyneuropathy
  C. Porphyric polyneuropathy
  D. Tick paralysis
  E. Critical illness polyneuropathy

II. Acute or subacute sensorimotor neuropathy[b]
  A. Deficiency states (alcoholism, beriberi, pellagra, vitamin B_{12})
  B. Toxic polyneuropathy

[a] Although acute motor weakness is the most prominent symptom in these conditions, sensory symptoms such as pain, paresthesias, or sensory loss commonly occur as well. See text for details.
[b] Either motor or sensory symptoms may predominate; the clinical picture varies from one syndrome to another and may vary among patients with the same condition. See text.

These can be difficult to distinguish from one another clinically, but the differences are of little importance to the acute care physician.

The major clinical symptom of GBS is progressive weakness. This usually begins in the lower extremities and may spread to involve the upper extremities, the trunk, the cranial muscles and sometimes even the eye muscles. Bilateral facial weakness develops in approximately 50% of cases. The weakness may be mild or may progress to total motor paralysis. Approximately 30% of patients develop marked weakness of respiratory muscles and thus require ventilator support. Reflexes are markedly reduced and frequently absent, even relatively early in the clinical course when weakness may be mild. Aching pain, especially in the thighs and back, is common. Some sensory loss is also common but is often overlooked since position and vibration sensation are more likely affected than pain sensation. The symptoms usually evolve over a few days to a week or so; in some cases maximal weakness may not be evident for several weeks. In rare instances, severe weakness may develop in less than a day. Autonomic symptoms, such as tachycardia, bradycardia, labile hypertension and hypotension, and hyperthermia, are common and potentially life threatening.

The key to the diagnosis is recognition by an alert physician. In patients with the typical clinical syndrome, the diagnosis is usually straightforward. The differential diagnosis includes the other entities listed in Table 6-2. Variant forms of the syndrome also occur and may pose a diagnostic challenge. In some cases, the initial symptoms may be pain in the back and legs with only mild or minimal weakness; these patients may be erroneously diagnosed with muscle strain, acute viral illnesses, and other conditions. Rarely, the muscles of the face, neck, and upper trunk are affected first. In the so-called Fisher variant, the initial symptoms are complete ophthalmoplegia, limb ataxia, and areflexia. In these patients, such conditions as brainstem strokes, myasthenia gravis, or botulism may be suspected initially.

The differential diagnosis is fairly broad. Diphtheria and acute intermittent porphyria can cause acute generalized weakness essentially identical to that caused by AIDP; both are quite rare. In diphtheria, mild weakness of cranial muscles may be present during the acute phase of the illness, but the polyneuropathy may not develop until some 6 to 8 weeks later. Treatment is supportive. Acute intermittent porphyria is characterized by recurrent attacks of colicky abdominal pain and vomiting, sometimes associated with confusion and delirium; attacks may be precipitated by a wide variety of drugs and other causes. The clinical picture of the polyneuropathy is very similar to that of AIDP, although the facial and cranial muscles are less likely to be affected. Treatment is directed at the porphyria, and treatment of the neurologic disorder is supportive. Other considerations include acute viral illnesses such as West Nile virus and arbovirus infections; these are typically associated with signs of encephalitis as well. Toxic neuropathies can cause a very similar picture and are discussed later.

Routine laboratory studies are of little help in diagnosis, but may help to exclude other diagnoses. The classic cerebrospinal fluid (CSF) formula is characterized by elevated protein with only minimal or no pleocytosis, but this finding is often absent early in the course of the disease and may not develop until several days or more after onset. Accordingly, normal CSF studies do not exclude the diagnosis. Even when present, the elevation of CSF protein is too nonspecific to be considered diagnostic. Respiratory function should be assessed as soon as the diagnosis is suspected and should be followed closely. Inspiratory pressure and vital capacity are useful measures that can be easily assessed at the bedside. A downward trend in vital capacity is an ominous sign; intubation is indicated if vital capacity falls to 12 to 15 mL/kg (25%–35% of normal).

Virtually all patients with suspected GBS should be admitted to the hospital, usually to an ICU or other setting where close observation of vital signs and respiratory function can be provided. The only exceptions are those patients with normal respiratory function and very mild weakness that has been present for a week or more and that is clearly stable, and who can be closely watched by a responsible person who can immediately return them to the hospital if there is any deterioration. Severe hypotension should be managed with volume expansion and with pressors if necessary; severe hypertension should be managed with short-acting agents that can easily be titrated since blood pressure may be very labile, and elevated pressures may suddenly fall. Specific treatment with either plasma exchange (200–250 mL/kg over four to six treatments) or intravenous immune globulin (0.4 g/kg each day for 5 days) has been shown to shorten the duration of ventilator support and hospitalization and to hasten recovery. Corticosteroids are of no benefit. Otherwise, care is largely supportive. Long-term prognosis is generally good, with 85% to 90% of patients eventually making a good functional recovery.[1,2]

Tick paralysis is a relatively rare syndrome of acute ascending weakness caused by a toxin secreted by the bite of a female tick (most often *Dermacentor* or *Ixodes*). The identity of the toxin and its mode of action remain obscure; the clinical syndrome is virtually indistinguishable from AIDP except that there are no sensory symptoms and the CSF protein remains normal. The weakness can be profound and can cause respiratory failure and death. The disease is more common in children (perhaps because of their relatively smaller body mass) and occurs during seasons when ticks are active. Diagnosis depends on finding the tick; there is no other diagnostic test. A careful search for ticks should be made in all patients with suspected GBS during appropriate seasons. Treatment consists of removal of the tick; improvement is rapid and complete recovery is expected. Treatments used for AIDP are ineffective in tick paralysis.[3]

Polyneuropathies may be caused by a bewildering variety of environmental and occupational toxins, plant and animal poisons, and drugs.[4-6] A partial list of potential neurotoxins is given in Table 6-3; the list is by no means complete and is intended to give the physician some indication of the variety of possible offending substances. The keys to

TABLE 6-3
NEUROTOXIC SUBSTANCES

Heavy metals
Arsenic
Lead
Thallium
Mercury

Chemical compounds
Acrylamide
Allyl chloride
Carbon disulfide
Chlorinated phenoxy herbicides
Ethylene oxide
Hexacarbons
Methyl bromide
Organophosphate esters
Polychlorinated biphenyls
Trichloroethylene
Vacor

Plant and animal toxins
Tick toxin
Snake and sea snake venoms
Ciguatera
Paralytic shellfish poison
Neurotoxic shellfish poison
Puffer fish (*Fugu*) poison
Buckthorn poison

Drugs
Antibiotics
　Isoniazid
　Ethambutol
　Nitrofurantoin
　Metronidazole
　Chloramphenicol
　Dapsone
Antineoplastic agents
　Vinca alkaloids
　Cisplatin
　Thalidomide
　Doxorubicin
Others
　Phenytoin
　Pyridoxine
　Nitrous oxide
　Tacrolimus
　Colchicine
　Disulfiram
　Procainamide
　Amiodarone
　Gold
　Antiretroviral agents

the correct diagnosis are a high index of suspicion and a history of exposure to an appropriate toxin. Obtaining an adequate history may involve considerable detective work since patients may be unaware of their exposure or, in the case of some toxins, unwilling to admit their exposure.

Toxic neuropathies are often subacute or chronic in onset but can present acutely. In fact, the clinical picture of an acute, rapidly progressive mixed sensory and motor neuropathy should suggest the diagnosis. The clinical picture is highly variable; a given neurotoxin may cause quite different clinical syndromes in different patients.

Toxic neuropathies are commonly characterized by both motor and sensory symptoms, although either may predominate. Pain is common. The symptoms most often begin in the distal parts of the extremities and spread proximally. In their more chronic forms, toxic neuropathies may be difficult to distinguish from chronic congenital or metabolic disorders (such as diabetes), but this is unlikely to be an issue in the acute care setting. A few representative toxic neuropathies are reviewed here.

Arsenic is an occasional cause of acute polyneuropathy. Arsenic may be encountered in industrial settings and in some insecticides and is occasionally used with suicidal or homicidal intent. Acute ingestion of arsenic causes severe abdominal pain, vomiting, and diarrhea and may be rapidly fatal. If the patient survives the acute exposure, the acute symptoms resolve, to be followed within a few days or weeks by the neuropathy. This commonly takes the form of an acute, rapidly progressive, often very painful motor and sensory neuropathy that begins in the feet and spreads proximally. It can be mistaken for GBS, especially early in the course. The diagnosis depends on a high index of suspicion; high levels of arsenic in the urine, hair, and fingernails confirm the diagnosis. The classic findings of arsenic intoxication (Mees lines in the nails, pigmented dermatitis, and others) may not occur for several weeks. Poisoning with thallium, lead, and mercury may cause a similar syndrome.

Chemical neuropathies may result from exposure to a wide variety of industrial and domestic chemicals; some seemingly exotic chemicals can be easily encountered in the everyday environment. Ethyl alcohol may cause polyneuropathy either directly or as a consequence of prolonged nutritional deficiency. Trichloroethylene is used in the dry cleaning industry, and ethylene oxide is used in gas sterilization systems. Hexacarbon solvents are the cause of the neuropathy and encephalopathy encountered in glue sniffers. Organophosphate compounds, employed as insecticides, cause acute neuromuscular blockade (see later) but may also be associated with a delayed peripheral neuropathy. The list of potential chemical toxins is large and constantly growing; appropriate references, material safety data sheets, and poison control centers should be consulted as needed.[5-7]

Animal and plant venoms and toxins can cause a variety of neuropathic syndromes. Tick paralysis has already been discussed. Some snake venoms, such as that of the eastern coral snake, and the Southern Pacific rattlesnake are neurotoxic and can quickly cause paralysis and death. Treatment consists of supportive care and administration of the appropriate antivenin; a poison control center should be consulted. Many species of marine fish and shellfish produce neurotoxins; clinically these cause a combination of gastrointestinal, autonomic, and neurologic symptoms. Treatment is mostly supportive.

Drug-induced neuropathies are fairly common and may be due to a wide variety of agents. Most often these conditions follow a subacute or chronic course and are unlikely to require emergency diagnosis or management. When more rapid in onset, they may present in the acute care setting and may be confused with GBS or other acute neuropathy; unfortunately, there are no reliable clinical findings specific to these syndromes. Usually, a careful history will reveal that the clinical symptoms began well before and evolved slowly; the patients present when their symptoms become noticeable or intolerable. Treatment is largely supportive; the offending substance should be withdrawn if possible. Agents such as amitriptyline or gabapentin may help to relieve the discomfort.

Critical illness polyneuropathy is an important cause of acute weakness, admittedly unlikely to present in the usual acute care setting. However, it is important for primary care physicians to be aware of this syndrome. It typically occurs in critically ill patients in ICUs, especially patients with sepsis and multiple organ failure. It is characterized by an acute axonal neuropathy, primarily affecting motor function; it may cause profound and prolonged weakness, delaying weaning from ventilator support. There is no specific treatment, and recovery is very prolonged.

Neuromuscular Junction Disorders

The neuromuscular junction is a highly specialized structure at which acetylcholine (ACh) is released from a nerve terminal in response to a nerve action potential and

TABLE 6-4

NEUROMUSCULAR JUNCTION DISORDERS

Myasthenia gravis
Lambert-Eaton myasthenic syndrome
Drugs and toxins
    Botulism
    Tetanus
    Black widow spider bite
    Strychnine poisoning
    Organophosphate poisoning
    Drug-induced neuromuscular blockade

diffuses across a narrow synaptic cleft to interact with receptors on a specialized area of muscle membrane (the motor end plate). In response to this chemical stimulus, a muscle action potential is generated that results in contraction of the muscle fibers. Clinical disorders that impair or prevent the release of ACh or interfere with its effective binding to the muscle receptors thus prevent normal muscle contraction and result in weakness of the affected muscles. As noted earlier, there are no sensory symptoms, and reflexes are generally preserved. Disorders of neuromuscular transmission that may be seen in the acute care setting are listed in Table 6-4.

Myasthenia gravis (MG) is the most important primary disorder of neuromuscular transmission. MG is an autoimmune disorder in which antibodies are produced that bind with ACh receptors on the motor end plate. Those receptors occupied by antibody are unable to bind ACh; although normal amounts of ACh are released into the synaptic cleft, the lack of adequate receptor sites results in failure of neuromuscular transmission and causes muscle weakness. Over time, permanent structural changes occur in the motor end plate leading to chronic weakness.

The cause of MG remains unknown. It may appear in isolation or in association with other autoimmune disorders such as Graves' disease or systemic lupus erythematosus. The peak age of onset is between 20 and 30 years in women and between 50 and 60 years in men. Often the onset is insidious, and many patients will have consulted several physicians before a diagnosis is made. In a few cases the onset is quite abrupt, and such patients may well present to acute care settings. Also, some patients with well-established and treated MG may experience periodic crises of markedly increased weakness and will present to the acute care setting.

The cardinal symptom of MG is fluctuating weakness; repeated use of an affected muscle results in progressive weakness and exhaustion, whereas rest often results in at least partial recovery. Weakness of the extraocular muscles and levator palpebrae (causing ptosis) is a common presenting symptom and eventually occurs in more than 90% of patients. Other bulbar muscles (facial expression, mastication, speech, and swallowing) are affected in 80%. Skeletal muscles may be affected as well. Although proximal muscles are more often and more severely affected than distal muscles, virtually any pattern of muscle weakness can be seen. The degree of weakness can be severe, with compromise of respiration, inability to swallow or speak, and other symptoms.

MG should be considered in any patient who presents with weakness of sudden onset, especially if the weakness is variable. The presence of weakness affecting the face, the levator palpebrae, and extraocular movements with sparing of the pupils is virtually diagnostic. If the patient can cooperate, repeat testing of an affected muscle may result in worsening weakness and rest results in improvement; when present, this finding is diagnostic. A common maneuver is to ask the patient to count backward from 100 until her speech is slurred and indistinct; a short period of rest will restore normal speech. In patients with diplopia, sustained gaze in one direction will result in worsening diplopia; allowing the patient to rest for several minutes with the eyes closed will temporarily restore normal vision. The diagnosis can be confirmed with the edrophonium test (Table 6-5); a positive test confirms the diagnosis, but a negative test does not exclude MG.

Treatment of MG is complex and should usually be managed by a neurologist. Severely affected patients should be admitted to the hospital, and a neurologist should be consulted. Patients with significant impairment of respiration or at risk for aspiration may require intubation and ventilator support until their condition improves. Once the airway is secured, definitive treatment can be delayed until expert help is available. Either plasma exchange or intravenous immune globulin may be used to manage severe myasthenia.[7,8] For patients with less severe symptoms, treatment with pyridostigmine 30 to 90 mg PO q6h may provide symptomatic relief until they can be seen by a neurologist. A common starting dose is 60 mg PO q6h. If desired, the response to pyridostigmine can be assessed by giving the first dose IM or IV using 1/30 of the PO dose (i.e., 1–2 mg).

TABLE 6-5

THE EDROPHONIUM TEST[a]

1. The strength of several affected muscles should be assessed as objectively as possible, e.g.:
   Measure the palpebral fissures in patients with ptosis.
   Observe the severity of ocular misalignment in patients with diplopia.
   Have the patient count out loud until unable to continue.
   Measure grip strength with a dynamometer; clinical assessment is less reliable.
   Assess respiratory function—maximum inspiratory force and vital capacity.
2. Administer 10 mg (1 mL) edrophonium chloride intravenously:
   Give 1 mg (0.1 mL) initially; observe for improvement or side effects.
   Give 3–6 mg (0.3–0.6 mL); observe for 45 seconds for improvement or side effects.
   If no effect, give the remainder; observe for improvement or side effects.
3. A *positive* result is objective improvement in the strength of one or more of the muscles assessed. There should be complete resolution of diplopia or ptosis and a measurable increase in muscle strength or respiratory function. Subjective improvement or equivocal results are not reliable.

[a] Side effects of edrophonium include nausea, vomiting, sweating, salivation, and occasionally bradycardia and hypotension. These can be prevented by pretreatment with atropine 0.4–0.8 mg SC. There is a very small risk of cardiac standstill, especially in older patients; facilities for resuscitation should be available.

TABLE 6-6

DRUGS THAT MAY WORSEN MYASTHENIA GRAVIS[a]

Neuromuscular blocking agents
Aminogycoside antibiotics
Tetracyclines[b]
β-blockers[b]
Antiarrythmics
Calcium channel blockers
Magnesium
Procaine, lidocaine
Iodinated contrast agents
Corticosteroids[c]
Statins

[a] This is not an exhaustive list. Drugs are listed by class to give the reader a sense of the wide variety of agents that may exacerbate myasthenia. Any new drug should be used with great caution in patients with myasthenia.

[b] The agents may exacerbate myasthenia even when used as topical agents (e.g., eye drops).

[c] Although corticosteroids are used in the treatment of myasthenia, they may cause temporary worsening, especially if introduced at full doses. A common strategy is to introduce corticosteroids at very low doses and titrate the dose upward as tolerated.

A special problem in the acute care setting concerns those patients with established myasthenia who present with abrupt worsening of their symptoms (myasthenic crisis). This is most often due to worsening of their disease and may result from intercurrent illness (often a respiratory or other infection), from treatment with certain drugs (Table 6-6), or from no evident cause. If these patients are not taking anticholinesterase drugs, a trial of pyridostigmine (see earlier in the chapter) may be helpful. Patients with myasthenic crisis may progress rapidly to severe weakness and respiratory collapse and should be hospitalized, preferably in the ICU, until their condition has been stabilized. Endotracheal intubation should be carried out as needed.

In myasthenic patients treated with anticholinesterase drugs, a similar clinical syndrome of progressive weakness can result from drug toxicity (cholinergic crisis). A common clinical scenario is that of the patient who experiences worsening of her myasthenic weakness and attempts self-treatment by increasing the dose of anticholinesterase medication. Excess cholinergic effect causes further weakness, leading to a vicious circle. Weakness due to excess cholinergic effect may be difficult to distinguish from myasthenic weakness, although the presence of miosis and increased secretions suggests excessive cholinergic effect. Unfortunately, both myasthenic and cholinergic weakness can coexist in the same patient, further complicating both diagnosis and treatment. Although small doses of edrophonium can be used to distinguish the two syndromes (cholinergic weakness will get worse and myasthenic weakness may improve), this approach may be quite hazardous, leading to increased pharyngeal secretions and respiratory collapse simultaneously. The safer course in such cases is to be certain that the airway is secure, by intubation if needed and stop all cholinergic (anticholinesterase) medications until the patient is stable (as the effects of the drugs wear off). Treatment is then cautiously restarted and titrated to good effect. Hospital admission to an acute care unit is necessary.

In summary, MG is an important cause of acute weakness in the acute care setting. The acute care physician should remember the following points:

1. Myasthenia gravis should be considered in all patients who present with acute weakness. A positive edrophonium test confirms the diagnosis; a negative or equivocal test does not exclude the diagnosis.
2. Severe myasthenic weakness, especially when the muscles of the pharynx or respiratory muscles are involved, is a medical emergency. The focus of initial management is to protect the airway and ensure adequate respiration.
3. Myasthenic patients with abrupt worsening may have either myasthenic or cholinergic crises; these are difficult to distinguish on clinical grounds. The safest approach is to withhold medication, protect the airway and respiration, and wait for the situation to stabilize.

Lambert-Eaton myasthenic syndrome (LEMS) is another cause of muscle weakness that worsens with progressive exercise. The onset is usually subacute; in contrast to MG, the weakness in LEMS most commonly initially affects the proximal muscles of the legs, trunk, and shoulders rather than the bulbar muscles. Strength may actually increase with the first few contractions of an affected muscle, but this is often difficult to detect on clinical examination. Autonomic symptoms (impotence, dry mouth, difficult urination) are common. There is little or no response to anticholinesterase drugs (edrophonium, neostigmine, or pyridostigmine). LEMS occurs most commonly in association with small cell carcinoma of the lung; it may appear before the underlying tumor is detectable and may also occur in the absence of cancer. No emergency treatment is available.

Botulism is a rare cause of acute muscle weakness. It is caused by an exotoxin of *Clostridium botulinum*, an anaerobic bacterium. There are at least eight serotypes of the toxin; types A, B, and E and occasionally F, cause disease in humans. The toxin is heat labile and is inactivated by adequate cooking. The toxin acts at the neuromuscular junction to prevent the release of acetylcholine, thus blocking neuromuscular transmission. The effect on the nerve terminal is irreversible, and recovery depends on sprouting of new nerve terminals.

Patients most often encounter the toxin by ingesting improperly preserved foods, but botulism may also occur from wound infections with the organism, and occasionally (usually in infants) from intestinal colonization with the organism. There have been several reports of wound botulism following surgical procedures or trauma, and as a result of "skin-popping" drugs such as heroin. Because *C. botulinum* does not elicit any inflammatory reaction, the wound may appear benign and may be easily overlooked. Another potential method of exposure is the release of the toxin in aerosolized form as a bioterrorism or biowarfare agent. Finally, there are rare reports of clinical botulism related to therapeutic uses of the toxin.

Clinical symptoms typically begin within 12 to 36 hours after ingestion of the contaminated food. The first symptoms usually involve the extraocular, facial, and pharyngeal muscles; ptosis, blurred vision, diplopia, facial weakness, dysarthria, dysphasia, and hoarseness may all occur. These early symptoms are similar to those of MG except that in botulism the pupillary reflexes are affected early; the pupils are rarely affected in MG. The weakness spreads rapidly to the muscles of the trunk and extremities and may progress to complete paralysis. As the weakness advances, it can be mistaken for

Guillain-Barré syndrome. In botulism, however, there are no sensory symptoms and reflexes are preserved. There is no response to edrophonium. Diagnosis and treatment are based on the clinical picture; assays for the toxin and attempts to recover the organism are not entirely reliable and the results are too delayed to be useful in the acute care setting.

Treatment is largely supportive; botulism antitoxin (obtained from the Centers for Disease Control and Prevention in Atlanta, Georgia) may shorten the course of the clinical illness. Recovery is very prolonged. Botulism is a reportable disease, and local health authorities should be notified.[9,10]

Tetanus, although technically not a disorder of peripheral neuromuscular transmission, is included here because, like botulism, it is caused by a bacterial exotoxin produced by an anaerobic bacterium. The toxin, *tetanospasmin*, is produced by *Clostridium tetani*. The spores of *C. tetani* are widespread in the environment, especially in soil; introduced into a wound with suitable anaerobic conditions, the spores become vegetative and elaborate the toxin. As with *C. botulinum*, there is no inflammatory reaction and the wound may appear benign. The toxin acts in the brain and spinal cord to block inhibitory the inhibitory neurotransmitters γ-aminobutyric acid and glycine.

The clinical illness begins with a sensation of stiffness and cramping in the muscles of the jaws and face. Weakness is not prominent, but the stiffness may be initially described as weakness by the patient. As the disease advances, severe, prolonged, and very painful muscle spasms develop and spread to involve the neck, the trunk, and proximal extremities. The hands and feet are relatively spared. These symptoms can progress to a state of generalized rigidity with respiratory failure, autonomic instability, and death. The differential diagnosis includes poisoning from strychnine or black widow spider bite, neuroleptic malignant syndrome (see Chapter 7), and malignant hyperthermia.[11]

Treatment for tetanus includes administration of tetanus antitoxin. Subsequent care is largely supportive; sedation, muscle relaxants (such as benzodiazepines), and neuromuscular blockade may be used; ventilator support is almost always required. Local wound care (debridement, antibiotics, and other measures) can prevent further toxin production. Of course, tetanus is a preventable disease, hence the emphasis on the regular use of tetanus toxoid. An attack of tetanus does not confer immunity and regular immunization is required.

Black widow spider venom acts at nerve terminals to provoke rapid release of acetylcholine, initially causing severe painful cramps, spasms, and muscle rigidity. As the supply of ACh becomes depleted, muscle weakness and paralysis develop and may be severe. The disorder can be fatal, especially in children (presumably because of their smaller body mass). Treatment is usually supportive; an antivenin is available. Complete recovery can be expected with proper supportive care.

Organophosphate compounds are widely used as insecticides; they can be used as chemical warfare and bioterrorism agents as well. These agents act by inhibiting the enzyme acetylcholinesterase, which is necessary to terminate the effect of ACh at synapses and at the neuromuscular junction; in effect, they act as cholinergic agents. Symptoms of acute organophosphate poisoning develop immediately after exposure and include nausea and vomiting, abdominal cramps and diarrhea, increased salivation and lacrimation, bronchospasm, and muscle weakness. The pupils are usually miotic. In severe cases, death results from respiratory paralysis. The clinical picture is similar to that resulting from overdose of antimyasthenic drugs such as edrophonium, neostigmine, and pyridostigmine.

Treatment with pralidoxime (2-PAM) can reverse the effect of the toxin if administered within 24 to 48 hours of exposure. After that time, binding between the toxin and the acetylcholinesterase becomes irreversible, and recovery depends on the synthesis of new enzyme, a process that may take weeks or months. Treatment with anticholinergic drugs such as atropine will reverse the effects of excessive cholinergic stimulation of muscarinic receptors (salivation, lacrimation, GI symptoms, and others) but will *not* reverse the skeletal muscle weakness (resulting from involvement of nicotinic receptors). With appropriate support and treatment, full recovery can be expected.[12]

Drug-induced neuromuscular blockade is sometimes seen in the acute care setting. Neuromuscular blocking agents are widely used in the acute care and intensive care settings and are not ordinarily a cause of diagnostic confusion. However, these drugs may occasionally be given in error, or with homicidal intent; possible intoxication with these agents should be suspected in a patient who abruptly develops generalized flaccid weakness. The clinical picture is similar to that of MG except for the abrupt onset of the symptoms. Use of these drugs in patients with MG (even in very mild or unsuspected cases) can result in prolonged paralysis and very delayed recovery.

A wide variety of other drugs can induce some degree of neuromuscular blockade (Table 6-6). These drugs do not cause clinically significant weakness in most patients but can potentially cause significant weakness in patients with MG. Treatment in these cases consists in withdrawal of the offending agent and supportive care as outlined for MG.

Finally, a similar picture can be seen with many environmental toxins including bites from coral snakes and the Pacific Coast rattlesnake, and from food-borne toxins such as puffer fish (*fugu*) and paralytic shellfish poisoning. The history will usually suggest the correct diagnosis on such cases, and the physician should consult a regional poison control center and appropriate references for advice on specific diagnosis and management.

Acute Disorders of Muscle

As with peripheral nerve diseases, many of the disorders of skeletal muscle are chronic and slowly progressive. Although not rare, chronic diseases such as the muscular dystrophies and most metabolic myopathies are unlikely to present in the acute care setting, except perhaps as the underlying cause of an acute disorder such as pneumonia. In general, no specific therapy for these conditions is available. There are however a few skeletal muscle disorders that may present with weakness of acute onset (Table 6-7).

The clinical hallmark of muscle disease is symmetric weakness, usually affecting proximal more than distal muscles. Although pain and muscle tenderness may be present, sensory symptoms are absent, and reflexes are often preserved unless the weakness is very severe. Elevation of muscle enzyme levels (CK, aldolase, SGOT) in the serum indicates necrosis of muscle fibers and is a common finding in acute myopathic disorders. Necrosis of muscle cells (rhabdomyolysis) liberates myoglobin; high concentrations of myoglobin in the serum can result in acute renal failure, and aggressive treatment to maintain high urine volumes is necessary. The presence of myoglobin in the urine results in dark discoloration that can be mistaken for blood; laboratory tests can confirm the presence of myoglobinuria even if blood is also present.

TABLE 6-7 ————————————————————————

MUSCLE DISORDERS CAUSING ACUTE WEAKNESS

Inflammatory disorders
Polymyositis/dermatomyositis
Trichinosis

Drugs and toxins
Alcohol (may be associated with both acute and chronic weakness)
Cholesterol-lowering drugs (statins, clofibrate, gemfibrozil)
Cocaine
Zidovudine
Colchicine
Vincristine (may also cause peripheral neuropathy)
Amiodarone
Cyclosporine
Chloroquine
Corticosteroids
Amphotericin
Rifampin
Venoms
Mushroom poisoning (*Amanita phalloides*)

Metabolic disorders
Electrolyte disorders
   Hyperkalemia/hypokalemia
   Hypercalcemia (malignancies, hyperparathyroidism)
   Hypermagnesemia
Periodic paralyses
Cushing's syndrome
Thyrotoxicosis

Note that many of the agents in this table associated with myopathic disorders are also listed in Tables 6-3 and 6-6, associated with neuropathic disorders and myasthenia gravis.

Polymyositis is characterized by muscle weakness that usually develops over several weeks or longer. As is typical for muscle disease, the weakness affects the proximal muscles more than distal muscles; the face is often spared. The weakness is usually painless but some aching, especially in the thighs and hips, may occur. The erythrocyte sedimentation rate (ESR) is usually but not always elevated, and the serum CK is elevated. MRI demonstrates inflammation in affected muscles and may serve to direct a muscle biopsy to confirm the diagnosis. Unless the weakness is very severe, urgent treatment is not necessary, and the patient may be referred to a neurologist or rheumatologist for further evaluation and management.

Dermatomyositis is clinically similar to polymyositis, with the addition of a skin rash on the extensor surface of the joints and often a purple or "lilac" (heliotrope) rash over the face. Dermatomyositis has been variably associated with an increased risk of systemic cancer, and an extensive workup may be appropriate.

Trichinosis is a parasitic disorder rare in the United States; it occurs occasionally as a result of eating improperly cooked pork or wild game. The encysted larvae of the parasitic nematode *Trichina spiralis* mature in the gut after ingestion by the host; the mature nematodes lay eggs and the resulting larvae then spread throughout the body where they induce an intense inflammatory reaction. Clinical symptoms begin a week or so after ingestion and consist of fever, muscle pain and swelling, weakness, and malaise. Laboratory studies reveal an elevated ESR and marked eosinophilia. Thiobendazole, given early in the course of the disease, or even before symptoms occur in cases of known exposure, may prevent production of larvae and reduce the severity of the disease. Prednisone at 40 to 60 mg/day may give symptomatic relief. The symptoms may last for many weeks, but complete recovery can be expected.

Toxic myopathies may be caused by a wide variety of drugs and poisons (see Table 6-7 for examples). Curry et al. identified a long list of drugs and toxins causing rhabdomyolysis.[13] The muscle weakness and other symptoms may be indolent or subacute or acute and fulminating. *Steroid-induced* myopathy may occur in patients treated with corticosteroids, particularly after prolonged use. A similar picture can be seen in patients with Cushing's disease. Patients present with slowly evolving weakness primarily involving proximal muscles; muscle enzyme levels are normal, and myoglobinuria is not present. Diagnosis depends greatly on clinical suspicion, and it may be difficult to distinguish weakness due to corticosteroid therapy from weakness due to an underlying disorder such as polymyositis. A careful drug history and a careful search through drug information resources can suggest the diagnosis. Treatment consists in withdrawal of the offending substance. A similar picture can be seen in association with thyrotoxiocosis.

Toxic myopathies with an acute or fulminating course may present with severe weakness and rhabdomyolysis, dramatic elevation of muscle enzyme levels, hyperkalemia, myoglobinuria, and renal failure. Potential causes include alcohol, many drugs, including statins and other lipid-lowering agents, and toxins from snakebites, mushroom poisoning, and others. A similar clinical picture with acute weakness and rhabdomyolysis can be caused by strenuous exercise, especially in patients with preexisting congenital muscle diseases. Rhabdomyolysis may result from pressure necrosis in patients with prolonged immobility or crush injuries, in cases of the neuroleptic malignant syndrome (see Chapter 7) and malignant hyperthermia (see later). In all these cases, diagnosis depends on recognition of the general clinical syndrome and on a careful search for potential causes. Treatment is largely supportive and includes withdrawal of the offending substance, aggressive hydration to maintain urine output, and other care as indicated.

Malignant hyperthermia is a rare and potentially catastrophic disorder associated with the use of some inhalational anesthetics (especially halothane) and neuromuscular blocking agents such as succinylcholine, which may be used in the acute care setting. Symptoms usually develop shortly after exposure to the causative agent but may begin several hours later. Initial symptoms are tachycardia and tachypnea, followed by dramatic muscle rigidity and severe hyperpyrexia. The syndrome is due to the sudden release of calcium from the sarcoplasmic reticulum, resulting in sustained muscle contraction. Treatment is aggressive management of the hyperpyrexia and administration of dantrolene 1 mg/kg IV initially, with additional doses as needed to maintain muscle relaxation. The syndrome is nearly always fatal if not recognized and treated immediately. Susceptibility to this disorder is inherited as an autosomal dominant trait, so a family history may be available. In potentially susceptible individuals, a muscle-biopsy-based laboratory test may be used to estimate risk prior to elective procedures.

Electrolyte disorders are an infrequent but important cause of acute muscle weakness. Either hyper- or hypokalemia by any reason can cause muscle weakness; serum potassium levels below 2 mEq/L or above 7 mEq/L can cause flaccid arreflexic paralysis similar to that seen in the Guillain-Barré syndrome. This is distinct from the genetic syndromes of periodic paralysis described later. Severe hypercalcemia, hypophosphatemia, and hypermagnesemia can cause a similar picture. Abnormalities in serum potassium are likely to be detected in "routine" blood work often obtained in the acute care setting, but their significance as a cause of severe generalized weakness may be overlooked. Other electrolyte abnormalities may be found only if specifically sought. Treatment consists of correction of both the acute electrolyte abnormality and the underlying cause.

The unusual disorders termed periodic paralysis syndromes are examples of a much larger group of muscle diseases collectively referred to as channelopathies. They are caused by mutations in the genes that control the structure of various ion channels (chloride, sodium, and calcium) in skeletal muscle. The periodic paralysis syndromes, as the name implies, are characterized by acute attacks of muscle weakness; between attacks the patients are clinically normal. Because these disorders are inherited as autosomal dominant traits, a family history is often present.

Hypokalemic periodic paralysis, the most common and best known of these disorders, is caused by a genetic defect in the calcium channel. The first attacks usually occur before age 20. Attacks often develop during sleep, especially after strenuous exercise or a meal rich in carbohydrates. Patients awaken with generalized muscle weakness that may be severe enough to prevent the patient's getting out of bed or even calling for help. The muscles of the face and trunk are usually spared so that respiration is not compromised. Reflexes may be diminished or lost, but sensation is preserved. Diagnosis depends first on a high index of suspicion and a positive family history. Laboratory studies usually reveal low levels of potassium, but the reductions need not be profound. If untreated, attacks may last from hours to days; administration of supplemental potassium (orally or IV) leads to rapid improvement. Regular administration of supplemental potassium may prevent subsequent attacks.

Hyperkalemic and *normokalemic* periodic paralyses are less common than hypokalemic periodic paralysis. The genetic defect is in the sodium channel. The clinical attacks are relatively brief (less than 1 hour) and typically occur after exercise. The cranial muscles and trunk muscles are usually spared. In mild attacks, no treatment is required, and the clinical symptoms may have resolved by the time the patient is evaluated. In patients with severe weakness, intravenous calcium gluconate (1–2 g) or intravenous glucose may be helpful.

Summary

Acute generalized weakness can result from disorders involving any level of the nervous system. Accurate diagnosis and appropriate treatment depend first and foremost on accurate localization of the likely lesion within the nervous system; accurate localization, in turn, depends on the results of the history and physical examinations. A careful search should be made for any alteration of consciousness, behavior, or mentation that suggests brain disease, or for any localizing signs, no matter how subtle, suggesting lesions of the brainstem or spinal cord (see Chapters 3 and 4). If there are no signs of a central nervous system disorder, then a disorder of peripheral nerves, the neuromuscular junction, or the muscles should be considered.

The initial assessment of a patient with acute generalized weakness has several goals:

1. Ensure that the patient's airway is secure and that respiratory function is adequate. Remember that early mortality in these patients is most often the result of ventilatory failure. Other vital functions should be assessed and stabilized as needed.
2. Determine whether the likely cause affects the peripheral nerves, the neuromuscular junction, or the muscles; determine the likely diagnosis, and obtain the necessary laboratory studies to secure the diagnosis.
3. Decide whether emergency treatment is required, either for the primary disorder (e.g., myasthenia gravis or Guillain-Barré syndrome) or for secondary effects (e.g., myoglobinuria in patients with rhabdomyolysis).
4. Initiate appropriate management and referral.

It is important to recall that many of the disorders causing acute weakness, such as the Guillain-Barré syndrome, can progress rapidly to severe weakness and respiratory failure even though the initial symptoms are quite mild. Accordingly, hospital admission and close observation should be considered even for patients with relatively mild symptoms, until the diagnosis is secure and until it is clear that the patient's condition has been stabilized.

REFERENCES

1. Lunn MPT, Willison HJ. Diagnosis and treatment in inflammatory neuropathies. *J Neurol Neurosurg Psychiatry.* 2009;80:249-258.
2. Pritchard J. What's new in Guillain-Barré syndrome? *Postgrad Med J.* 2008;84:532-538.
3. Edlow JA, McGillicuddy DC. Tick paralysis. *Infect Dis Clin North Am.* 2008;22(3):397-413.
4. Spencer PS, Schaumberg HH, eds. *Experimental and Clinical Neurotoxicology.* 2nd ed. New York: Oxford University Press; 2000.
5. Goldfrank LR, ed. *Goldfrank's Toxicologic Emergencies.* 6th ed. Stamford, CT: Appleton & Lange; 1998.
6. Aminoff MJ. Effects of occupational toxins on the nervous system. In: Bradley WG et al., eds. *Neurology in Clinical Practice.* 3rd ed. Boston, MA: Butterworth-Heinemann; 2000:1511-1599.
7. Gold R, Schneider-Gold C. Current and future standards in treatment of myasthenia gravis. *Neurotherapeutics.* 2008;5(4):535-541.
8. Bershad EM, Feen ES, Suarez JI. Myasthenia gravis crisis. *South Med J.* 2008;101(1):63-69.
9. Davis LE, King MK. Wound botulism from heroin skin popping. *Curr Neurol Neurosci Rep.* 2008;8(6):462-468.
10. Dembek ZF, Smith LA, Rusnak JM. Botulism: cause, effects, diagnosis, clinical and laboratory identification, and treatment modalities. *Disaster Med Public Health Prep.* 2007;1(2):122-134.
11. Farrar JJ et al. Tetanus. *J Neurol Neurosurg Psychiatry.* 2000;69:292.
12. Walter C Robey III, Meggs William J. Insecticides, Herbicides, Rodenticides. In: Tintinalli JE, Kelen GD, Stapczynski JS, Ma OJ, Cline DM, eds. *Tintinalli's Emergency Medicine: A Comprehensive Study Guide.* 6th ed. New York: McGraw Hill; 2004 http://www.accessmedicine.com/content.aspx?aID=603498.
13. Curry SC, Chang D, Connor D. Drug and toxin-induced rhabdomyolysis. *Ann Emerg Med.* 1989;18:1068-1084.

MOVEMENT DISORDERS

Much of the territory of the central and peripheral nervous systems is devoted to the initiation and control of voluntary movement. As a result, abnormalities of movement are among the most common symptoms of disorders of the nervous system. For practical purposes, neurologic disorders affecting movement are sometimes divided into two broad groups. The first group includes those that are conditions characterized by weakness or paralysis of movement (discussed in Chapters 5 and 6). The second group includes multiple heterogeneous disorders characterized primarily by decomposition and disorganization of motor control rather than by weakness or paralysis. These disorders are often referred to collectively as "movement disorders" and are attributed to abnormalities of the so-called extrapyramidal motor system, which includes parts of the frontal lobes of the brain, the basal nuclei (or basal "ganglia"), the cerebellum, and related structures. Symptoms of these disorders include the following:

1. Abnormalities of muscle tone (rigidity or hypotonia).
2. Slowing or paucity of spontaneous movement (bradykinesia or akinesia).
3. Involuntary movements.
4. Inhibition of normal postural reflexes.

Some of these disorders are quite rare but a few, such as essential tremor and Parkinson's disease, are quite common. They are commonly insidious in onset and only slowly progressive, so they do not often present as the primary problem in the acute care setting. Nevertheless, there are several reasons why acute care physicians should have a working knowledge of these conditions. First, a few of these disorders, such as the neuroleptic malignant syndrome or the serotonin syndrome, may present as true medical emergencies. Second, movement disorder symptoms may worsen abruptly in the face of an acute medical illness or on exposure to some drugs, prompting a visit to the emergency department or other acute care setting. Third, one of the more common causes of movement disorders of acute onset is reaction to medications, including drugs commonly used in acute care medicine. Potential causative drugs include such diverse agents as antipsychotic drugs, antidepressants, lithium, metoclopramide, and drugs used to treat Parkinson's disease. Finally, the tremors, muscle stiffness, or other symptoms of movement disorders may complicate the assessment of other disorders.

CLINICAL ASSESSMENT

The clinical findings in patients with movement disorders may be quite subtle and can be easily overlooked, particularly in supine patients in busy emergency departments. Also, laboratory and imaging studies are usually of little help in these patients, so the clinician must rely on the time-honored techniques of the history and physical examination. Careful observation, rather than direct examination, is often the key to recognizing movement disorders.

History

The clinical history should seek to obtain as accurate a description as possible of the patient's symptoms. Many of the symptoms of the movement disorders may be more apparent to family members than to the patients themselves. Frequently, patients are unaware of involuntary movements that are obvious to everyone around them, and some patients even flatly deny their obvious involuntary movements. The physician should inquire about the onset and progression of the symptoms as well as about the extent to which the symptoms have interfered with the patient's regular function. It is important to know how the symptoms are affected by sleep, fatigue, and anxiety as well as by any drug or alcohol. A detailed drug history is very important and is frequently diagnostic. Can the patient exert any control over the movements, even for a short time? Have any family members had the same or a similar disorder?

Physical Examination

In addition to the usual general physical and neurologic examinations, there are several observations of special importance. The patient should be carefully watched for any involuntary movements or abnormal or bizarre postures of the trunk or extremities, both when the patient is at rest and when engaged in some activity such as walking or talking. Note should be made as well of any evident decrease or absence of normal spontaneous movements. In Parkinson's disease, for example, there is often a striking lack of spontaneous movements such as patients crossing and uncrossing their legs or adjusting the posture of their trunk or extremities. Patients often have a reduced blink rate, and there may be little or no movement of the face when they are speaking. Special attention should be paid to the patient's gait and to control of fine movements (finger–nose–finger, heel–knee–shin, finger-tapping movements, and others). Muscle tone should be assessed. Relevant findings are often quite subtle, and their recognition requires an examiner with skill and experience. The physician should try to characterize the findings in detail, as this will often be the key to differential diagnosis.

SYMPTOM DEFINITIONS

Movement disorders are characterized by a wide variety of abnormal motor phenomena, denoted by sometimes obscure and confusing terms. Some of the more important ones are defined here for the convenience of the reader.

Abnormalities of Muscle Tone

Rigidity and *spasticity* refer to increased resistance of resting muscle to passive movement. In awake patients, normal muscles are never completely flaccid, and there is some slight resistance to passive movement by the examiner. With rigidity, the increased tone is not dependent on the rate at which the muscles are moved. The increased tone may be constant (sometimes called "lead-pipe" rigidity) or may have a curious ratcheting quality ("cogwheel" rigidity). Muscle stretch reflexes are usually normal. With spasticity, the increased tone is rate-dependent. If the affected muscles are moved slowly, the increased tone may be minimal or absent. When the muscle is stretched quickly, there is a sudden "catch," which suddenly disappears if the tension is maintained (the "clasp-knife" phenomenon). Spasticity is generally associated with increased muscle stretch reflexes. Rigidity is characteristic of movement disorders, whereas spasticity is more characteristic of weakness due to disorders affecting upper motor neurons (see Chapter 4).

Slowing or Absence of Spontaneous Movements

Bradykinesia is a slowing down of spontaneous or voluntary movements. Patients seem to move slowly and deliberately. Spontaneous movements such as blinking, swallowing saliva, facial expressions, and gesticulating with the hands while speaking are reduced both in frequency and in speed. Movements such as handwriting, doing and undoing buttons, etc., may be agonizingly slow. The virtual absence of such movements is termed *akinesia*. This can be very dramatic in patients with Parkinson's disease and related disorders who may sit virtually immobile, with a fixed, expressionless, unblinking "reptilian" stare.

Involuntary Movements

The most familiar, obvious, and characteristic symptoms of the movement disorders are involuntary movements. They are referred to by the collective term dyskinesias and are identified by classical terminology that may create the impression that the various movements are separate and distinct. In fact, there is considerable overlap among the various kinds of involuntary movements. The dyskinesias share some features in common; they are generally worsened by anxiety and stress and generally disappear with sleep. They can often be temporarily suppressed by the patient but will eventually recur despite the patient's efforts to prevent them. In the past, these movements were often considered to be psychogenic in origin, but it is now clear that they are definitely "organic." It should be noted that psychologically based movement disorders do occur quite commonly, and assessment by a movement disorders specialist may be needed to distinguish them from organic disorders.

Although certain kinds of movements have been classically associated with specific diseases, there is considerable overlap. This section will briefly define the various symptoms of the movement disorders; the following section will consider some of the more important clinical conditions associated with these symptoms.

Tremor is defined as a rhythmic, regular, purposeless, oscillating movement that may involve the extremities, the trunk, and the head and neck. Most individuals experience tremor at some time, usually when anxious or fatigued or in association with alcohol, caffeine, or medications; such tremors are usually self-limited and such individuals do not seek medical attention. In other individuals, tremor may be much more persistent and severe and may cause considerable personal distress and functional impairment.

Tics are repetitive twitching or jerking movements that may involve the head and face, the trunk, or the extremities. Tics may involve the coordinated movement of multiple muscles and may resemble voluntary movements. A given patient may have one or more different tics, each of which follows a fixed pattern from one occurrence to the next. Tics can usually be temporarily suppressed by the patient, who will then gradually develop an irresistible urge to perform them.

Akathisia is a state of motor restlessness; patients have a constant urge to move some part of the body and find it impossible to relax and remain still. Patients constantly shift position; they may constantly move their legs or bodies or get up and walk about. They find the sensation difficult to describe but usually distressing. Akathisia is a common side effect of many drugs (see below). It is often unrecognized or mistaken for anxiety or agitation.

Chorea is characterized by irregular, purposeless, brief movements that often flow randomly from one part of the body to another. They often involve the distal extremities but may also involve the tongue and face, the head, or the trunk; they are not stereotyped and are more prolonged than tics. They may be modified by patients into apparently purposeful movements. The movements frequently disrupt normal activity such as speaking, writing, and walking. Slower, more sinuous movements are described by the term *athetosis*; there is considerable clinical overlap, and the term *choreoathetosis* is often used to refer to this group of abnormal movements.

Ballism refers to wild flinging or flailing movements, usually of one or both extremities on one side of the body (*hemiballismus*). The movements can be continuous and quite violent and may result in injury. Ballism is considered by many researchers to be a variant of chorea.[1] Ballism is classically associated with isolated lesions of the subthalamic nucleus of Luys, usually due to lacunar infarctions. Fortunately quite rare, it is one of the more dramatic of involuntary movements.

Dystonic movements are slower and more prolonged than choreic or athetoid movements, with which they may coexist. Dystonia may result in prolonged abnormal or even bizarre postures of individual muscles, groups of related muscles, or even the entire body.

Myoclonus consists of very brief lightning-like jerking movements that may involve individual muscles, groups of related muscles, or even major portions of the body. The movements are strong enough to move joints and may be very vigorous and dramatic. The jerks may be isolated or recurrent and may be confined to small groups of muscles or may flit randomly from one body region to another. Unlike tics, which they may superficially resemble, myoclonic movements are not stereotyped.

Asterixis, in contrast to the involuntary movements described thus far, is characterized by sudden brief lapses in tonic muscle contraction. Thus, when a muscle is held in a fixed position, there will be sudden movements as the muscles suddenly lose their contraction. This is best seen when the hands are held outstretched with the wrists extended; the sudden loss of strength results in an irregular peculiar "flapping" movement of the hands. Asterixis is considered by some to be a variant of tremor or of myoclonus and by others to represent an entirely distinct phenomenon.[1,2] Asterixis may be seen in a variety of toxic metabolic encephalopathies and is characteristic of hepatic encephalopathy.

Fasciculations are brief spontaneous contractions of groups of muscle fibers; they may produce visible twitching in the skin overlying the muscle but are not strong enough to actually move joints. They may occur in normal individuals, especially after vigorous exercise, and are characteristic of diseases affecting anterior horn cells. As a rule, fasciculations that occur chronically in the absence of weakness, muscle atrophy, or other abnormalities on neurologic examination may be regarded as benign.

Spasm is a nonspecific term that refers to any sustained contraction of muscle. Painful spasms are referred to as cramps.

Impairment of Postural Reflexes

In normal individuals, upright posture is maintained in part by very rapid-acting *postural* or *righting reflexes*, which compensate for any deviations from normal position. In patients with some movement disorders, such as Parkinson's disease and related conditions, these reflexes are impaired and patients are therefore very susceptible to falls. Even a minor push or stumble may result in a fall; protective reflexes, such as stretching out the arms to break a fall, are impaired as well and these patients are at risk for severe injury as a result.

CLINICAL SYNDROMES

Tremor

Tremor is an extremely common symptom, which most people experience at one time or another, usually in association with anxiety or fatigue, use of caffeine or other stimulant drugs, or following excessive alcohol use. Most tremors are benign and self-limited, cause no significant functional impairment, and only rarely lead to medical attention. In some patients, however, tremor is severe and persistent and may cause embarrassment, social disablement, or even substantial functional impairment. Some varieties of tremor, especially resting tremor or intention tremor, may be signs of severe underlying disease such as Parkinson's disease or cerebellar disorders.

Tremors are classified as either action tremors or resting tremors, depending on when they are most evident. Action tremors are most evident when the involved extremity is active in some way, and they improve or may disappear at rest. Action tremors encountered in clinical practice include physiologic tremor, essential tremor, and intention tremor. Resting tremor, as the name implies, is most evident when the involved extremity is at rest and it is often partially or completely suppressed by voluntary movement. The distinction between resting and action tremors is not absolute, and more than one variety may be present in a given individual.

Physiologic tremor can be detected in virtually everyone. It is a low-amplitude, rapid (8–12 Hz) tremor most evident in the hands. Physiologic tremor can be embarrassing but usually does not cause significant functional impairment. It may be exacerbated by a wide variety of drugs and other influences (Table 7-1), and it is commonly present in patients with thyrotoxicosis and other metabolic disorders. A similar tremor is seen in patients withdrawing from alcohol, benzodiazepines, and other drugs. Treatment of simple physiologic tremor consists of reassurance, and reduction or elimination of offending

TABLE 7-1

FACTORS ACCENTUATING PHYSIOLOGIC TREMOR

Anxiety
Fatigue
Weakness
Hypercapnia
Drug withdrawal
Hypocalcemia
Hypoglycemia
Hypomagnesemia
Uremia
Severe liver disease
Heavy metal intoxication
Drugs (catecholamines, theophylline, caffeine, lithium, tricyclic antidepressants,
    steroids, antipsychotic drugs, sodium valproate, antihistamines,
    amphetamines)
Thyrotoxicosis
Hysteria

substances. In patients whose tremor is associated with intense anxiety, occasional use of anxiolytic drugs may be helpful.

Essential tremor is a low- or medium-amplitude tremor that may occur in the hands, the legs, or the head and trunk. It is most evident in distal muscles such as in the fingers, hands, and wrists. It is generally lower in frequency compared to physiologic tremor (5–10 Hz). It is increased by sustained contraction of muscles and often interferes with fine movements such as writing, eating, sewing, or playing musical instruments. Essential tremor is common in older persons but can develop at any age, and, once present, tends to worsen slowly as the patient ages. Essential tremor can be worsened by the same factors that worsen physiologic tremor and the two tremors sometimes cannot be easily distinguished. Essential tremor is often relieved by even small amounts of alcohol; this should not be taken to mean that the tremor is the result of excess drinking. Because of their concern about this implication, patients will often not mention the fact that their tremors improve after drinking. In older patients, essential tremor is sometimes referred to as senile tremor; in patients with a family history of similar tremor, it is called familial tremor.

Apart from the tremor itself, the neurologic examination of patients with essential tremor should be normal. A careful search should be made for signs of Parkinson's disease (see below), both to avoid missing that diagnosis and to reassure those patients who do not have that condition. Clinical features that help differentiate essential tremor from parkinsonian tremor are listed in Table 7-2. Of course, essential tremor and Parkinsonism disease can coexist.

Acute treatment for essential tremor is rarely needed. Patients may find that a glass of wine will suppress the tremor enough that they can enjoy social situations without embarrassment. Anxiolytics can also be helpful, but of course both alcohol and anxiolytics carry risks of increasing dependence. For many patients with more

TABLE 7-2

ESSENTIAL TREMOR VERSUS PARKINSONIAN TREMOR

Clinical Feature	Essential Tremor	Parkinsonism
Onset	Bilateral	Unilateral
Frequency	3–6 Hz	5–10 Hz
Movement	Flexion–extension	Pronation–supination
Most evident	With movement	At rest
Involves head	Yes	No
Involves voice	Yes	No
Abnormal examination	No	Yes
Relived by alcohol	Yes	No

severe tremor who need regular medication, propranolol may be helpful. Primidone can also be helpful, but sedation is often limiting. For patients with severe tremor, referral to a neurologist is appropriate since more aggressive treatment, including deep brain stimulation, can provide dramatic relief to more severely affected patients.

Intention tremor is the least common form of tremor but frequently the most disabling. It is typically higher in amplitude and lower in frequency (3–5 Hz) than other action tremors. As the name implies, it is usually most evident when the patient reaches out to grasp or touch an object, particularly near the end of the movement. There may be little or no tremor at the beginning of the movement, but as the moving finger nears its target, the tremor becomes increasing severe and may prevent the patient from completing the movement. On examination it is often best demonstrated by the classic tests of coordination such as the finger–nose–finger maneuver. The tremor tends to involve more proximal joints such as the elbows or shoulders rather than more distal joints such as the wrists and fingers. Intention tremor is classically associated with cerebellar disorders; in younger patients, injury of the cerebellar peduncles or cerebellum from multiple sclerosis is a common cause. However, intention tremor may also result from drug intoxication, especially anticonvulsant drugs and alcohol, or from lesions as diverse as stroke or peripheral neuropathy affecting the motor and sensory pathways. Accordingly, the presence of intention tremor indicates the need for a comprehensive neurologic evaluation. Treatment depends on the underlying disorder; the results are frequently disappointing.

Resting tremor, as the name implies, is most evident when the involved extremity is in repose; it is suppressed and may disappear entirely with movement. It is not unusual to see patients with quite severe resting tremor who can nonetheless perform the finger–nose–finger maneuver or even drink a cup of coffee without difficulty. Resting tremor is characteristic of parkinsonism (see below). These patients may exhibit a pronation–supination movement of the hands and fingers (the pill-rolling tremor) or more commonly will have flexion–extension movements of the fingers, wrists, or elbows. The tremor is usually asymmetric and may be entirely confined to one side or the other. The tremor rarely involves the head. Careful examination of these patients will usually reveal other signs of parkinsonism (see later in the chapter). Treatment is discussed below.

Tics

Tics can range from very simple movements such as eye blinking, shoulder shrugging, or head jerking through much more complex movements involving multiple muscles or large portions of the body. Vocal tics may occur as well and may range from simple grunts or barks through words or short phrases. The movements are apparently purposeless and inappropriate to the situation but sometimes can be modified by the patient into an apparently purposeful movement. Simple motor tics are quite common in childhood and often resolve with maturation. As noted above, the tics can often be temporarily suppressed by the patient, who will then experience a steadily mounting, and eventually irresistible, urge to perform the movement. A given patient may exhibit only one or a few simple motor tics or may have multiple motor tics and vocal tics (Gilles de la Tourette syndrome). Tics often occur in association with other conditions such as obsessive–compulsive disorder or the attention-deficit/hyperactivity disorder.[3] Like the other movement disorders, tics are frequently increased with stress and anxiety; they are absent during sleep. Management is difficult and frequently requires the use of neuroleptic drugs; treatment is not required in the acute care setting.

Akathisia

The term *akathisia* refers to a sense of motor restlessness; patients feel an irresistible urge to move. These patients are in constant motion—standing up and sitting down, rubbing various parts of their bodies, picking at their clothing, fidgeting, etc. The sensations are very distressing to patients (and others) and sometimes painful. Akathisia occurs most often as a complication of neuroleptic drug use and may occur in 30% to 40% of patients on these agents. It is a common side effect of drugs such as prochlorperazine, which is often used in the acute care setting to manage nausea and vomiting. It may also occur in patients taking selective serotonin reuptake inhibitors (SSRIs). The syndrome is thought to be quite common but very often unrecognized. It may respond to β-blockers, diphenhydramine, and benzodiazepines.[4–7]

Choreoathetosis

Choreiform movements may occur in a wide variety of neurologic disorders (Table 7-3). Most of these are chronic disorders, with the abnormal movements developing gradually. Accordingly, these patients will rarely present to the acute care setting for their initial evaluation. There are a few situations in which choreiform movements may develop acutely, and these will be discussed briefly.

   Levodopa and other dopaminergic drugs used in the management of Parkinson's disease are common causes of choreoathetoid movements. The movements can develop quite abruptly, especially after dose adjustment or after an accidental or deliberate overdose. The abnormal movements are usually more distressing to family members or other observers than to the patient, who may be unaware of even quite dramatic involuntary movements. In fact, many Parkinson's disease patients feel at their best when their dose of levodopa is at the point where they develop some choreiform movements. The movements may affect the extremities, the head and trunk, the face and voice, or any combination of these. A similar clinical picture may result from drugs such as neuroleptics (tardive dyskinesia) or from other drugs such as amphetamines and tricyclic antidepressants. Treatment is withdrawal of the offending substance (when possible).

TABLE 7-3 ——————————————————————————

CAUSES OF CHOREA

Drugs (levodopa, other dopaminergic agents, neuroleptics, amphetamines, tricyclic antidepressants, and others)
Pregnancy (chorea gravidarum) and oral contraceptives
Toxic/metabolic disorders (carbon monoxide, anoxia, hypomagnesemia, electrolyte derangements, hypo- and hyperglycemia, and others)
Huntington's disease, Wilson's disease, other hereditary and degenerative disorders
Rheumatic fever
Lupus erythematosus
Vascular disease (particularly lacunar infarction)
Senile chorea

Rarely, acute chorea may be seen in pregnant patients or those on oral contraceptives (chorea gravidarum). This syndrome has become exceedingly rare with the virtual disappearance of Sydenham's chorea. The abrupt onset of chorea in children should suggest Sydenham's chorea, one of the major manifestations of rheumatic fever, now extremely rare in the United States.[1,8]

Dystonia

Like other involuntary movements, dystonia may occur in a wide variety of primary and secondary neurologic disorders, many of which are quite rare and few of which are likely to be encountered in the acute care setting. Acute dystonias do occur, most often as a consequence of neuroleptic drug treatment. Because these agents are often used in the management of nausea and vomiting, the acute care physician should be familiar with these unusual but dramatic events. Patients may present any of a wide variety of bizarre movements or postures such as forced deviation of the eyes and head, twisting the face and slurred speech, torticollis, hyperextension of the head and trunk (opisthotonus), and choreoathetoid movements. Despite their often bizarre (and sometimes painful) postures, patients remain awake and alert with normal mental function. The diagnosis can be confirmed (and the symptoms relieved) by giving diphenhydramine 25 to 50 mg IV or IM or benztropine 1 to 2 mg IM. This will result in rapid, often spectacular, resolution of the abnormal posture and movements. Because the duration of action of the offending drug may be quite long, repeat treatment may be needed.

Myoclonus

As noted above, myoclonus may involve single muscles, groups of related or adjacent muscles (termed segmental myoclonus), or even the entire body. The movements may be isolated or recurrent; they are usually irregular but may occur in rhythmic bursts. They may occur spontaneously or in response to tactile stimulation or attempts to move the affected body part. As with other involuntary movements, myoclonus is nonspecific and may occur in a wide variety of neurologic conditions, including many chronic

TABLE 7-4

CAUSES OF MYOCLONUS

Benign myoclonus—sleep starts, hiccoughs, exercise-induced
Drug-induced—tricyclics, penicillins, meperidine, tacrolimus, many others
Toxic-metabolic encephalopathies—especially hypoxia/ischemia, heat stroke,
    electric shock, hepatic and renal failure, dialysis, heavy metal poisoning
Encephalitis—herpes simplex, other viral encephalites, Creutzfeldt-Jakob disease,
    and others causes
Epileptic myoclonus
Degenerative diseases of the central nervous system (multiple)

disorders (Table 7-4). Several causes of myoclonus are more likely to be seen in the acute setting and these are discussed briefly.

Benign myoclonus is common. The most familiar form is "sleep starts," the sudden jerks that occur just as one is falling asleep. These are occasionally mistaken for seizures and can be a source of anxiety. Exercise-related myoclonus is another benign phenomenon; as with exercise-related fasciculations, this can safely be ignored if the neurologic examination and history are otherwise unremarkable. Finally, myoclonus occasionally occurs in association with syncope, especially if the patient is held upright and cannot fall to a supine position. Myoclonus in this setting can easily be mistaken for seizure activity.

Myoclonus is a feature of a wide variety of toxic and metabolic encephalopathies, including drug intoxication, hypoxia, hyponatremia, and others. Multifocal myoclonus is common following hypoxic ischemic injury (as in cardiac arrest) and may be difficult to distinguish from seizure activity. Multifocal myoclonus is also prominent in intoxication with tricyclic antidepressants and SSRIs (see below). In patients receiving repeated doses of meperidine, especially in the face of renal insufficiency, accumulation of normeperidine, a toxic metabolite, may cause encephalopathy and dramatic myoclonus. A similar picture has been seen in patients treated with tacrolimus (Prograf and others) following organ transplantation.

Myoclonus per se does not cause any alteration of consciousness. Patients and witnesses should be questioned carefully in the case of episodic myoclonus—if there is any alteration of consciousness, myoclonic seizure activity should be suspected.

Spasms and Cramps

Most muscle spasms result from local irritation or injury of muscle. Pain from any cause may create reflex spasm in local muscles, as is commonly seen near sites of injury such as fracture. Muscle spasm may also occur spontaneously or as a result of some activity; when prolonged and painful, these spasms are called cramps. Spontaneous cramps are particularly common in the elderly patients; these do not indicate any serious disease, but can cause considerable distress and may disturb sleep. During the cramp, the muscle will be very hard to palpation. The cramp can usually be overcome by massage and passive forceful stretching; it will often recur if the muscle is allowed to relax too soon. Treatment is directed at the underlying injury, if any. Analgesics and anti-inflammatory agents and muscle relaxants may be helpful. In elderly patients with recurrent nocturnal cramps, quinine sulfate 300 mg PO at bedtime may be useful.

Irritation or injury to peripheral nerves may cause spasm of isolated muscles or groups of muscles. Hemifacial spasm is characterized by repetitive twitching of the muscles on one side of the face and may occur as a primary process or following Bell's palsy. Injury to other peripheral nerves may result in similar spasms in affected muscles, especially during recovery.

Muscle spasm may result from a variety of electrolyte abnormalities. Hypocalcemia, hypomagnesemia, and other electrolyte abnormalities can result in muscle cramps. Hyperventilation, by causing an abrupt fall in ionized calcium, can cause muscle spasm and cramp. The classic clinical sign of hypocalcemia is Chvostek's sign, in which tapping the facial nerve at the angle of the jaw induces reflex spasms of the facial muscles.

More ominous acute causes of muscle spasm include tetanus and strychnine poisoning. The diagnosis of tetanus must be based on clinical suspicion. Common early symptoms of tetanus include jaw tightness, irritability, and headache. Later, more pronounced spasm of the masseter muscles (*trismus*) prevents jaw opening (*lockjaw*) and tonic contraction of facial muscles causes a fixed facial grimace (*risus sardonicus*). The painful spasms spread progressively, eventually leading to complete rigidity and immobility. The spasms are intensified with any external stimulation. Treatment is complex and requires intensive nursing and medical care (see also Chapter 5).

Strychnine is found as a common adulterant in many street drugs and in products used to kill animal pests; it is occasionally taken intentionally. It can produce symptoms within 15 to 30 minutes of ingestion. Initial restlessness and agitation may be followed by heightened auditory and visual acuity. Usually spasms and convulsions lasting up to 2 minutes occur, followed by periods of relaxation. Extensor muscle spasm may produce opisthotonus, and risus sardonicus may occur. These are often accompanied by convulsions, hyperthermia, lactic acidosis, and rhabdomyolysis. At onset the differential diagnosis centers around the spasms; however, later in the course, the picture resembles repetitive seizures but with preservation of consciousness during the paroxysms.

Parkinsonism

The most common clinical syndrome associated with disease of the basal nuclei and extrapyramidal motor system is parkinsonism. Although not usually a medical emergency, the syndrome is common, especially in older patients, and all physicians should be familiar with its major features. Patients often consult several physicians before receiving a correct diagnosis, and as a result, may have had several trials of inappropriate and ineffective treatment. The symptoms include slowing or paucity of movement (bradykinesia/akinesia), increased muscle tone (rigidity), tremor or other involuntary movements, and impaired posture and gait. The early symptoms are gradual in onset, mild, and nonspecific, and unexplained falls are a common presenting symptom. Patients and their families report that patients seem dull and lifeless, with decreased interest in their daily activities. Their gait is slow, shuffling, and unsteady, with frequent falls. Other common early symptoms include very small handwriting (micrographia), and soft, slurred speech. Patients often have trouble sleeping; a common complaint is difficulty turning over in bed, difficulty getting into and out of bed, and difficulty getting up from soft low chairs. Not surprisingly, these patients are often misdiagnosed as depressed or "senile," or given a meaningless diagnosis such as "ministrokes."

TABLE 7-5

CAUSES OF PARKINSONISM

Parkinson's Disease

Secondary parkinsonism
Drugs and toxins
   Phenothiazines, butyrophenones, other neuroleptics
   Lithium, metoclopramide, etc.
   Manganese, mercury, ethanol, methanol, etc.
Vascular disease—small vessel vasculopathies, multiinfarct state
Structural lesions—head injury, neoplasms, hydrocephalus
Anoxic/ischemic—cardiac arrest, carbon monoxide
Degenerative diseases—multisystem atrophies, Lewy body disease, cortical-basal
   ganglionic degeneration, progressive supranuclear palsy, etc.

The most common cause of the parkinsonism syndrome is Parkinson's disease, but a similar clinical picture can result from a wide variety of other conditions (Table 7-5). For the acute care physician, perhaps the single most important aspect of the disorder is that it be recognized, particularly in its early stages. Once it is familiar to the physician, the syndrome of bradykinesia and increased muscle tone, often with "cogwheeling," is virtually unmistakable. Parkinson's disease should always be considered in an older patient with abnormal gait and frequent falls. Note that resting tremor, although common, is not always present. Although the disease cannot be cured, patients with Parkinson's disease may have a dramatic response to treatment and their distress can be greatly reduced. Emergency treatment is not necessary. Since the effective management of Parkinson's disease requires a long-term commitment from both physician and patient, referral to a neurologist is usually the best course.

The acute care physician should also be aware that choreiform and dystonic movements are common side effects of anti-Parkinson's drugs. These symptoms may develop abruptly and may provoke a visit to the acute care setting. Confusion and hallucinations may also occur, especially with some of the newer agents such as ropinirole (Requip) and pramipexole (Mirapex). Episodes of syncope should suggest autonomic insufficiency or postural hypotension, possibly exacerbated by medications. Later in the course of Parkinson's disease, patients may experience "on–off" symptoms: sudden and dramatic fluctuations in motor function or "freezing" episodes of sudden immobility. Cognitive disturbances are also common, and 30% of patients with Parkinson's disease will have a dementia. All these complications are difficult to manage and require referral to the patient's treating physician. Another "complication" of Parkinson's disease is the presence of deep brain stimulation equipment (increasingly used in the treatment of this disease). These can be easily overlooked on a casual examination but their presence means that patients are not candidates for MR imaging.

It is important to remember that not all "parkinsonism" is due to Parkinson's disease. A similar clinical syndrome may be seen in many other degenerative disorders of the central nervous system (Table 7-4). It is often difficult to distinguish among these conditions, especially early in their courses, and a convincing diagnosis can sometimes be made only after prolonged observation. Most important in the acute care setting is parkinsonism caused by specific, sometimes treatable causes, primarily drugs and toxins. Parkinsonism is common and well known in patients treated with neuroleptics, but can also result from drugs such as lithium and metoclopramide (Reglan). Possible toxins include manganese, mercury, carbon disulfide, and alcohols, among others. A complete list is obviously impossible; a physician confronted with a patient with recent onset of parkinsonian symptoms should obtain a detailed history of drug use and exposure to toxins. Treatment is withdrawal, if possible, of the offending agent.

Neuroleptic Malignant Syndrome

The neuroleptic malignant syndrome is a rare but potentially lethal disorder characterized by muscle rigidity, hyperpyrexia, altered mental status, and autonomic dysfunction. It is a rare complication of neuroleptic drug use (phenothiazines, haloperidol, and others) but also occur in association with lithium, antidepressants, and metoclopramide, and rarely following sudden withdrawal of agents such as levodopa. It has occurred with all of the antipsychotic drugs including the newer atypical antipsychotics, though the newer agents appear to carry a substantially lower risk. It may occur following a single dose of the inciting agent, but more commonly occurs after more prolonged exposure. The clinical picture is characterized by muscle rigidity that can be focal or generalized, elevation of temperature ranging from mild to extreme ($>42°C$), altered mental status ranging from mild confusion to coma, and autonomic disturbances including tachycardia, labile blood pressure, and profuse sweating. If muscle rigidity is severe and generalized, rhabdomyolysis may occur, with elevation of serum creatine kinase (CK) levels sometimes elevated to spectacular levels. The syndrome should be suspected in patients taking neuroleptic drugs who develop increasing agitation, muscle stiffness, and fever. Treatment includes stopping the inciting drug and providing supportive care. Other measures of unproven effectiveness include aggressive use of benzodiazepines to manage muscle rigidity, neuromuscular blockade, and dopaminergic drugs such as bromocriptine (5–20 mg via NG tube q8h). These patients require intensive management in a critical care unit.[7,9]

The differential diagnosis includes heat stroke and poisoning with anticholinergic drugs, both of which are associated with flaccid muscles and dry skin.

Serotonin Syndrome

A wide variety of serotonergic drugs are employed in modern clinical practice. These include many antidepressant medications such as the tricyclic antidepressants (amitriptyline and others), SSRIs such as fluoxetine and citalopram, and serotonin norepinephrine reuptake inhibitors (SNRIs) such as duloxetine and venlafaxine. Other serotonergic agents include monoamine oxidase inhibitors and drugs such as buspirone and trazodone, and a variety of illicit agents. Any of the drugs, particularly when used at higher doses or when used in combination, can cause the serotonin syndrome. The clinical features include agitation and confusion, tremor, myoclonus, and increased reflexes, and autonomic disturbances (sweating, fever, and tachycardia). Coma and muscle rigidity may be seen in very severe cases. In severe cases, rhabdomyolysis, seizures, and disseminated intravascular coagulation can occur. Treatment includes withdrawal of serotonergic drugs and management of individual symptoms as needed. Cyproheptadine, a serotonin antagonist, may be beneficial.[7]

TABLE 7-6

MOVEMENT DISORDERS—EMERGENCY CONDITIONS

Acute dystonic reactions to neuroleptics and other drugs
Neuroleptic malignant syndrome
Serotonin syndrome
Muscle cramps and spasms due to tetanus, strychnine poisoning
Myoclonus due to electrolyte abnormalities, drug toxicity, and hypoxemia

Summary

It is common to think of movement disorders as uncommon and unusual conditions rarely seen in the emergency department. However, involuntary movements occur in a wide variety of common disorders and are common side effects of many drugs and toxins (Table 7-6). Effective treatment may be possible in many of these patients. Confronted by a patient with an apparent movement disorder, the acute care physician should first try to classify the involuntary movements, since correct classification often will suggest the correct diagnosis. Second, it is important to obtain a detailed history of drug use (both prescribed and otherwise) and toxin exposure. Except in the case of common "repeat offenders," it may be necessary to look up each drug in an up-to-date reference source because even common agents familiar to the physician may cause rare side effects. Finally, the physician should recall that bizarre and incomprehensible movements and behaviors even in a patient with a known psychiatric disorder need not indicate a psychiatric condition. Careful assessment may disclose a specific treatable "organic" condition.

References

1. Lang AE. Movement disorder symptomatology. In: Bradley WG et al., eds. *Neurology in Clinical Practice*. 3rd ed. Boston: Butterworth-Heinemann; 2000.
2. Victor M, Ropper AH. *Adams and Victor's Principles of Neurology*. 8th ed. New York: McGraw-Hill; 2001.
3. Weiner WJ, Lang AE. *Movement Disorders: A Comprehensive Survey*. Mt Kisco, NY: Futura; 1989.
4. Bakheit A. The syndrome of motor restlessness—a treatable but unrecognized disorder. *Postgrad Med J*. 1997;73:529.
5. Weiden PJ et al. Clinical nonrecognition of neuroleptic induced movement disorders; a cautionary study. *Am J Psychia*. 1987;144:1148-1153.
6. Vinson DR, Drotts DL. Diphenhydramine for the prevention of akathisia induced by prochlorperazine: a randomized, controlled trial. *Ann Emerg Med*. 2001;37:125-131.
7. Haddad PM, Dursun SM. Neurological complications of psychiatric drugs: clinical features and management. *Hum Psychopharmacol Clin Exp*. 2008;23:15-26.
8. Shoulson I. On chorea. *Clin Neuropharmacol*. 1986;9:585.
9. Lavonas EJ, Ford MD. Antipsychotics. In: Marx JA et al., eds. *Rosen's Emergency Medicine: Concepts and Clinical Practice*. 5th ed. St Louis: Mosby; 2001:2174-2179.

The evaluation of headache is a common task for any physician working in the acute care setting. Sorting the benign from the serious causes of headache is often a challenge because of the nonspecific nature of headache pain and the wide variety of systemic and intracranial disorders that can cause headache, and the frequency of headache as a complaint. Generally, headaches are not due to serious disease, but rarely they do indicate a severe systemic or intracranial process.[1,2] Patients often regard pain in the head as potentially more significant than pain elsewhere, with brain tumor being a common but frequently unexpressed fear.

Headache is the ninth most common cause of physician visits and one of the most common causes (5%)[3] for emergency department visits. Ninety-nine percent of women and 94% of men will experience headache in their lifetime. Although muscle contraction and migraine are the most common causes of headache, the potential list of causes is extensive.

This chapter will discuss an approach to the headache patient. Because physicians practicing acute care medicine will see headache problems that encompass the entire spectrum, from acute to chronic, many etiologies will be covered. Some will simply be listed to serve as a reference starting point and to keep some uncommon etiologies under consideration. Some etiologies will be dealt with in more detail because of their frequency or seriousness.

HISTORY

The history may serve as the sole basis for a diagnosis, because objective physical signs, laboratory abnormalities, or imaging findings are frequently lacking or are nonspecific. A focused workup starts with a careful clinical history. Table 8-1 lists numerous historical factors that may aid in diagnosis. Of those listed, the temporal relationships and associated symptoms are most important. A headache that begins and becomes maximal in an instant ("thunderclap") suggests causes that are vastly different from those with a vague,

TABLE 8-1

HEADACHE HISTORY

- Temporal relations: Time of day, time to maximum intensity, frequency, duration
- Associated symptoms: Fever, nausea, vomiting, loss of consciousness, flushing, lacrimation, neck stiffness, photophobia, dizziness
- Pattern profile: Prodrome, correlation with medications, menstruation, activities
- Site of pain: Unilateral, bilateral, frontal, occipital, facial, and radiation
- Quality of pain: Pulsatile, steady, shocklike, tightness
- Intensity
- Precipitating or aggravating factors: Exertion, position, foods, drugs, weather, anxiety
- Relieving factors: Darkroom, position, pressing on scalp, medication
- Medical history: Drugs, hypertension, cancer, travel, trauma
- Family history
- Occupational history: Solvents, vapors, chemicals

poorly defined onset. The significance of these historical clues will be covered in the individual discussions of headache etiologies. Some of these historical aspects warrant brief discussion.

The intensity of the pain does not necessarily correlate with the severity of the causative illness. Sudden excruciating pain, however, suggests an acute subarachnoid hemorrhage (SAH). Many of the symptoms associated with headache may implicate a specific entity, e.g., lacrimation is associated with cluster headaches. Sudden loss of consciousness should always be considered serious because it suggests important etiologies, such as SAH or a third ventricular tumor (e.g., colloid cyst) obstructing the ventricular system.

A travel history may cause one to suspect etiologies not common in North America, such as parasitic infection or other tropical illness. A history of multiple patients or family members with a similar illness might prompt consideration of carbon monoxide poisoning in the appropriate setting.

When taking a family history, one should beware of patients labeling chronic-recurrent headaches as "sinus" and try to seek details of the headaches themselves. Frequently in layman's terms any commonly occurring headache is mislabeled as sinus,[4] and any intense headache as migraine. Many patients in the general population with significant headaches have migraines, despite the lack of a formal diagnosis by a physician.[5]

"Red flags" that may point to a serious underlying etiology of a headache include a very sudden onset of symptoms, an accelerating pattern of systemic illness, the presence of an associated stiff neck, new onset after age 50, known underlying cancer or HIV/AIDS and, most importantly, associated focal neurologic findings. New abnormalities on mental status testing or on evaluation of extraocular movements or pupils, should prompt consideration of serious underlying pathology (Table 8-2). In addition to the routine vital signs, and the results of a patient's general physical and neurologic examinations, some specific clinical findings may be very helpful. Scalp artery tenderness may occur with cranial (temporal) arteritis. Scalp tenderness may also accompany unrecognized trauma, cranial neuralgias, or underlying infection. Meningeal signs such as stiffness of the neck

TABLE 8-2
"RED FLAGS" IN THE HEADACHE PATIENT

1. Focal neurologic findings
2. New mental status changes
3. New ocular movement abnormalities
4. Instantaneous onset of symptoms
5. Accelerating pattern of systemic illness
6. Meningismus
7. New onset after age 50
8. Cancer
9. HIV/AIDS

(nuchal rigidity), Kernig's sign (meningeal irritation resulting in hamstring pain upon leg extension of a patient who is lying in the supine position with hips and knees flexed), or Brudzinski's sign (meningeal irritation resulting in hip and knee flexion when the neck of a supine patient is flexed) are commonly present in patients with meningitis. While mild, objective nuchal rigidity may be found on passive neck flexion in patients with early disease, Kernig's and/or Brudzinski's signs typically occur only in advanced cases. Examination of the fundus should be performed with the patient seated, because venous pulsations can be lost in the supine position.

PROCEDURES AND LABORATORY EVALUATION

A previously unsuspected diagnosis in the headache patient is seldom made by laboratory evaluation alone. Several exceptions occur and should be kept in mind. A markedly elevated sedimentation rate (SR) virtually always occurs in temporal arteritis (giant cell arteritis) and should be considered in patients over the age of 55 when the clinical scenario is suggestive, though an elevated SR is a very nonspecific finding. Carbon monoxide levels may be useful in the appropriate setting. Although anemia and anoxia can cause headache, it is unlikely that they would be present, but unsuspected clinically. Other blood chemistries usually do not provide a basis for an etiology. Rarely, when considering tropical diseases, a CBC may be helpful; in that a low platelet count may point toward further investigation for malaria or dengue as the cause of headache in the febrile international traveler.[6,7] A pregnancy test may be helpful, as venous sinus thrombosis may be a suspect diagnosis in the pregnant patient with sudden severe headache.

Of the studies that will provide the basis for or against a given diagnosis, lumbar puncture and noncontrast computed tomography (CT) scan are the most useful. The indications for an emergent lumbar puncture are a clinical suspicion of meningitis/encephalitis or subarachnoid hemorrhage, or rarely, to evaluate intracranial pressure (ICP). It should be noted that elevated intracranial pressure alone does not raise the risk of brain herniation, but when present in the setting of a unilateral supratentorial mass, hydrocephalus, or a posterior fossa mass, it can precipitate brain herniation syndromes.

It is uncommon for such patients with these structural lesions to present with the clinical picture suggestive of meningitis, which would necessitate obtaining a CT scan or other imaging study before a lumbar puncture was performed. Further discussion of this potential problem will be given at the end of this chapter.

When elevated intracranial pressure is found in isolation, one should still collect cerebrospinal fluid (CSF) for analysis.

One sometimes may need to begin urgent measures to reduce intracranial pressure, plan for an emergency CT scan (to rule out an intracranial mass, mass effect, or increasing intraventricular pressure), and/or call for neurosurgical evaluation.

If SAH is suspected clinically, but a CT scan is negative (or not available), and there are no imaging or clinical findings consistent with an intracranial mass effect, a lumbar puncture may still detect blood suggesting an underlying SAH hemorrhage, particularly if the hemorrhage occurred in the posterior fossa or upper cervical spinal canal.

When the suspicion of SAH is low but still must be excluded, lumbar puncture can be performed as the primary procedure in certain clinical settings.

CT scanning is the most useful tool for rapidly assessing for acute intracranial abnormalities in the headache patient. It should be performed, however, only on a selective basis when the clinical history and/or physical examination suggests the possibility of a SAH or other intracranial lesion, and not as a screening tool.[8] A nonenhanced CT is the imaging test of choice. It should be noted, however, that other less common, but still important, causes of headache in the acute care setting such as cortical or dural venous sinus thrombosis, hypertensive encephalopathy, or carotid/vertebral dissection will not be reliably detected on a noncontrast screening head CT and will usually require MRI, MRA, MRV, CTA, or CTV for definitive delineation (see Chapter 2). Finally, while acute hemorrhage and mass effects are well seen on most CT scans (and their detection is the primary concern in the acute care setting), the cause of a hemorrhage is rarely delineated on that CT scan and will require additional imaging such as MRI, MR angiography, CT angiography, or formal endovascular angiography to identify an underlying aneurysm, vascular malformation, dural fistula, or vasculitis. Similarly, small masses often require MRI for detection though such evaluation is usually not emergently indicated.

As suggested previously and also as reviewed in Chapter 2, it is important to remember that some CT scans will be falsely negative for pathologic processes. Small amounts of subarachnoid blood may not be demonstrated because of obscuring artifacts intrinsic to CT (such as proximity of the SAH to dense osseous structures), low iron content of the subarachnoid blood (from anemia), or suboptimal resolution of the CT scanner employed. Small amounts of subarachnoid blood from aneurysmal SAH can be subtle on CT. More chronic, larger "isodense" extra-axial collections of blood located over the cerebral convexities or in the posterior fossa, especially if present bilaterally (and therefore not associated with focal mass effects), may also be difficult to detect.

Osseous abnormalities such as basilar skull fractures may be missed if they are not clinically suspected and directed imaging to that region is not performed.

Plain skull x-rays now play only a minimal role in the evaluation of headache.[9] They may be useful in evaluating the extracranial portion of a ventricular shunt in a patient with suspected shunt malfunction. For other headache issues, the most they can do is lead one to do another imaging study (CT) and therefore should not be performed.

TABLE 8-3

CLINICAL CLUES TO HEADACHE SYNDROMES

Clue	Considerations
"Thunderclap"	Subarachnoid Hemorrhage
Dilated pupil	Posterior communicating aneurysm
Double Vision	Mass lesion, pseudotumor cerebri
Source of incomplete combustion	Carbon monoxide poisoning
Pregnancy	Eclampsia, cerebral venous thrombosis
Fever	CNS or systemic infection
Papilledema	Mass lesion, pseudotumor cerebri
Horner's syndrome	Carotid dissection
"Rheumatoid symptoms" in elderly	Temporal arteritis

Paranasal sinus radiographs may help confirm or exclude a diagnosis of sinusitis, but are frequently over- and underread. CT is rarely indicated to assess for sinus disease in the acute care setting and can be misleading as they will demonstrate sinus inflammation in many patients without a clinical syndrome of sinusitis. Clinical clues to specific headache syndromes are listed in Table 8-3.

Pain Mechanisms in Headache

Explanations for the pathophysiology of head pain are in constant evolution and revision, and do not impact the diagnostic evaluation of headache and will therefore not be discussed further here.

Initial Approach to the Headache Patient

Because of the wide range of etiologies of headache, one must develop an approach to narrow the diagnostic possibilities yet not overlook potential serious etiologies. Patients present to the emergency and outpatient facilities with acute headaches, chronic headaches, and acute exacerbations of chronic headache problems. Although it is not necessary, or even possible to achieve a final diagnosis on every patient on initial evaluation, certain etiologies require more acute diagnosis and treatment than do others.

One of the most important etiologies to consider in a patient with a sudden-onset severe headache is SAH. Though SAH is not a common cause of headache, its detection is important because morbidity and mortality increase when the diagnosis is missed.[10] Details on SAH are discussed later in the chapter.

Because of its potential for rapid progression and morbidity, meningitis should also be considered in the appropriate clinical setting in headache patients. Although in the past, most cases of meningitis occurred in the young age group and most presented with meningeal signs, strong exceptions to these generalities exist. These are discussed in more detail later.

HEADACHES IN CHILDREN AND ADOLESCENTS

Headaches are common in children and even more so in adolescents, with reports of headache prevalence in the 30% to 80% range by age 15. The approach to headaches in children is similar to that in adults. Evaluation begins with a focused history, physical and neurologic examination. Depending upon the age of the child, some elements of the history may be difficult to determine. As with adults, the results of the history and examination will determine the need for further investigation.[11] Variables tending to predict the presence of space occupying lesions (i.e., intracranial masses or mass effects) or other serious etiologies include an abnormal neurologic examination, particularly gait disturbances, headache of less than 1-month duration, seizures and acute systemic illness and no family history of migraine. Migraine is a frequent occurrence, and half of individuals who are ultimately determined to be migraineurs develop their respective migraine symptoms prior to age 20. In the acute care setting, upper respiratory tract infections are a common cause of headache, along with migraine and recent trauma. Meningitis, ventricular shunt malfunction, and posterior fossa tumors are also serious potential causes of headache to consider in the appropriate setting.[12–14]

SUBARACHNOID HEMORRHAGE

As mentioned earlier, although SAH is an uncommon cause for headache in the acute care setting (less than 1%),[15] it is a particularly important etiology to consider because of the devastating morbidity and mortality associated with missing a ruptured aneurysm as the cause of the SAH. The incidence of SAH increases after the third decade of life and peaks in the sixth decade. Spontaneous hemorrhage into the subarachnoid space usually results in a sudden cataclysmic headache ("thunderclap" headache), which maximizes quickly, usually over seconds. It is typically very severe, different from past headaches ("worst headache of my life"), and is of very sudden onset. It may occur during vigorous physical activity including sexual intercourse or it may occur at rest. SAH can be graded using the system proposed by Hunt and Hess (Table 8-4). Patients with grade I and II SAH have the best prognosis, and represent about one-half of all SAH patients but can be the most challenging in which to suspect SAH[16] as they have a normal neurologic examination. The pain associated with SAH spontaneously subsides over time, particularly with small hemorrhages. The typically severe headache of SAH may improve with both narcotic and nonnarcotic analgesics, and such improvement should not serve as the sole basis for excluding the diagnosis of SAH. Some patients present with a history of acute headaches that resolved spontaneously or with medication, though they were never formally evaluated. Some of these patients then present acutely with a large SAH at which time their underlying aneurysm is diagnosed. The initial headaches in such patients are sometimes attributed to "warning" or "sentinel" aneurysmal SAHs from an aneurysm that might have been detected, had a formal evaluation been performed at that time. While the diagnosis of a sentinel bleed can only be made, by definition, in retrospect, the concept that headache due to transient small aneurysm leaks, which improve spontaneously or with treatment can occur, is important to bear in mind.

Nausea and vomiting, photophobia, and stiff neck commonly occur with typical SAH. Obtundation is common within 15 minutes in one-fourth of patients and one-half

TABLE 8-4 ——————————————————————————
HUNT AND HESS CLASSIFICATION OF SAH

Grade 1. Asymptomatic, or minimal headache and slight nuchal rigidity
Grade 2. Moderate to severe headache, nuchal rigidity; no neurologic deficit other than cranial nerve palsy
Grade 3. Drowsiness, confusion, or mild focal deficit
Grade 4. Stupor, moderate to severe hemiparesis, possibly early decerebrate rigidity and vegetative disturbances
Grade 5. Deep coma, decerebrate rigidity, moribund appearance

will lose consciousness, with 10% to 30% experiencing unconsciousness at the outset.[17] Unless the hemorrhage has entered the brain substance, there are usually no focal neurologic signs. Posterior communicating artery aneurysms, either ruptured or unruptured, can compress the third nerve locally and cause a dilated pupil and/or other features of third nerve palsy. Later, vasospasm can produce focal cerebral ischemia and deficits in almost any portion of the brain. Meningeal irritation from SAH and/or sudden elevated ICP causes the headache in these patients. Pain may radiate into the neck and rarely to the low back, occasionally causing sciatica. Fever may develop. Hypertension is common at the time of presentation either as a result of hemorrhage or as a predisposing factor. Seizures may occur at the time of hemorrhage and recur with rebleeding. Subhyaloid hemorrhage (see Glossary) may occasionally be seen on examination of the fundus. Electrocardiographic (ECG) changes, usually diffuse nonspecific T-wave changes, may occur. These and other concomitants are listed in Table 8-5. Of patients with "thunderclap" headaches with normal neurologic examinations, only a minority will be found to have SAH.[18] However, given the worse prognosis with missed SAH, investigation is usually warranted.

Several symptoms usually found with SAH may rarely be absent. Meningeal signs may be absent. Neck or back pain may be the sole complaint, raising suspicion of spinal etiology of a SAH, such as an arteriovenous malformation.

Spontaneous SAH is most commonly caused by an aneurysm, except in patients under age 20, in whom arteriovenous malformations are more common. Patients with polycystic kidney disease or who have immediate relatives with intracranial aneurysms have an increased risk of such aneurysms.[19]

Other causes for spontaneous intracranial hemorrhage are distinctly uncommon. Cortical or dural venous sinus thrombosis may cause cerebral infarction with associated hemorrhage, which can extend to the subarachnoid space. Thromboembolism with cerebral infarction and intracerebral hemorrhage for any reason can extend to the subarachnoid space. Tumors (e.g., in the pituitary region) may bleed into the subarachnoid space. Other rare causes of subarachnoid bleeding include coagulopathies, mycotic aneurysms, and metastatic tumors. Blunt trauma, with or without resultant cerebral cortical contusion or penetrating trauma, may cause bleeding into the subarachnoid space.

In up to 10% of cases, no cause for the SAH is found and the prognosis is usually good.

As mentioned previously and in Chapter 2, the diagnostic modality of choice for detection of SAH is a noncontrast CT scan as it will detect most recent intracranial hemorrhages,

TABLE 8-5

POTENTIAL FEATURES OF SUBARACHNOID HEMORRHAGE

- Headache
- Loss of consciousness
- Obtundation
- Meningeal signs
- Seizures
- Nausea
- Vomiting
- Dizziness
- Neck or back pain
- Paralysis or pareses; visual field defects
- Cranial nerve palsies III, VI
- Fever
- GI bleeding
- Pulmonary edema
- Syndrome of secretion of inappropriate antidiuretic hormone
- ECG changes
- Visual blurring
- Subhyaloid hemorrhage
- Papilledema

depending upon the amount of blood and other factors (as discussed earlier). Note again is made of the fact that the yield of CT diminishes over time (on the order of days; see Chapter 2). The concept of spectrum bias, the test being more likely to be positive at one extreme of the spectrum of disease being investigated (in the case of SAH, the volume of blood), is particularly applicable to CT for SAH. The small bleeds, and those evaluated many hours or days after the event, are the most likely to be missed by CT.

As mentioned previously, a lumbar puncture should be performed even if the CT scan is negative in the clinical setting of persistent suspicion of SAH or if no CT scan is available and there are no clinical signs present to suggest an intracranial mass effect or increased intracranial pressure (e.g., decreased level of consciousness or focal neurologic deficit, abnormal funduscopic examination).[20,21] When clinical suspicion is very low for hemorrhage but one still wishes to exclude it in the face of a normal examination, one might proceed directly to a lumbar puncture. In most cases of SAH, many thousands of red cells are seen on microscopic evaluation of the CSF. There is, unfortunately, no particular threshold below which SAH is excluded, and very rare cases with only a few hundred cells may occur. Red blood cells should appear in the lumbar subarachnoid space within the time frame in which clinical and radiographic evaluation can occur. A "traumatic" lumbar puncture is particularly problematic in suspected SAH patients, and it may be difficult or impossible in selected patients to determine whether the red blood cells in the CSF are from a pathologic SAH or due to the lumbar puncture itself. Xanthochromia may not occur for many hours after a pathologic SAH and is variably detectable by the laboratory and/or clinicians and has no commonly accepted "gold standard."[22] In this patient group, or in patients whose primary SAH may have occurred days or weeks ago, or in patients who have contraindications to a lumbar puncture, there may still be a role for more definitive vascular imaging, such as cerebral angiography, CT angiography, or MR angiography, sometimes on an urgent basis.

Neurologic decompensation following the hemorrhage may be caused by elevated intracranial pressure, hydrocephalus, cerebral vasospasm, or repeat hemorrhage. Patients with established, common headache syndromes such as migraine may also have intracranial aneurysms. Cerebral aneurysms are present in 3% to 6% of the population, depending upon age and method of detection.[23] Thus, a significant change in the nature of a headache in a patient with recurrent headaches presents a serious challenge to the clinician. Dramatic symptoms such as syncope, seizures, abrupt onset, or, if associated with meningismus, should prompt further evaluation.

Meningitis and Encephalitis

Meningitis, representing as it does a potentially treatable medical emergency, bears consideration in patients with headache. The classic symptoms and signs of malaise, headache, fever, photophobia, meningeal signs, nausea and vomiting, and obtundation may be only incompletely present or conspicuously absent. Bacterial meningitis can occur without stiff neck, particularly in infants but rarely in older adults. Most adults have fever, and the absence of altered mental status and nuchal rigidity argues strongly against bacterial meningitis. Nuchal rigidity is best tested as a resistance to passive neck flexion with the patient supine. The classic Kernig's and Brudzinski's signs (see "History") are insensitive early on in the course of bacterial meningitis. The accompanying mental status changes range from irritability, restlessness, confusion, and hallucination to coma, but each of these findings may be absent. Seizures are not common in adults.

In infants, the diagnosis can be difficult because of the lack of meningeal signs and the nonspecificity of manifestations (fever, vomiting, irritability, and anorexia). Drowsiness is common, and seizures are much more common than they are in adults. In infants, a bulging fontanel with the patient upright (when not crying or straining) can indicate elevated intracranial pressure.

The clinical suspicion of bacterial meningitis should prompt administration of antibiotic therapy and examination of the cerebrospinal fluid. Contraindications to lumbar puncture (e.g., presence of an intracranial mass, intracranial mass effects, or hydrocephalus) usually will not be present because such patients usually present with different clinical findings. The rare patient in whom these two possibilities exist presents a particularly difficult problem (discussed later in the chapter). One should bear in mind that a posterior fossa mass causing cerebellar tonsillar herniation can cause a stiff neck and is also considered a contraindication to lumbar puncture.

Appropriate antimicrobial regimens for meningitis change with time and drug availability and current references, including local drug sensitivity reports that should be used to guide initial therapy. Examination of the cerebrospinal fluid for the antigens of *Haemophilus influenzae*, *Neisseria meningitidis*, and *Streptococcus pneumoniae* may be useful, if positive, in patients previously treated with antibiotics, but are not reliable enough, if negative, to exclude a bacterial etiology. Blood cultures may also yield the offending organism.

Some conditions predispose the patient to meningitis. These include CSF leak, in which *Streptococcus pneumoniae* is the most common pathogen. Infections near the meninges, such as sinusitis, mastoiditis, and otitis media, may lead to meningitis. Defects in the coverings of the nervous system, either surgical or congenital as in dermal sinuses, increase the risk. Systemic infections such as bacterial endocarditis and systemic conditions such as sickle cell anemia are also predisposing factors for meningitis, as is a history of splenectomy. Patients with systemic malignancy or previous transplant (who may or may not be currently treated with immunosuppressive therapy) are at risk for a wide variety of unusual infections such as *Cryptococcus*. Other organisms such as viruses, spirochetes, rickettsiae, fungi, and protozoa may cause meningitis. Detection of these organisms will depend on special techniques of evaluating the cerebrospinal fluid. Thus, having clinical suspicion and obtaining sufficient cerebrospinal fluid remain the best ways to detect less common or less easily diagnosable entities, expeditiously.

Meningitis, inflammation of the meninges, usually also elicits an inflammatory response in contiguous brain (encephalitis) resulting in meningoencephalitis. Some disease entities, such as herpes virus, tend to affect brain tissue primarily and less so the meninges.

Encephalitis presents as headache with dramatic mental changes including drowsiness, delirium, stupor, coma, and irritability. Photophobia, seizures, malaise, fever, nausea, and vomiting also commonly occur. Encephalitis is further discussed in Chapters 4 and 5. The potential etiologies of encephalitis are many and include many virus infections, parasitic infections, bacterial and rickettsial diseases, and spirochetal disease. Clinical suspicion of herpes virus encephalitis, one of the few viral encephalitides with a specific treatment, should prompt initiation of antiviral therapy (see Chapter 5). Children may present with a clinical picture resembling meningoencephalitis (headache, confusion, irritability, and vomiting) as a result of Reye's syndrome, a now rare condition. Fever is usually absent.

MIGRAINE

Migraine headache is one of the most common etiologies for headache in an acute care setting and in the population as a whole. One-third of the population will experience migraine in their lifetime. The prevalence of migraine in the general population is 18% among females and approximately 7% among males. In 1999 there were an estimated 28 million people with migraines in the United States. Five percent of the population suffers recurrent migraine. The character of the pain and not the intensity of the pain identifies a headache as migrainous, although most patients describe the pain as severe at a physician visit. A pulse-synchronous (often unilateral, about 60%) headache, worse with exertion, accompanied by nausea, vomiting, photophobia, and phonophobia is commonly reported. Factors that point strongly toward migraine headache and help distinguish it from tension headache are nausea, photophobia, phonophobia, and an increased intensity with physical activity.[24] The mnemonic *"pounding"* has been applied— *p*ulsatile quality, duration 4–72 h*o*urs, *u*nilateral location, *n*ausea or vomiting, *d*isabling intensity.[25]

In 15% of patients, classic migraine symptoms are preceded by a neurologic symptom, usually visual. This constellation of findings is now termed migraine with aura. The visual symptom is typically described as having a light of its own or being bright, scintillating, or zigzag with stars or flashes, and typically disappears as the headache begins. It may be described as a negative visual phenomena including scotoma or hemianopsia. The neurologic symptom most commonly occurs before the headache, but may occur during, or even after the headache phase. The pain may also be described as simply pressure and not pounding. Common migraine, now termed migraine without aura, is far more frequent than classic migraine; it lacks the neurologic symptoms and the pain is less commonly localized. The International Headache Society has developed a complex Headache Classification System that, while detailed with 128 distinct syndromes, is rarely used by clinicians.[26] The criteria are very rigid (Table 8-6) and may not be able to be applied in an ER setting.[27]

TABLE 8-6

ICHD HEADACHE CLASSIFICATION CODING CRITERIA

Migraine without aura (previously "common" migraine)
A. At least 5 attacks fulfilling B–D
B. Headache lasting 4–72 h (untreated or unsuccessfully treated, or in children under age 15 lasting 2–48 h)
C. Headache has at least two of the following characteristics
    a. Unilateral location
    b. Pulsating quality
    c. Moderate or severe intensity (interferes with daily activities)
    d. Aggravated by climbing stairs or similar activity
D. During headache, at least one of the following
    a. Nausea and/or vomiting
    b. Photophobia and phonophobia
E. At least one of the following
    a. History, physical, and neurologic examinations do not suggest other specified disorders or
    b. If suggested, the disorder was ruled out or
    c. Headache did not occur in close temporal relation to it

Migraine with aura (previously "classic" migraine)
A. At least 5 attacks fulfilling B
B. At least 3 of the following 4 characteristics
    a. One or more fully reversible aura symptoms indicating focal cerebral cortical and/or brainstem dysfunction
    b. At least one aura symptom develops gradually over more than 4 minutes or 2 or more symptoms occur in succession
    c. No aura symptom lasts more than 60 min
    d. Headache follows aura with free interval of less than 60 minutes, or begins before or simultaneously with the aura
C. At least one of the following
    a. History and physical and neurologic examinations do not suggest other specified disorders or
    b. If suggested, the disorder was ruled out or
    c. Headache did not occur in close temporal relation to it

Patients can experience both of the above-described types of migraine, and the individual characteristics of the headache may change from one episode to another. The diagnosis is solely made by history.

In hemiplegic migraine, the neurologic symptom is often weakness but may also be sensory or speech. Total hemiplegia may occur and may be ipsilateral to the side of the reported headache. Seizures and vertigo are rare. This variant of migraine is usually familial and occurs in a setting of other forms of migraine. Ophthalmoplegic migraine, where a third-nerve palsy is present, ipsilateral to the side of the headache, is extremely uncommon. Most cases of suspected ophthalmoplegic migraine are in fact due to other pathologic entities, particularly aneurysms. The diagnosis cannot be made without excluding aneurysms and other causes such as tumor, arteritis, and sinusitis.

In childhood migraine, the necessary history may be difficult to obtain, and the diagnosis may have to await the development of a recognizable pattern. Vomiting is very common as is motion sickness, and acute crises of abdominal pain ("abdominal migraine") or "migraine equivalent" can occur. The headache is usually brief, 1 to 6 hours. Epilepsy is common in patients with pediatric migraine and is unassociated with attacks of headache. Attacks may be triggered by trivial head trauma. Males are more commonly affected. Acute confusional states may also occur, simulating a toxic psychosis.

Many factors (Table 8-7) are felt to contribute to migraine. Some, such as relationship to menstrual cycle, are commonly accepted. Others, such as food sensitivity, are controversial. Other variants of migraine, such as cluster headache, are described in Table 8-8.

Many agents have been used in the treatment of migraine. Therapy with narcotic medications is the subject of controversy. Some physicians, wary of chronic headache patients as potential substance abusers, recognizing that narcotics do little to affect the underlying pathophysiology and having concern for perpetuating medication-overuse headaches and potential substance abuse, are reluctant to give narcotic analgesics. Guidelines usually discourage their use,[28] find little evidence to support their use,[29] or ignore their use.[30] Other physicians recognize the value of therapeutic doses of narcotic analgesics as rescue medications in the acute painful phase. The primary goal of therapy is elimination of the headache, not simply overpowering the pain with opiates. In general, nonnarcotic medications such as prochlorperazine, DHE, or triptans are used initially or in combination with narcotics, reserved for rescue in selected cases. However, many migraine

TABLE 8-7

FACTORS ASSOCIATATED WITH MIGRAINE

- Menstrual: First day of period or before; decreased headache after third-month pregnancy; rarely increased
- Photogenic: Flashing lights, glare
- Food: Alcohol, wine, chocolate, milk, cheese, fruit
- Weather: Approaching low pressure
- Psychological: Both "good" and "bad" events
- Excessive sleep
- Heredity

TABLE 8-8 —————————————————————————
OTHER MIGRAINOUS HEADACHES

Cluster headache: Male predominance, age of onset 10–60 years, rarely familial, attacks provoked by alcohol, nitrates, sudden agonizing unilateral pain deep to eye, restlessness
- Conjunctival injection, lacrimation, rhinorrhea, small pupil, ptosis (partial Horner's syndrome)
- 10–30 min for each attack, attacks may "cluster" for days or weeks and disappear for years

Basilar migraine
- Rare: Patient usually has other sudden visual symptoms of migraine, including cortical blindness followed by a combination of: vertigo, ataxia, dysarthria, tinnitus, paresthesia, and then gradual decreased level of consciousness or confusional state and severe pounding occipital headache, nausea, and vomiting; usually females, under 21 years, with family history of migraine

medication regimens exist because none are universally effective nor without their drawbacks. There are no studies comparing the effectiveness of every medication used for migraine against every other one, especially in the ER setting. The choice of medication will depend upon the patient's past medication use and experience, the preferred route of administration, and the cost; but the top performing parenteral medications, in rank order, seem to be prochlorperazine, metoclopramide, droperidol, and triptans.

Chronic prophylaxis against migraine now includes too vast an array of medications to be reviewed here. Local injections and nerve blocks may have their place in the management of difficult cases, but are seldom used in the acute care setting. Corticosteroids may be useful for prolonged migraine or to prevent recurrence. Triptans are useful and may be self-administered in some patients. Table 8-9 lists some of the medications and selected adult dosages that are used for treating migraines.

NONMIGRAINOUS VASCULAR HEADACHES

There are several other causes for headaches with "vascular" characteristics (i.e., pounding, worse with exertion, pulse-synchronous). The most common of these is "fever headache."

This pulsatile headache occurs in a variety of systemic syndromes and is so common that the headache is usually the feeling that causes people to believe their temperature is elevated. Some systemic illnesses such as shigellosis have headache as a prominent part of the symptom complex.

Other causes of nonmigrainous vascular headache are listed in Table 8-10. Only a few will be described here.

Carbon monoxide (CO) intoxication is an important cause of headache, which may be reported as episodic or completely resolved by the time a patient presents in the acute care setting. Carboxyhemoglobin blood values may also have returned to normal or be in

TABLE 8-9 ────────────────────────────

MEDICATION FOR MIGRAINE (WITH SELECTED ADULT SINGLE DOSAGES)

- Phenothiazines—prochlorperazine (2–10 mg IV/IM), chlorpromazine (0.1 mg/kg IV/IM)
- Butyrophenones—droperidol (2–5 mg IV/IM), haloperidol (5 mg IV/IM)
- Dihydroergotamine (DHE) (0.5–1 mg IM/IV, 0.5–1 mg intranasal × 2)
- Triptans—sumatriptan (6 mg SQ), naratriptan (1–2.5 mg PO), almotriptan (6.25–12.5 mg PO), zolmitriptan (1.25–2.5 mg PO), rizatriptan (5–10 mg PO), frovatriptan (2.5 mg PO), eletriptan (20–40 mg PO)
- Valproate sodium IV (500 mg IV over 15 min)
- Ketorolac (15–30 mg IM/IV)
- Metoclopramide (2–10 mg IV)
- Diphenhydramine (25–50 mg IV/IM)
- Corticosteroid—dexamethasone (10 mg IV)
- Opioids—hydromorphone, methadone, nalbuphine, butorphanol, meperidine, morphine, codeine
- Common analgesics—NSAIDs, aspirin, acetaminophen
- Caffeine

nondiagnostic ranges while some headache lingers. Assessing the patient's environment for potential sources of leakage of products of combustion may be reasonable and potentially lifesaving.

Hypertension

Hypertension is not a usual cause of headache. This commonly occurring medical condition may occur in patients with other common causes of headache. However, hypertension

TABLE 8-10 ────────────────────────────

NONMIGRAINOUS VASCULAR HEADACHES

- Fever: Pneumonia, tonsillitis, septicemia, typhoid fever, tularemia, influenza, measles, mumps, mononucleosis, malaria, shigellosis
- Substances: Carbon monoxide, lead, benzene, carbon tetrachloride, insecticides, nitrites ("hotdog headache"), toluene, nitrobenzene, hydrogen sulfide, methanol, monosodium glutamate ("Chinese restaurant syndrome"), alcohol
- Drugs: Nitrates, indomethacin, oral progestogens, vasodilators
- Withdrawal: Ergots, caffeine, amphetamines, many phenothiazines, alcohol, opioids
- Other: Hypoxia, hypoglycemia, hypercarbia, anemia, toxemia of pregnancy, hypertensive encephalopathy, hypothyroidism, hyperthyroidism, hypoadrenalism, vasomotor rhinitis, altitude, effort, cerebrovascular accidents (CVAs), coital headache

TABLE 8-11

POSTTRAUMATIC HEADACHE

- Chronic subdural hematoma
- Subdural hygroma
- Hydrocephalus
- Skull fracture
- Meningitis
- Brain abscess
- Subarachnoid hemorrhage
- Muscle contraction (tension)
- Neck trauma
- Psychogenic

itself is unlikely the etiology of headache even at moderately elevated blood pressure levels (180 mm Hg systolic, 110 mm Hg diastolic).[31] The role that hypertension plays in the generation of headache is controversial; however, many patients and their physicians assume that their headache is caused by hypertension because blood pressure may be elevated at the time of the headache. Ambulatory monitoring of moderate elevations of blood pressure, along with headache diaries, fails to establish a cause-and-effect relationship between blood pressure and headache. Finally, hypertensive encephalopathy is a more distinct syndrome than simple elevated blood pressure (see Chapter 4).

Cerebrovascular Accident

The three common pathologic processes usually encompassed in the nonspecific term cerebrovascular accident (CVA), also called "stroke" are embolism, thrombosis, and hemorrhage. Each may be associated with headache. The neurologic examination will form the basis for the diagnosis of CVA, but the presence of headache does not help to differentiate among these three processes. Dramatic, sudden onset headache should suggest SAH.

Posttraumatic Headache

After head trauma, headache is extremely common. It may be prolonged in a posttraumatic syndrome (see Chapter 10). Several other entities that cause sustained posttraumatic headache are listed in Table 8-11.

TEMPORAL ARTERITIS AND OTHER VASCULITIDES

Inflammation of the scalp and intracranial arteries is a cause for headache in the elderly and others with predisposing medical conditions. Left untreated, its consequences, particularly blindness, can be devastating. Temporal arteritis (TA) usually begins after age 55, with an average age of onset of 72 years, is more common in women, and can present without the classic accompanying jaw claudication, fever, malaise, weight loss, anemia, and polymyalgia rheumatica early on in its course that characterize the typical disease.

Tender, bulging temporal, or occipital arteries are not invariable findings, especially early on in the course of the disease. Jaw claudication and diplopia are the best historical predictors of TA, and a prominent, beaded or enlarged temporal artery is the most reliable physical examination finding. Elevated sedimentation rates almost invariably occur, but the specificity of this finding is low. However, a normal sedimentation rate makes TA extremely unlikely.[32] Definitive diagnosis by temporal artery biopsy need not always be performed in the acute setting in an obvious case and should not delay administration of corticosteroids to prevent visual loss (visual loss occurs suddenly in 50% of patients who ultimately develop visual loss). A brief course of corticosteroids will not obscure the pathologic findings on temporal artery biopsy specimens. However, biopsy is usually eventually done to be certain of the diagnosis, as long-term steroid administration can be problematic in elderly patients.

Other systemic vasculitides such as periarteritis nodosa, rheumatoid arthritis, scleroderma, polymyositis, dermatomyositis, erythema nodosum, and Sjögren's syndrome should bring vasculitis to mind as a cause of headache. Other causes of hypersensitivity vasculitis, such as drug reactions, systemic lupus erythematosus, Henoch-Schönlein purpura, etc., may be considered in the appropriate setting.

Uncommon Vascular Headaches

Several uncommon entities should be mentioned. Coital headache, a benign, well-described entity,[33] may begin during sexual arousal or at orgasm, or immediately after orgasm. The pain is sudden and usually occipital. Many patients with this condition also have a history of migraine headaches. Subarachnoid hemorrhage can also occur during sexual intercourse. Effort headache may occur with athletic efforts, such as running, but is also a well-described component of posterior fossa tumors, which rarely may need to be excluded. Cough headache is another similar entity, as is the headache that occurs after the exertional effort involved in sneezing and defecating. While these are usually benign, a history of recent increase in symptoms should prompt consideration of further evaluation.

HIGH CSF PRESSURE SYNDROMES AND TUMORS

Although headache is a common early symptom with posterior fossa tumors, it may not necessarily be an early sign with supratentorial tumors, except those lying adjacent to pain-sensitive (meningeal) structures (e.g., meningiomas). Intraventricular tumors, such as colloid cysts, may suddenly occlude the third ventricle by a ball valve action and cause a very sudden headache (classically when the patient is supine), and sometimes syncope or even sudden death.

Pituitary tumors may cause a sudden headache from hemorrhage or necrosis of the tumor. The resultant syndrome (pituitary apoplexy, visual loss, and bloody cerebrospinal fluid) may simulate SAH. The reaction in the CSF may also simulate meningitis as an aseptic reaction to tumor contents. Brain abscesses may act like tumors and may present with similar symptoms and a history of febrile illness, but may not demonstrate fever at presentation, making suspicion of an infectious etiology problematic. Children with

TABLE 8-12
HIGH INTRACRANIAL PRESSURE AND MASSES

- Tumors: Supratentorial—pituitary, meningiomas, gliomas; Posterior fossa; Metastatic
- Intraventricular
- Brain abscess
- Subdural hematoma
- Vascular malformations
- Pseudotumor
- Intracranial venous thrombosis
- Postpartum seizures
- Cerebral edema
- Hypertensive encephalopathy

headache secondary to brain tumor very commonly have abnormalities on neurologic and neuro-ophthalmologic examination, which is by far the best screening technique. Table 8-12 lists causes of high CSF pressure syndromes.

Pseudotumor Cerebri

Pseudotumor cerebri, a rare condition, is also termed idiopathic intracranial hypertension and refers to a condition characterized by elevated intracranial pressure, headache, and papilledema. Although it typically occurs in obese women in late adolescence or early adulthood, it may also occur in men and children. The headache typically develops over weeks to months and may wax and wane. The condition may last for many months. There are usually no neurologic findings other than papilledema, although sixth nerve palsy may occur. Symptoms include headache, nausea, vomiting, pulsatile intracranial noises, transient visual obscurations, and diplopia.[34] The cause of pseudotumor cerebri is unknown. Many factors have been implicated, often anecdotally, such as menstrual irregularities, pregnancy, corticosteroids, weight gain, hypervitaminosis A, oral retinoids, and tetracycline administration. Pseudotumor cerebri is a diagnosis of exclusion. By definition, one must exclude other causes for elevated intracranial pressure, principally those of mass effect, chronic meningitis, and intracranial dural or cortical venous thrombosis. A CT scan will rule out hydrocephalus and mass effects, but contrast-enhanced MRI, MRV, or CTV may be necessary to assess for dural venous sinus thrombosis or chronic meningitis.

In pseudotumor, the cerebrospinal fluid opening pressure at lumbar puncture is often between 250 and 400 mm H_2O, but CSF analyses should otherwise be normal.

LOW CSF PRESSURE

The headache of low CSF pressure is worsened by an upright posture and relieved by recumbency. The most common cause is post-lumbar puncture. Bed rest or the head-down position after lumbar puncture does not decrease the incidence of this problem.[35,36]

Spontaneous intracranial hypotension, a syndrome of spontaneously low CSF pressure with the characteristics of a post-lumbar puncture headache, has also been discussed. This syndrome is believed to be due to spontaneous CSF leaks somewhere in the spinal canal. The headache usually occurs within 15 minutes of being upright, but it may be delayed for hours. Headache relief with assuming a recumbent position usually occurs within 30 minutes. The CSF may have up to 200 cells/mm^3, usually lymphocytes and elevated protein. There are several distinct MRI findings including brain "sagging," abnormal meningeal enhancement, and chronic subdural hematomas. CSF pressure when measured with the patient supine is a low of 0 to 60 mm H$_2$O.[37]

Headaches related to a recent lumbar puncture or spontaneous CSF leak may respond to bed rest or a blood patch. While the use of caffeine (500 mg caffeine sodium benzoate in 1 liter fluid IV over 1 h) for postspinal headache is popular, the evidence supporting it is scant, suggests only short-term efficacy, and is of questionable quality.[38,39]

TENSION HEADACHE

Sustained scalp and neck muscle contraction may cause pain that outlasts the contraction. Whereas psychic tension may be the underlying cause, muscle tension is the final common pathway to a variety of conditions. It is one of the most common causes of headache. In its purest form, the pain is usually bilateral, dragging, or tight and bandlike in character; it is usually constant and decreases with sleep. It may encompass the entire head or only the back of the head or neck. It is not associated with nausea and vomiting, an associated prodrome, a pulsatile character and it is not exacerbated with exertion. Rarely, photophobia or phonophobia is present, but not both. Tension headache may coexist with, or be a secondary phenomenon in patients with other primary headache syndromes, such as migraine.

NEURALGIAS

The chief characteristics of the neuralgias are the sudden, brief, lancinating character of the pain, which are usually precipitated by a tactile stimulus. This stimulus may be cold air, touch, or shaving in trigeminal neuralgia (tic douloureaux), or swallowing, as in glossopharyngeal neuralgia. See Chapter 5 for additional comments on trigeminal neuralgia.

ARTERIAL DISSECTION

Nontraumatic or traumatic carotid or vertebral artery dissection may cause sudden severe headache, usually in addition to neck pain. Neck manipulation or injury, at times trivial, may be associated with vascular dissections,[40] and there may be a history of similar occurrences in family members. Vascular dissections also are associated with the presence of connective tissue disorders. Vascular dissections are rare conditions but can cause ischemic symptoms, particularly in young patients, due to thromboemboli arising at the site of dissection or due to frank occlusion of a cervicocranial blood vessel. The pain, however, may not be intense or different from other headaches; in such cases, the diagnosis can only be suspected once neurologic deficits occur, which may not be for days or weeks.[41] With carotid dissection, local involvement of the cervical sympathetic chain may cause an associated ipsilateral Horner's syndrome.[42] Although most causes of sudden severe headache, especially without an associated neurologic deficit, can be eliminated with a normal CT, lumbar puncture, and very few to no laboratory tests, arterial dissection cannot be ruled out with these tests. CT angiography and/or MR angiography have replaced formal endovascular angiography for the evaluation of the majority of patients in whom a vascular dissection is of clinical concern.

MISCELLANEOUS CAUSES OF HEADACHE

Other causes of headache, some common, such as sinusitis and others rare, such as Tolosa-Hunt syndrome, are listed in Table 8-13, along with selected diagnostic characteristics.

THE PATIENT WITH SUSPECTED MASS VERSUS MENINGITIS

An uncommon but difficult clinical scenario occasionally arises with clinical suspicion of an intracranial mass versus meningitis or brain abscess. Whereas in their respective pure forms these syndromes rarely overlap, the real world is full of contradictory examples.

TABLE 8-13

MISCELLANEOUS CAUSES OF HEADACHE

- Sinusitis
- Dental disease
- Temporomandibular joint (Costen's syndrome)
- Ocular: Iritis, orbital inflammation, cavernous sinus thrombosis, acute narrow-angle glaucoma
- Ice cream headache
- Postseizure
- Cervical spine disease
- Pheochromocytoma: Onset over minutes, bilateral, offset usually less than 1 h, throbbing, perspiration, palpitation, pallor, tremor, nausea, elevated blood pressure during paroxysm
- Tolosa-Hunt syndrome (painful ophthalmoplegia): Unilateral pain near eye, ophthalmoplegia (pupil usually spared), elevated sedimentation rate, optic involvement, steroid responsive, inflammatory process, etiology unknown
- Raeder's paratrigeminal syndrome: Rapid onset, severe frontotemporal burning, aching, ptosis, miosis with normal sweating, involvement of cranial nerves II, III, IV, V, and VI; multiple etiologies
- Reversible cerebral vasoconstriction syndrome
- Chiari malformations

For example, a patient may be postictal and have a focal neurologic deficit, confusion, and lethargy from a mass lesion and fever, from aspiration pneumonia or other cause. However, when practicing medicine prospectively, one may not have sufficient information to generate these diagnoses. However, the clinical presentation could also be one of postictal state and fever from meningitis alone. A clinically stiff neck may arise from a posterior fossa tumor and cerebellar tonsillar herniation, or a neck injury. Patients may have a coagulation defect, from either medication or a medical condition, which may predispose to a mass lesion such as subdural hematoma, which could represent a relative contraindication to lumbar puncture. In these cases, one is clinically pulled in different directions by opposing factors. Early lumbar puncture and immediate institution of antibiotics is called for with meningitis, but these measures may be dangerous in the presence of an intracranial lesion with mass effect. CT scans, if rapidly available, should be performed to rule out intracranial mass effects. However, in some settings, CT scanners are not always immediately available. One possible solution is to treat the patient as if meningitis were present with antibiotics appropriate to organisms common in that age group after obtaining blood cultures or other (but not CSF) cultures, while awaiting a definitive study to rule out an intracranial mass lesion. Once an intracranial mass lesion has been excluded, a lumbar puncture can then safely be performed, and the CSF characteristics of meningitis will not have been obscured, sometimes even after 48 hours of antibiotic treatment.[43] After this time, the value of the CSF culture may be lost. Antigen testing of cerebrospinal fluid for *Haemophilus influenzae, N. meningitidis,* and *Streptococcus pneumoniae* can be performed, but are rarely diagnostic; blood tests or other body fluid cultures may be helpful.

REFERENCES

1. Dickerman RL et al. Management of non-traumatic headache in university hospital emergency room. *Headache*. 1979;19:391.
2. Fitzpatrick R, Hopkins A. Referrals to neurologists for headaches not due to structural disease. *J Neurol Neurosurg Psychiatry*. 1981;44:1061-1067.
3. Vinson DR. Treatment patterns of isolated benign headache in US emergency departments. *Ann Emerg Med*. 2002;39(3):215-222.
4. Schreiber CP, Hutchinson S, Webster CJ, et al. Prevalence of migraine in patients with a history of self-reported or physician diagnosed "sinus" headache. *Arch Int Med*. 2004;164(16): 1769-1772.
5. Diehr P et al. Acute headaches: presenting symptoms and diagnostic rules to identify patients with tension and migraine headache. *J Chron Dis*. 1981;34:147-158.
6. Bottieau E, Clerinx J, Vander Enden E, et al. Fever after a stay in the tropics: diagnostic predictors of the leading tropical conditions. *Medicine*. 2007;86(1):18-25.
7. Wichmann O et al. Severe dengue virus infection in travelers: risk factors and laboratory indicators. *J Infect Dis*. 2007;195:1089.
8. Lipton RB et al. Migraine diagnosis and treatment: results from the American Migraine Study II. *Headache*. 2001;41:638-645.
9. Knaus W et al. CT for headache: cost/benefit for subarachnoid hemorrhage. *AJR Am J Roentgenol*. 1981;136:537.
10. Edlow JA Caplan LR. Avoiding pitfalls in the diagnosis of subarachnoid hemorrhage. *N Engl J Med*. 2000;342:29-36.

11. Lewis DW, Ashal S, Dahl G, et al. Practice parameter: evaluation of children and adolescents with recurrent headaches. *Neurology*. 2002;59:490-498.

12. Lewis DH, Qureshi F. Acute headache in children and adolescents presenting to emergency department. *Headache*. 2000;40(3):200-203.

13. Burton LJ, Quinn B, Pratt-Cheney JL, et al. Headache in a pediatric emergency department. *Pediatr Emerg Care*. 1997;13(1):1-4.

14. Kan L, Nagelberg J, Maytal J. Headaches in a pediatric emergency department: etiology, imaging and treatment. *Headache*. 2000;40(1):25-29.

15. Leicht MJ. Non-traumatic headache in the emergency department. *Ann Emerg Med*. 1980;9: 404-409.

16. Kowalski RG, Classen J, Kreiter KT, et al. Initial misdiagnosis and outcome after subarachnoid hemorrhage. *JAMA*. 2004;291(7):866-869.

17. Fontanarosa PB. Recognition of subarachnoid hemorrhage. *Ann Emerg Med*. 1989;18(11): 1199-1205.

18. Morgenstern LB, Luna-Gonzales H, Huber JC. Worst headache and subarachnoid hemorrhage: prospective, modern computed tomography and spinal fluid analysis. *Ann Emerg Med*. 1998;32(3)297-304.

19. Brisman JL, Song JK, Newell DW. Cerebral Aneurysms. *N Engl J Med*. 2006;355:928-939.

20. Schull MJ. Lumbar puncture first; an alternative model for the investigation of lone acute sudden headache. *Acad Emerg Med*. 1999;6:131-136.

21. Edlow JA, Panagos PD, Godwin SA, et al. Clinical policy: critical issues in the evaluation and management of patients presenting to the emergency department with acute headache. *Ann Emerg Med*. 2002;39(1):108-122.

22. Mark DG, Pines JM. The detection of nontraumatic subarachnoid hemorrhage: still a diagnostic challenge. *Am J Emerg Med*. 2006;24:859-863.

23. Wardlaw JM, White PM. The detection and management of unruptured intracranial aneurysms. *Brain*. 2000;123:205-221.

24. Smetana GW. The diagnostic value of historical features in primary headache syndromes. *Arch Int Med*. 2000;160:2729-2737.

25. Detsky ME, McDonald DR, Baerlocker MO, et al. Does this patient with headache have a migraine or need neuroimaging. *JAMA*. 2006;296(10):1274-1283.

26. Headache Classification Committee of the international headache society. Classification and diagnostic criteria for headache disorders, cranial neuralgias and facial pain. *Cephalgia*. 1988;8(suppl 7):1-96.

27. Friedman WB, Hochberg ML, Esses D, et al. Applying the International Classification of Headache Disorders the emergency department: an assessment of reproducibility and the frequency with which a unique diagnosis can be assigned to every acute headache patient. *Ann Emerg Med*. 2007;49(4):409-419.

28. Ducharme J. Canadian Association of Emergency Physicians guidelines for the acute management of migraine headache. *J Emerg Med*. 1999;17(1):137-144.

29. Members of the task force: Evers S, Afra J, Frese A, et al. EFNS guideline on the drug treatment of migraine—report of an EFNS task force. *Eur J Neurol*. 2006;13:560-572.

30. Lewis D, Ashwal S, Hershey A. Standards Subcommittee and the Practice Committee of the Child Neurology and adolescents: report of the American Academy of Neurology Quality Practice Parameter: pharmacological treatment of migraine headache in children. *Neurology*. 2004;63:2215-2224.

31. Karras DJ et al. Lack of relationship between hypertension-associated symptoms and blood pressure in hypertensive ED patients. *Am J Emerg Med*. 2005;23(2):106.

32. Widico CR, Newman DH. Does this patient have temporal arteritis? *Ann Emerg Med*. 2005;45:85-87.

33. Porter M, Jankovic J. Benign coital cephalalgia: differential diagnosis and treatment. *Arch Neurol*. 1981;38:710-712.

34. Wall M. Idiopathic intracranial hypertension. *Neurol Clin*. 1991;9(1):73-95.

35. Handler CE et al. Posture and lumbar puncture headache—a controlled trial in 50 patients. *J R Soc Med*. 1982;75:404.

36. Carbaat PAT, Van Crevel H. Lumbar puncture headache: controlled study on the preventive effect of 24 hours of bedrest. *Lancet*. 1981;2:1133.

37. Schievink WI. Spontaneous spinal cerebrospinal fluid leaks and intracranial hypotension. *JAMA*. 2006;295(19)2286-2296.

38. Halker RB, Demaerschalk BM, Wellik KE, et al. Caffeine for the prevention and treatment of postdural puncture headache: debunking the myth. *Neurologist*. 2007;13(5):323-327.

39. Frank RL. Lumbar puncture and post-dural puncture headaches: implications for the emergency physician. *J Emerg Med*. 2008;35(2):149-157.

40. Showalter W et al. Vertebral artery dissection. *Acad Emerg Med*. 1997;4:991-995.

41. Yoshimoto Y, Wakai S. Unruptured intracranial vertebral artery dissection. *Stroke*. 1997;28:370-374.

42. Stapf C, Elkind MS, Mohr JP. Carotid artery dissection. *Annu Rev Med*. 2000;51:329-347.

43. Blazer S et al. Effect of antibiotic treatment on cerebrospinal fluid. *Am J Clin Pathol*. 1983;80:386.

C H A P T E R

9

ACUTE DOUBLE VISION, BLINDNESS, AND ABNORMAL PUPILS

In emergency and urgent care settings, complaints of sudden decrease in visual acuity or diplopia are not common, but when they occur they may be symptoms of both serious and eminently treatable disease. The initial evaluation of such complaints should establish the difference between structural and nonstructural visual system disease and permit the physician to proceed with a rapid, specific diagnosis and appropriate treatment.

HISTORY

The historical features needed to diagnose acute visual problems are specific but few in number (Table 9-1). The term *blurred vision* is used by patients in such a broad manner that it must be clarified before further history or physical examination is undertaken.

Lateralization

The first question is to determine whether a visual problem is monocular or binocular. A patient can usually tell through simple observation whether one or both eyes are involved. As a general rule, visual problems such as monocular decreased vision or monocular diplopia represent structural disease lying anterior to the optic chiasm or disease involving the eye. Bilateral visual problems usually involve diffuse toxic, infectious, or metabolic processes; posterior circulation; or vascular occlusions. Rarely, structural lesions in the area of the pituitary gland will cause bilateral visual loss.[1,2]

Rate of Onset

Decreased vision that occurs within a matter of minutes represents vascular disease or retinal problems.[3] This may be in the form of embolic or hemorrhagic lesions and may involve

TABLE 9-1

HISTORICAL FEATURES OF
NEURO-OPHTHALMOLOGIC SYMPTOMS

Lateralization (right/left or both visual fields)
Associated symptoms
Rate of onset
Drugs/medications
Pain and trauma

only the visual system or larger areas of the brain.[4] Other disease processes will have time courses that will help to differentiate their various etiologies, i.e., infection, trauma.

Associated Symptoms

Sudden changes in visual acuity or diplopia associated with headache should be considered an urgent neurologic condition. The visual system from the retina moving posterior is essentially insensitive to pain unless meningeal irritation is also involved.[5] Any lesion that will give immediate eye symptoms and severe pain should be considered to be involving the pain-sensitive structures of the eye and head. Pain-sensitive structures from the retina forward to the cornea should be visible and/or testable on physical examination. Other acute painful lesions with visual change should be considered vascular in etiology until proven otherwise.

Trauma

Trauma from the front of the globe to the occipital cortex can affect visual acuity and coordinated eye movements. Along with globe and orbit evaluation, attention should be paid to signs of trauma to the areas of the posterior skull and neck.

Drugs

Heavy use of alcohol and tobacco should be noted along with the patient's over-the-counter medications and prescription drugs, including eye drops. It may be necessary to ask specifically about the use of vitamins, laxatives, pain medications, and tranquilizers. Crack cocaine and even excessive licorice ingestion have been associated with acute visual changes.[6,7]

Pain

Pain in the eye is generally a local phenomenon. If anesthetic drops relieve the pain, it is generally a conjunctival or corneal problem. If pain persists despite topical anesthesia, an intraocular process must be considered.

GENERAL EXAMINATION

The general physical examination of the patient with visual complaints should be centered around the head and neck region and the cardiovascular system (Table 9-2).[8] The general

TABLE 9-2 ——————————————————————————————

EXAMINATION OF ACUTE VISUAL COMPLAINTS

1. General physical examination, including general eye; slit lamp, and funduscopic examination as appropriate
2. Neurologic examination, including visual acuity, extraocular movements, pupils
3. Specific neuro-ophthalmologic testing as appropriate:
   a. Marcus Gunn pupil
   b. Optokinetic nystagmus
   c. Red glass test

appearance of the patient, with particular attention to focal symmetry, position, and prop-tosis, should be noted. Evidence of trauma should be sought. The position of the eyes within the head and their relationship to the orbital rims (exophthalmus, enophthalmos) should be noted. Palpation of the orbital rims and skull is necessary in traumatic situations.

The neck should be evaluated for signs of trauma or mass lesions. In cases of sudden monocular visual loss, the neck should be examined for bruits. Palpation of the arteries of the head, particularly the temporal arteries, should be performed in elderly patients with a sudden loss of vision.

Ophthalmologic Examination

For a summary of the examination, see Table 9-2.

Visual Acuity

The most important part in examining an eye complaint is visual acuity testing. If cor-rective lenses are generally worn, the patient should be examined while wearing them in order to obtain the best corrected vision. If the patient has relatively poor visual acuity or the corrective lenses are not available, the pinhole technique can be employed.[9]

Pinhole testing is performed by having the patient read the eye chart while looking through a card with small holes in the center. Pinhole testing cuts down all extraneous visual input and allows the patient to focus light only on the fovea. Pinhole vision is gen-erally the best vision one can hope to get with corrective lenses. A patient whose vision improves substantially by use of the pinhole has a refractive error and not a neurologic decrease in vision.

Visual Fields

In the acute care setting, visual field testing can be done most simply by the confronta-tion[9] method (Fig. 9-1). The patient should look at the examiner while the examiner's fin-gers are moved simultaneously in the major visual quadrants. Each eye is tested sepa-rately. If the patient detects simultaneous movement of two fingers moved on opposite sides of the body, little else need to be done. If the patient fails to recognize one of the moving fingers, then the stimuli must be given independently. If the patient can recognize stimuli given independently but cannot detect movement done simultaneously, then he/she is illustrating visual suppression or extinction. This is usually a sign of nondominant

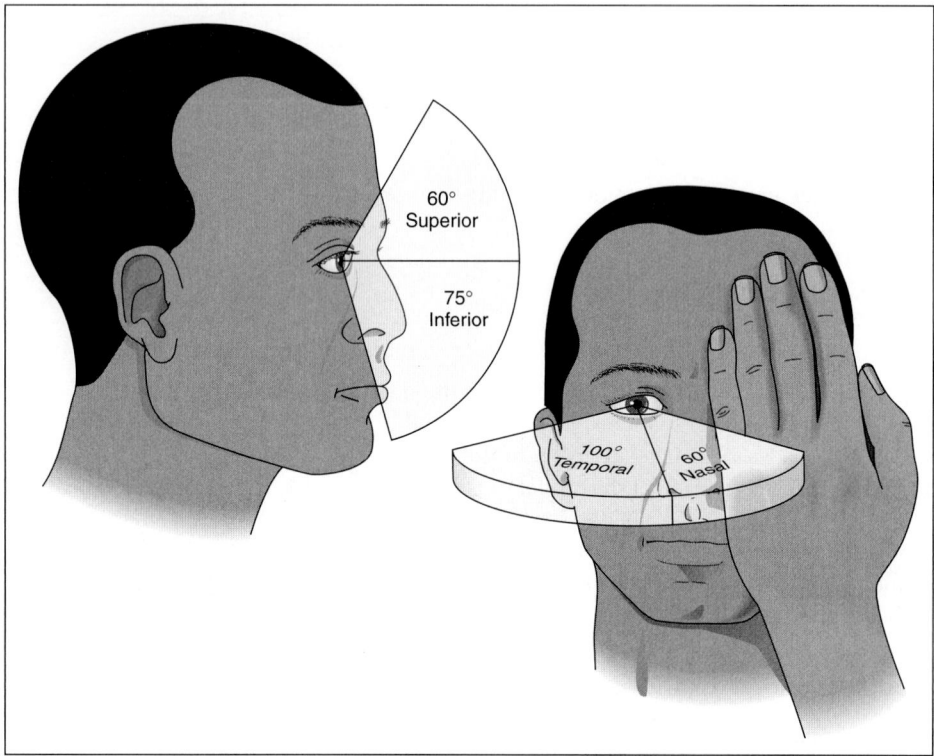

FIGURE 9-1 **Normal limits of the visual field.** (Reproduced with permission from Simon et al. *Clinical Neurology.* 7th ed. New York, NY: McGraw-Hill; 2009.)

parietal lobe disease, as opposed to an involvement of the visual system per se. This finding can be checked by giving other sensory stimuli simultaneously on other portions of the patient's body and noting whether a consistent lateralization of such suppression exists. Sophisticated visual field testing with various-sized objects and tangent screens is not usually available or necessary in the acute care setting. Visual field testing should be reserved for patients with a segmented or partial visual loss.

Slit Lamp and Funduscopic Examination

Most causes of decreased vision involve only the eye and are not related to nervous system elements. Careful slit lamp examination, with particular attention to the cornea, anterior chamber, and lens abnormalities, is helpful. Funduscopic examination to view the condition of the vitreous body, retina, and optic nerve head may also be important.

Intraocular Pressure

Intraocular pressure recording with a Schiotz instrument, an applanation tonometer, or other appropriate measuring device should be performed in cases of decreased vision in which glaucoma may be suspected due to pain, conjunctival injection, and decreased movement of the pupil.

Neuro-ophthalmologic Testing

Basic neuro-ophthalmologic testing can be done in the emergent or urgent setting with relative ease and little special equipment. The following three tests may prove particularly useful in the evaluation of selected acute visual complaints.

Marcus Gunn Pupil

The Marcus Gunn pupil sign, or the swinging flashlight sign, should be elicited in patients with decreased vision. The midbrain nuclei sense the total amount of light received through both eyes to set pupillary size. The Marcus Gunn pupil response tests to see whether a decrease in total light is actually being perceived by an eye. An intense light is shined in the affected eye, and the size and reactivity of the pupils are noted. The light is then moved to the supposedly good eye, and the pupils are again observed. The light is then moved back to the involved eye, and the size of pupils is checked. As one moves from the eye with poor vision to the eye with normal vision, the pupils should constrict. As the light is moved from the eye with good vision to the eye with poor vision, the pupils should dilate because less total light is actually reaching midbrain nuclei. The Marcus Gunn pupil sign is nonspecific but extremely sensitive. A disease process seriously decreasing vision that is anterior to the optic chiasm should have a positive Marcus Gunn pupil sign. By definition, a positive Marcus Gunn sign is when the light source is moved from the good eye to the eye of decreased visual acuity and both pupils dilate. This test is not helpful if both optic nerves are equally involved. A positive Marcus Gunn test is pathognomonic for optic or retrobulbar neuritis.

Optokinetic Nystagmus

Optokinetic nystagmus (OKN) is a simple yet effective test to distinguish cortical from noncortical blindness. OKN can be induced in normal subjects by continuous movement of a series of visual targets across the visual field. This is usually accomplished using paper with narrow lines or a rotating drum with stripes. Normal eyes will fix on a stripe, involuntarily following this target for a short distance, and then quickly return to primary gaze, where they will pick up another target to follow. On a repeated basis, this results in nystagmus. OKN can be induced in any direction. The presence of intact OKN means that the visual input from the eyes has reached the occipital cortex and from there has gone to connections in the brainstem and back to the extraocular control centers of the eyes through the third, fourth, and sixth cranial nerves. These deviations have been monitored by anterior cortical visual centers and corrective instructions sent to the brainstem by the cortex. The presence of OKN virtually ensures that the patient is not blind.[8]

The absence of OKN with preservation of the pupillary light reflex in the face of sudden visual loss is strongly suggestive of cortical blindness involving the occipital lobes. Note that a very small group of people who do repetitive spinning and whirling motions (i.e., professional ice skaters, roller skaters, and others) have suppressed their OKN and so it will not be present.[8]

Red Glass Testing

Red glass testing is done to separate double images in patients complaining of binocular diplopia. The test is performed by having a colored lens placed over one eye with a white light used for testing. The covered eye will then have a colored image, and the uncovered

Right		Left
Right upward gaze Right superior rectus Left inferior oblique	Upward gaze	*Left upper gaze* Left superior rectus Right inferior oblique
Right lateral gaze Right lateral rectus Left medial rectus	Primary gaze	*Left lateral gaze* Left lateral rectus Right medial rectus
Right downward gaze Right inferior rectus Left superior oblique	Downward gaze	*Left downward gaze* Left inferior rectus Right superior oblique

FIGURE 9-2   Muscle pairs in extraocular movements.

eye will have a white image. Extraocular movement testing is then performed. In all nine regions tested (Fig. 9-2) in the normal patient, there will be one image that will represent the fusion of the white and colored light. If these colors are not perfectly fused, separate images will be present, indicating diplopia. If the colored image appears on the same side as the eye being tested, this is considered uncrossed diplopia. A sixth nerve palsy would be considered an example of such a diplopia (Fig. 9-3).

If the image appears on the opposite side of the white light from that of the eye being tested with the colored lens, this is termed a crossed diplopia, a type seen with third nerve palsies.

It is important to remember that diplopia will be at its maximum when the field of action of the involved nerve or muscle is to be maximally tested. For example, if a right sixth nerve palsy is present, looking laterally to the left would cause no diplopia, since the right lateral rectus muscle is not involved in this action. Looking laterally to the right, however, which is the principal area of action of the involved muscle, will produce the maximum diplopia.[8]

The second basic rule of the test is that when diplopia exists, the most lateral or outside image is always the false image. One can determine which eye is creating the false image merely by having the patient shut one eye at a time. When one eye is closed and the most lateral image disappears, that is the eye of neurologic involvement.

The third rule of diplopia testing is simply to record what the patient sees in various positions of gaze and then try to relate it to classic patterns. Third, fourth, and sixth nerve palsies have specific patterns of diplopia. If multiple muscles or nerves are involved, testing patterns can be considerably more complex and difficult to analyze.

SPECIFIC COMPLAINTS

Ptosis

Ptosis, drooping of the upper eyelids, is a rare complaint that may be found in a patient presenting with visual problems. Unilateral ptosis may be seen with involvement of third nerve lesions, but pupillary and eye movement motor findings are virtually always seen in conjunction with such a problem.[10] Myasthenia gravis may present unilaterally, and a seventh nerve palsy may, on occasion, involve the upper lid more than the lower. Unilateral ptosis is

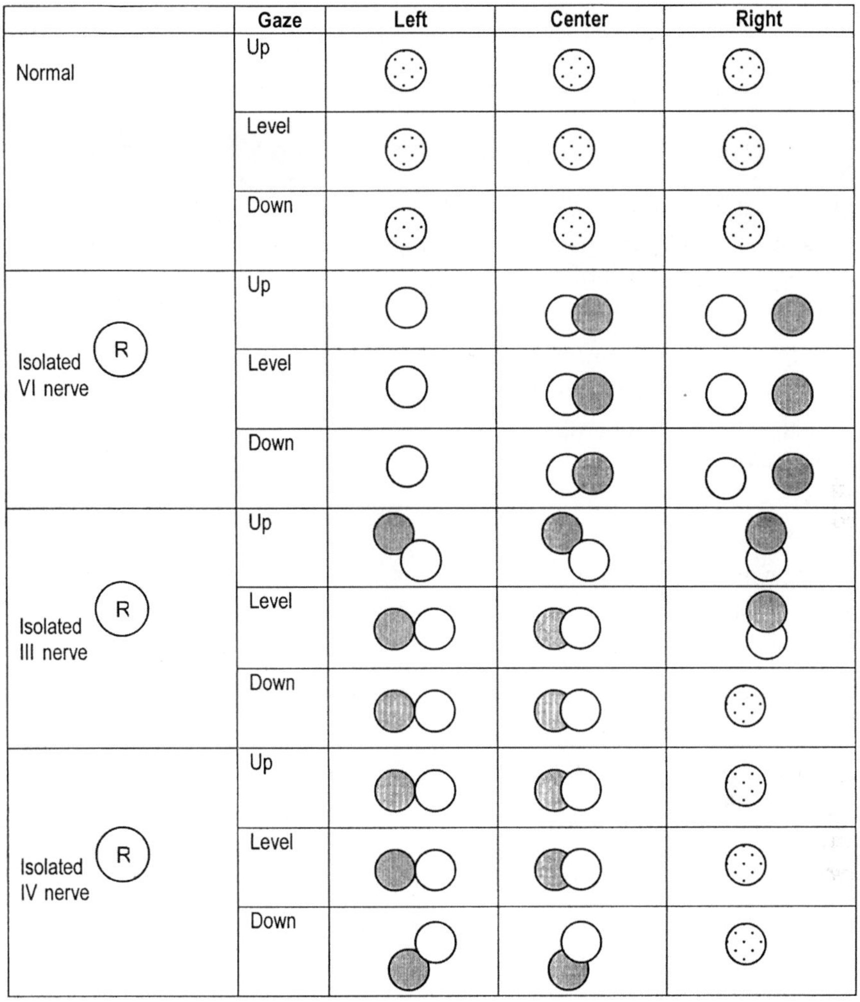

	Gaze	Left	Center	Right
Normal	Up	⊙	⊙	⊙
	Level	⊙	⊙	⊙
	Down	⊙	⊙	⊙
Isolated (R) VI nerve	Up	○	○●	○ ●
	Level	○	○●	○ ●
	Down	○	○●	○ ●
Isolated (R) III nerve	Up	●○	●○	⊛
	Level	●○	●○	⊛
	Down	●○	●○	⊙
Isolated (R) IV nerve	Up	●○	●○	⊙
	Level	●○	●○	⊙
	Down	●○	●○	⊙

FIGURE 9-3 Patterns of specific nerve dysfunctions on red glass testing. ® = red glass covers eye in all testing.

almost always a sympathetic chain or third nerve pathology. Although the seventh nerve also innervates the eyelid, isolated ptosis without involvement of other facial muscles is not seen.

Bilateral ptosis is usually from myasthenia gravis or age-related skin changes with redundant tissue. In advanced cases, hypothyroidism, electrolyte abnormalities, and other myopathies can cause bilateral ptosis. Rare sporadic cases of oculopharyngeal dystrophy have been reported, but these are generally slowly progressive problems.

Abnormal Pupils

Pupillary changes, although rarely the presenting complaint of a patient, may be an important part of any neuro-ophthalmologic problem. Multiple factors can affect pupillary

TABLE 9-3

DRUGS AND TOXINS CAPABLE OF PRODUCING
CONSTRICTION–DILATION OF PUPILS

Parasympathetic Stimulator (Cholinergics)	Sympathetic Inhibitors (Antiadrenergics)	Parasympathetic Inhibitors (Anticholinergics)	Sympathetic Stimulators (Adrenergics)
Acetylcholine	Guanethidine	Botulinum toxin	Cocaine
Nicotine	Bretylium	Hemicholine	Amphetamine
Tetraethyl ammonium	Reserpine	Pentolinium	Ephedrine
Bromides	Alpha-methyl-dopa	Atropine-like	Adrenalin drugs
Physostigmine	Monoamine oxidase inhibitors	Scopolamine	Neosynephrine
Neostigmine		Homatropine	Tyramine
Pyrophosphates	Dibenzylines	Eucatropine	
Carbachol	Narcotics	Over-the-counter sleep medications	
Mecholyl		Toadstool toxin	
Pilocarpine		Jimson weed	
		Wild sage	

size, because pupils are susceptible to both topical medications and trauma as well as influences through the sympathetic and parasympathetic nervous systems.[11] As a general rule, bilateral pupillary findings such as extremely large or extremely small pupils are on a centrally mediated basis from either structural or chemical causes (drugs and chemicals ingested or placed directly into the eye). Anisocoria (unequal pupils) may represent a lateralized nervous system problem or a local effect on nervous elements supplying that particular eye or it may be the consequence of topical drugs or local ocular disease (Tables 9-3 and 9-4).

Large Pupils

The unilateral, large, poorly reactive pupil can be the result of parasympathetic denervation, sympathetic excess, or end-organ blockade by drugs instilled into the eyes. Figure 9-4 illustrates a system for deciding the cause of a large pupil. The first chemical instilled in the eye is 2% mecholyl. This drug stimulates acetylcholine that is released by the parasympathetic nerve system. If the pupil constricts with mecholyl, the problem is generally one of parasympathetic denervation. An example of parasympathetic denervation would be compression of the third cranial nerve. In this case both the pupillary finding (large pupil) and motor finding (eye deviated laterally and slightly down) should be present.[12]

If the pupil does not respond to 2% mecholyl, pilocarpine can be instilled. Pilocarpine will overcome the effects of sympathetic excess in the eye.[13] Sympathetic excess

TABLE 9-4

CAUSES OF MYDRIASIS (LARGE PUPIL)

Unilateral
1. Topical medications (antiparasympathetic blockade; see Table 9-3)
2. Parasympathetic denervation; uncal herniation, diabetes mellitus, aneurysm
3. Sympathetic excess (stimulation); the "fight-or-flight response"
4. Dilation phase of Adie's pupil
5. Unilateral blindness when the normal eye is covered (Marcus Gunn phenomenon)
6. Ophthalmoplegic migraine
7. Trauma and posttraumatic synechiae

Bilateral
1. Systemic drugs and chemicals (see Table 9-3)
2. Thyrotoxicosis
3. Bilateral parasympathetic paralysis, i.e., bilateral uncal herniation, etc.
4. Blockade at neuromuscular junction, i.e., botulism
5. Neuropathy involving cranial nerve III; diabetes mellitus, diphtheria
6. Cheyne–Stokes respirations
7. Asphyxia

may be due to systemic chemicals or increased outflow from the stellate ganglion. When a pupil does not become smaller with mecholyl or pilocarpine, end-organ blockade with a parasympathetic blocking drug, such as an atropine-like drug placed in the eye, is strongly suggested.

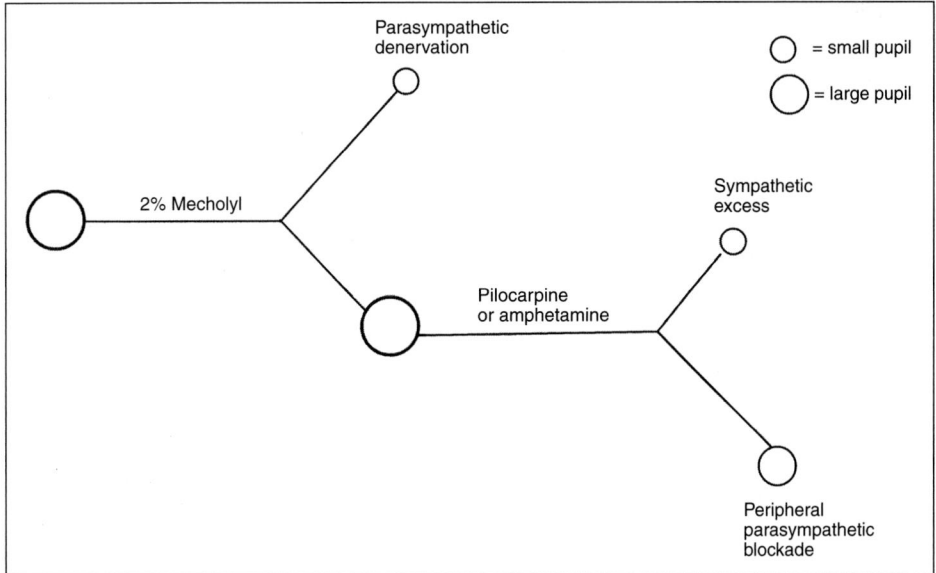

FIGURE 9-4   Evaluation of the large pupil.

Small Pupils

The causes of unilateral or bilaterally small pupils are many (Table 9-5). A system is needed to evaluate the unilateral, nonreactive small pupil (Fig. 9-5). Homatropine can be instilled in the eye. If dilation occurs quickly, a parasympathetic excess from systemic medications or the central nervous system nuclei should be suspected. If the pupil remains small, 4% cocaine may be instilled. The cocaine acts as a sympathetic nervous system transmitter; dilation of the pupil would indicate dysfunction of the peripheral sympathetic system. The small pupil that responds to neither homatropine nor cocaine should be considered to have a peripheral sympathetic block such as a pupillary constricting drop that was placed in the eye.

Bilateral midposition pupils that are poorly reactive to either light or dark stimuli in an otherwise awake patient should be considered a normal variant.

Adie's Pupil (Myotonic or Tonic Pupil)

Adie's pupil is a syndrome that may be either bilateral or unilateral. In this condition, the pupil is usually dilated, sometimes oval, and apparently fixed to both light and convergence. On other occasions, it may be small and apparently unreactive to light.[8]

Careful testing reveals that patients with this syndrome have a delayed or slow pupillary constriction and dilation. Adie's pupil is usually considered to be part of a wider dysautonomia including abnormalities with sweating and orthostatic hypotension. The patients may also manifest decreased reflexes, insensitivity to pain, and

TABLE 9-5

CAUSES OF MIOSIS (SMALL PUPIL)

Monocular

1. Topical drugs; peripheral sympathetic blockade (see Table 9-3)
2. Interruption of sympathetic fibers; central sympathetic failure, i.e., lateral medullary syndrome, ciliary migraine (cluster), pontine hemorrhage, disease of the lung (Pancoast's tumor), trauma, carotid aneurysm, cavernous sinus fissure, cavernous sinus thrombosis
3. Parasympathetic irritation; purulent meningitis, arachnoiditis, compression of third nerve (very early phase)
4. Syphilis (unilateral Argyll Robertson pupil)
5. Constriction phase of Adie's pupil
6. Histamine cephalgia (cluster headache)
7. Anisocoria
8. Acute or chronic iritis

Binocular

1. Central or topical effects of drugs (see Table 9-3)
2. Pontine hemorrhage
3. Pineal tumor
4. Apneic stage of Cheyne–Stokes respirations
5. Syphilis (bilateral Argyll Robertson pupil)

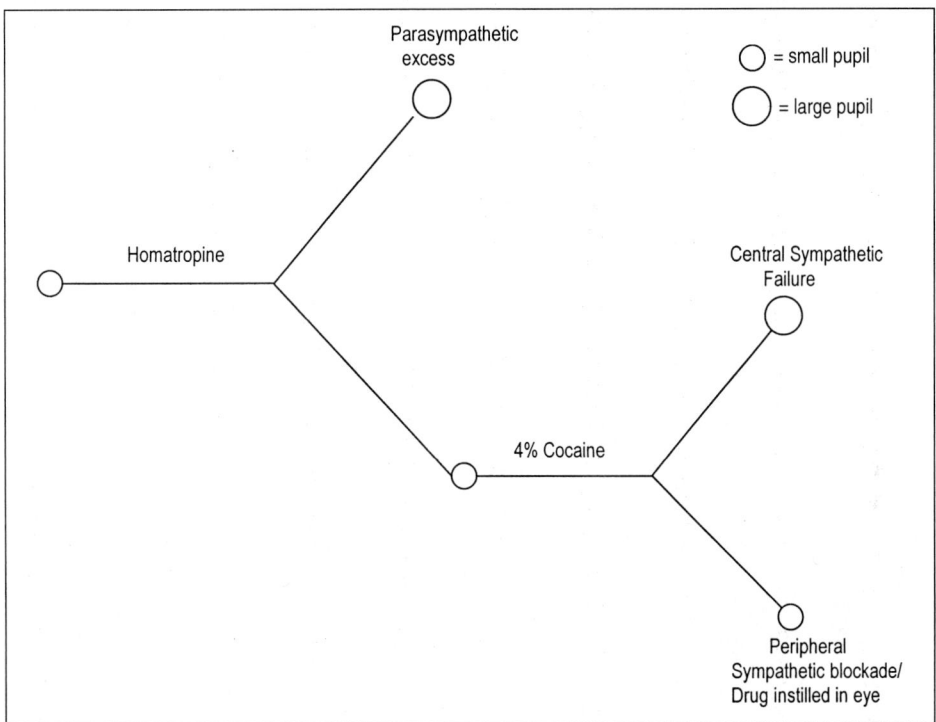

FIGURE 9-5   Evaluation of the small pupil.

generalized slowness in all reactions. A patient with the findings of Adie's pupil and no other visual or neurologic complaint should be considered to have a normal variant.

In the evaluation of pupillary size and reactivity, some general rules should be followed. The pupils are smaller at the age extremes of life. The very young and the very old tend to have smaller and less reactive pupils. Pupils generally become smaller when individuals are looking at near objects and dilate when they are looking at far objects, the so-called divergence–convergence response. Large refraction errors of vision may also influence pupil size. Patients with myopia have slightly larger pupils than do patients with hypermetropia.

ACUTE VISUAL FIELD DEFECTS

The anatomy of the visual system is such that the optic nerves from each eye join at the optic chiasm (Fig. 9-6). From here the fibers recombine so that the right half of each eye (i.e., the temporal fibers of the right eye and the nasal fibers of the left eye) combine and then again divide into superior fibers passing through the parietal lobe and inferior fibers passing through the temporal lobe to arrive in the occipital cortex (Fig. 9-7).[4]

Monocular Visual Loss

Monocular losses of vision must be located anterior to the optic chiasm before the fibers have recombined (Fig. 9-8) or in the eye itself (Figs. 9-6 and 9-7).

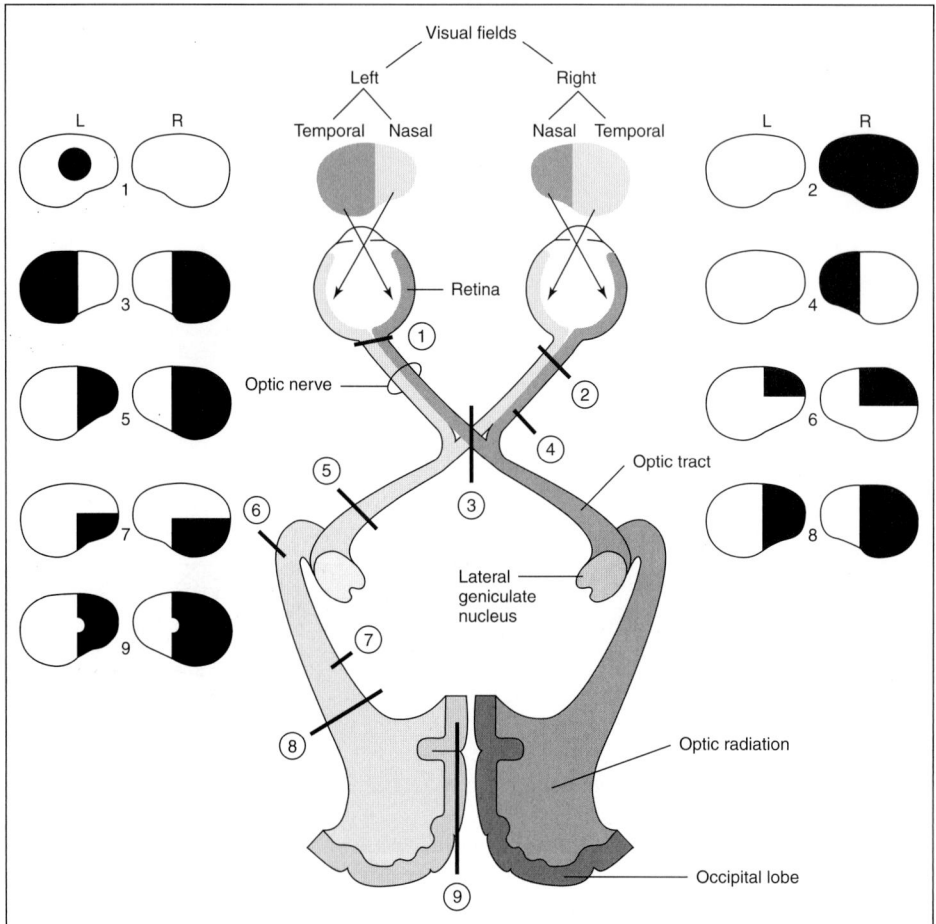

FIGURE 9-6 Common visual field defects and their anatomical bases. 1. Central scotoma caused by inflammation of the optic disc (optic neuritis) or optic nerve (retrobulbar neuritis). 2. Total blindness of the right eye from a complete lesion of the right optic nerve. 3. Bitemporal hemianopsia caused by pressure exerted on the optic chiasm by a pituitary tumor. 4. Right nasal hemianopsia caused by a perichiasmal lesion (e.g., calcified internal carotid artery). 5. Right homonymous hemianopsia from a lesion of the left optic tract. 6. Right homonymous superior quadrantanopsia caused by partial involvement of the optic radiation by a lesion in the left temporal lobe (Meyer loops). 7. Right homonymous inferior quadrantanopsia from a complete lesion of the left optic radiation. (A similar defect may also result from lesion 9.) 9. Right homonymous hemianopsia (with mascular spring) resulting from posterior cerebral artery occlusion. (Reproduced with permission from Simon et al. *Clinical Neurology.* 7th ed. New York, NY: McGraw-Hill; 2009.)

Bitemporal Hemianopsia

Bitemporal hemianopsia (losing vision in both lateral eye fields), an extremely rare condition, indicates that the medial fibers from each optic nerve are involved (Figs. 9-6 and 9-7). The only place that such a lesion can sit is at the optic chiasm.[2] Pituitary lesions, both hemorrhage and tumors, represent the most common causes of bitemporal hemianopsia.

Interpretation of field defects		
Defect	Pattern	Possible Diagnosis
1. Monocular blindness	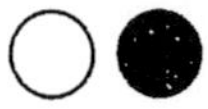	Primary eye disease Optic neuritis Optic neuropathy Retinal arteritis Toxins, trauma
2. Bitemporal hemianopsia	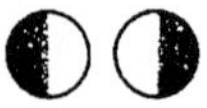	Aneurysm-anterior circulation Tumors-pituitary-meningioma Pituitary infarct or apoplexy Third ventricular cysts, arachnoiditis
3. Homonymous hemianopsia	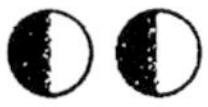	Vascular disease involving parietotemporal lobe or occipital lobe, large hemispheric mass Trauma, demyelinating disease
4. Homonymous quadrantanopsia	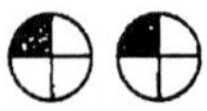	Occipital lobe vascular lesion, temporal lobe vascular lesion, tumor, parietal lobe lesion
5. Altitudinal defect	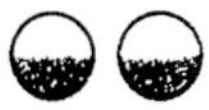	Occipital lobe trauma, inflammatory or destructive process. Both hemispheres above or below calcarine fissure
6. Sparing central vision	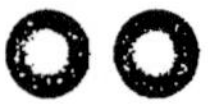	Toxic—metabolic bilateral neuritis, occipital lobe lesions
7. Sparing peripheral vision	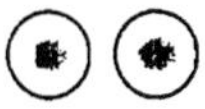	Toxic—metabolic

FIGURE 9-7   Interpretation of field defects.

Homonymous Hemianopsia

Homonymous hemianopsia involves the loss of vision in either the right or left visual field in each eye (Figs. 9-6 and 9-7). A full homonymous hemianopsia must involve the optic tract shortly after leaving the optic chiasm or must include an extremely large lesion affecting both sets of fibers both superiorly and inferiorly passing through the temporal and parietal lobes or involve both superior and inferior areas of the occipital cortex.[14] Partial hemianopsia is much more common than full hemianopsia.

Quadrantanopsia

More common than full homonymous hemianopsias are homonymous quadrantanopsias (Figs. 9-6 and 9-7). These are the result of involvement by either superior or inferior visual fibers.[15] Minor quadrantanopsias are usually detected as part of the complete neurologic examination in a patient showing other evidence for a cerebral vascular cortical lesion. Frequently the patient is unaware of a quadrantanopsia.

Altitudinal Defects

Altitudinal defects are those that involve the upper or lower half of both visual fields (Figs. 9-6 and 9-7). Lesions producing this type of defect most commonly involve the occipital lobes above or below the calcarine fissure bilaterally.[14]

Central Visual Sparing

Preservation of central vision with marked reduction in peripheral vision has usually been associated with quinidine-type drugs or bilateral optic neuritis.[16] Testing needs to be done carefully so as not to mistake this finding for a psychiatric problem (Fig. 9-7).

Peripheral Sparing

Certain visual field defects are more likely to be on a metabolic or toxic rather than on a structural basis. Central visual loss with sparing of peripheral vision may, in rare instances, be caused by lesions in the calcarine cortex (Fig. 9-7).[14] Such defects are usually, however, the result of toxins such as methanol.

ACUTE VISUAL DETERIORATION OR LOSS

The etiologies of acute visual loss can in general be divided between entities causing monocular blindness and those causing binocular blindness (Fig. 9-8). It should be

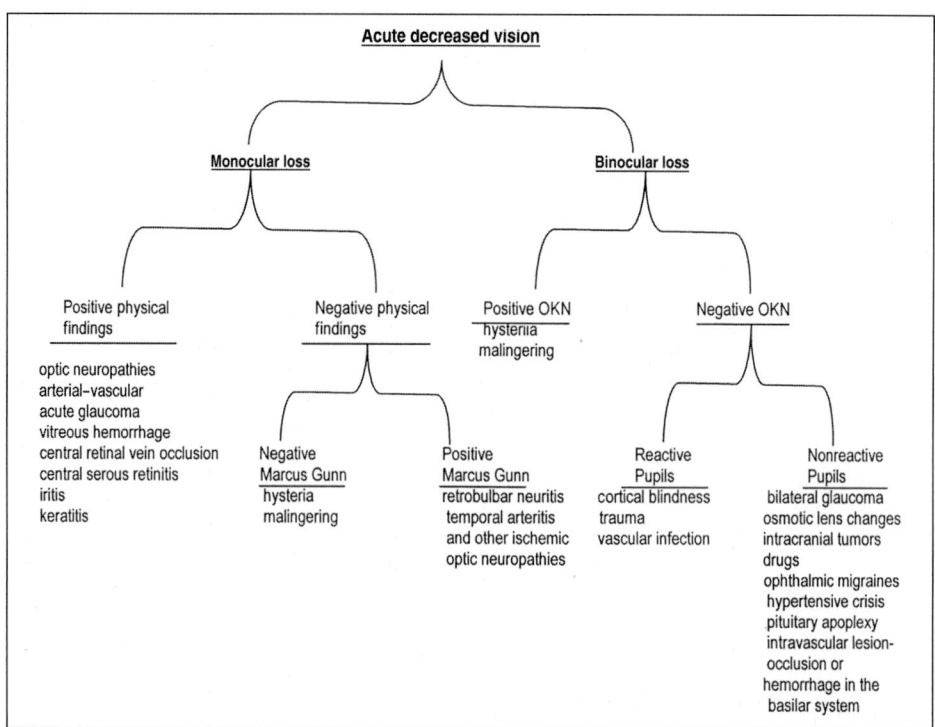

FIGURE 9-8   Acute decreased vision. OKN, optokinetic nystagmus.

pointed out that certain disease entities such as temporal arteritis and retrobulbar neuritis may be present as either unilateral or bilateral processes (Fig. 9-8).[17]

Monocular Visual Loss

Patients with monocular visual loss basically can be divided into those who have obvious physical findings, i.e., retinal detachments, central retinal artery occlusions, anterior eye disease, etc., and those who do not.

Optic Neuropathy

Optic neuropathic processes affect the visual system. Papillitis causes swelling and edema of the nerve head that can be easily mistaken for papilledema (Table 9-6). Unlike patients with papilledema, patients with papillitis generally have a marked decrease in vision without other indications of increased intracranial pressure. Papillitis is also usually a monocular process, whereas papilledema, except in rare instances, is bilateral.

Papilledema refers to edema of the optic nerve head by various causes. The current theory about the underlying mechanism of all forms of papilledema relates to axoplasmic transport or to the flow of cytoplasmic material along the nerves resulting in swelling of the axon. From a practical consideration, papilledema should be thought of as being from one of four causes: (1) increased intracranial pressure, (2) intraorbital disease, (3) intraocular disease, and (4) systemic disease affecting the eyes. Table 9-7 details the multiple causes of papilledema. Except for increased intracranial pressure, all other forms are rare.

Besides papillitis, or inflammation of the optic nerve head, other entities may also cause blurring of the optic disc margins, which may be interpreted as papilledema. Table 9-8 details disease entities that may be mistaken for either papilledema or papillitis on general physical examination.

Ischemic Optic Neuropathy

Acute ischemic optic neuropathies are associated with temporal arteritis, anemia, polycythemia, and carotid artery stenosis. The ischemic optic neuropathies should show pale

TABLE 9-6

DIFFERENTIAL DIAGNOSIS OF BLURRED OPTIC DISKS

Finding	Papilledema	Papillitis	Pseudopapilledema
Pupils	Normal	If unilateral + Marcus Gunn	Normal
Vision	Without change	Reduced—variable amount	Normal
Fields	Enlarged blind spot	Central decrease or scotoma	Normal
Other	Hemorrhage occasionally around disk	Frequent hemorrhage	No hemorrhage
Focally	Usually bilateral	Frequently unilateral	Variable

TABLE 9-7

CAUSES OF PAPILLEDEMA

1. Intrancranial
    a. Masses
        (1) Epidural, subdural, intracranial, hemorrhage
        (2) Brain tumor, brain abscess, hydrocephalus
    b. Intracranial hypertension
        (1) Intracranial thrombosis (sinus thromboses)
        (2) Drugs: vitamin A, tetracycline, nalidixic acid
        (3) Pseudotumor cerebri
    c. Hydrocephalus
    d. Meningitis
    e. Arachnoiditis
    f. Cranial suture stenosis
2. Orbital disease
    a. Tumors of the optic nerve
    b. Retroorbital tumor
    c. Thyroid ophthalmopathy
3. Ocular disease
    a. Acute glaucoma
    b. Trauma
    c. Surgery
    d. Uveitis
4. Systemic disease
    a. Malignant hypertension
    b. Anemia
    c. Hypovolemia
    d. Anoxia
    e. Guillain–Barré syndrome
    f. Sarcoidosis
    g. Various poisons

TABLE 9-8

CAUSES OF PSEUDOPAPILLEDEMA

More common
1. Myelinated nerve fiber
2. Gliosis
3. Hyperopia
4. Hyaline bodies (drusen)

Rare
1. Occular crescents
2. Neoplasm of disk
3. Colomboma

Retroorbital fibroplasia

fundi, but the findings may be so subtle as to be nonexistent. Objective evidence of the fact that there is decreased vision in the eye affected, however, is established by the positive Marcus Gunn pupil sign and decreased visual acuity. Such patients should receive consultation with an ophthalmologist on an urgent basis.

Arterial Vascular Causes

Arterial vascular lesions, both occlusion and hemorrhage, affect the ophthalmic artery in the same manner as they do all arteries of the internal carotid system. Emboli may occlude the ophthalmic artery from (1) primary cardiac causes such as endocarditis or arrhythmias, (2) carotid artery disease, (3) aortic aneurysms, and (4) arterial thrombus. A sudden loss of vision as a result of an arterial vascular accident is most often monocular, and the site of the occlusion and areas of decreased arterial flow generally follow the vascular anatomy.[18]

Occlusive diseases on an embolic basis tend to involve more than peripheral retinal arteries, causing branch occlusions of the retinal artery. The onset is acute, and usually some vision is preserved. The retina may take on a diffuse cloudiness and paleness in the area of the branch artery that has been occluded.

Central retinal artery occlusion, on the other hand, is generally the result of a thrombosis of the central retinal artery. This usually occurs in elderly patients and may be preceded by amaurosis fugax.[18] It is generally sudden in onset with a complete or nearly complete monocular visual loss. The retina quickly takes on a diffuse paleness while retaining a red center, which is the "cherry red" portion of the macula. After only a few days of occlusion, pronounced optic atrophy will be visible.

Treatments for acute retinal artery occlusions have basically been ineffective. It is believed that treatment delayed beyond 6 hours reduces the likelihood that any meaningful vision will be returned to areas involved. Emergency management of the patient with a branch or central retinal artery occlusion is essentially anecdotal. There are no controlled studies that have compared various methods in the management of such occlusions. In recent years, retrobulbar injection of 2% xylocaine and 200 mg acetylcholine has been tried with limited success. Low-molecular-weight dextran infusions, manual intermittent compression–decompression of the eyeball, and the use of acetozalamide, carbon dioxide, and steroids have all been advocated but never proven in any series. At this point in time no clear preference for one method or another can be shown.

Acute Glaucoma

Both narrow- and open-angle glaucoma can result in rapid decrease in vision. Immediate changes in intraocular pressure, however, generally cause pain as well as irritation, with pronounced conjunctival infection. Acute narrow-angle glaucoma is almost always associated with a clouding of the cornea and anterior chamber and relative midposition fixation of the pupil. The sudden onset of decreased vision, eye and head pain, and nausea and vomiting should prompt investigation for glaucoma. Checking the intraocular pressure is the test of choice. Management of acute glaucoma is beyond the scope of this book but acute lowering of intraocular pressure and involvement of an ophthalmologist are essential when vision is threatened.

Vitreous Hemorrhage

Hemorrhage into the vitreous body should be readily diagnosable by funduscopic examination. Acute systemic diseases that affect bleeding, as well as intracranial and intraocular

TABLE 9-9

CAUSES OF ACUTE VITREOUS HEMORRHAGE

1. Clotting disorders
2. Arterial hypertension
3. Venous hypertension
4. Vasculitis
5. Atriovenous malformation
6. Trauma
7. Retinal detachment
8. Neovascularization; bleeding
9. Choroid degeneration
10. Postoperative intraocular surgery
11. Tumor mass of the eyeball

problems, can cause vitreous hemorrhage. Table 9-9 lists the multiple causes of vitreous hemorrhage. Hemorrhage into the vitreous body is an emergent situation and requires consultation with an ophthalmologist.

Central Retinal Vein Occlusion

Multiple underlying disease entities can progress to cause central retinal vein occlusion. This presents a dramatic funduscopic appearance, with multiple areas of hemorrhage and engorgement of the veins of the retina. No specific treatment is available except that of managing the underlying disease (Table 9-10).

Space-Occupying Intracranial Disorders

An intracranial mass lesion lying anterior to the optic chiasm, such as a meningioma or malignant tumor, and causing enough pressure to decrease vision generally has positive neurologic findings. Such disease entities occupying the superior orbital fissure and sphenoid ridge may involve the cranial nerves that pass into the orbit along with the optic

TABLE 9-10

CAUSES OF CENTRAL RETINAL VEIN OCCLUSION

1. Diabetes mellitus
2. Polycythemia
3. Multiple myeloma
4. Hyperglobulinemias
5. Sickle cell disease
6. Infections
7. Tuberculosis
8. Sarcoidosis
9. Continuous inflammation
10. Trauma

nerve. Pressure sufficient to decrease vision usually results in papilledema. With the Foster–Kennedy syndrome, optic atrophy may be noted in the involved eye and papilledema in the opposite eye.

Retinal Detachment

Retinal detachment may present as either a gradual or a sudden deterioration of vision. The disease process involved is actually a separation of the two layers of the retina. The pigmented layer remains attached to the fibrous underlying choroid, and the sensory retina separates and falls away. The amount of vision lost is proportional to the areas of detachment involved. The more central the detachment, the more involvement of macular fibers and the greater the decrease in vision there is. Severe trauma has been associated with both acute and delayed retinal detachments. Patients usually complain of decreased vision over minutes to hours; blurred vision, flashes of light, or hazy clouds are often described. In older patients, the so-called secondary retinal detachment may be due not to a primary ocular process but to a metastatic tumor of the choroid layer. Acute retinal detachment is a medical urgency requiring timely involvement of ophthalmology.

Iritis

Iritis may be a unilateral or bilateral disease. Trauma, infectious disease (i.e., sarcoidosis), collagen vascular disease, degenerative processes, and idiopathic ocular disease may all lead to iritis. A typical history includes a deep ocular pain with tearing but no discharge. Unlike conjunctivitis, the pain is not relieved with topical anesthetics. The typical physical findings include perilimbal injection of the iris and the classic finding of cells in the anterior chamber of the eye on slit lamp examination. After the process has become established, proteinaceous material is also seen in the anterior chamber and is referred to as a cell and flair reaction when seen on slit lamp examination. Medical management will depend on the underlying disease entity.

Keratitis

Keratitis, inflammation of the corneal stroma, may also be unilateral or bilateral. It may be the result of trauma or an infectious process, but it involves irritation and infiltration of a cloudy proteinaceous material into the layers of the cornea. The differential diagnosis of keratitis is extensive, and an ophthalmologic consultation should be sought before starting therapy.

Retrobulbar Neuritis

In patients with monocular visual loss who do not have an obvious physical finding, a positive Marcus Gunn pupillary reaction is a strong indication that the patient's visual acuity is decreased, from either ischemic optic neuropathy with extremely subtle findings or retrobulbar neuritis. Retrobulbar neuritis is classically considered the disease in which the patient sees nothing and the doctor sees nothing on physical examination of the eye. Such visual loss may come on over hours to days and is usually painless. A young person with monocular visual loss and without ocular findings should be considered to have retrobulbar neuritis. Retrobulbar neuritis may be considered a manifestation of multiple sclerosis. Some 70% of young patients with retrobulbar neuritis will carry the diagnosis of multiple sclerosis within 2 years.

Steroids have been the mainstay of therapy and should be considered in conjunction with ophthalmology or neurology.

Chorioretinitis

Acute inflammation of the choroid or retinal layers in the region of the macula may cause sudden decrease in vision over a few days. Autoimmune disease, toxoplasmosis, histoplasmosis, bacterial and viral infections, AIDS, and idiopathic inflammation have all been suspected in this disease process. In the majority of cases, no underlying disease etiology is ever found.

The principal symptoms are decreased vision and a feeling of heaviness or fullness in the eye. On slit lamp examination, the anterior chamber of the eye may not show any sign of inflammation. Ophthalmoscopic examination may reveal a cloudy vitreous that may be elevated and may occasionally have small hemorrhages. Treatment of chorioretinitis can be a medical emergency. Specific therapy should be aimed at any underlying disease entities discovered, but the majority of cases are idiopathic.

Psychiatric Causes

Patients who complain of a significant monocular visual loss but who have no positive physical findings and a negative Marcus Gunn pupil test generally have a psychiatric base for their complaint. The differential diagnosis between the hysterical patient and the malingering patient will be based principally on the occupational and social milieu of the patient and the potential secondary gains involved (see Chapter 10).

Binocular Visual Loss

The patient complaining of severely decreased vision or blindness bilaterally may represent a serious medical emergency (Fig. 9-8). A patient who lacks OKN is likely to have an organic lesion. Patients complaining of binocular blindness or severe visual loss who maintain normal OKN and pupillary responses have a high probability of hysteria or malingering. Pupillary responses become important in determining the location of the lesion. Patients without OKN who maintain normal pupillary light reflexes should be considered to have a cortical type of blindness.[4] Trauma to the occipital lobes and vascular hemorrhage or insufficiency involving the posterior cerebral arteries are the most common causes of cortical blindness. Ophthalmic migraine with binocular visual loss should also be considered in this group. Focal infections involving the occipital regions have been rarely reported to cause a similar type of cortical blindness.[8] Patients with binocular visual loss, lack of OKN, and decreased pupillary reaction to light stimulus must have as the basis of their disease a process that involves both visual pathways anterior to the optic chiasm or a diffuse metabolic or vascular process.

Bilateral keratitis, iritis, and papillitis, as well as intraocular bleeding, should all be readily diagnosable by standard ocular examination. Pituitary apoplexy can certainly result in bilateral blindness.[2] Pituitary apoplexy is a catastrophic medical condition caused by hemorrhage into the pituitary gland. This may be on a vascular basis or hemorrhage into a preexisting tumor. Pituitary apoplexy usually causes alterations in consciousness, and other neurologic findings will usually take precedence over the visual loss in determining the diagnostic workup.

Retrobulbar neuritis and the ischemic optic neuropathies may present as bilateral disease, particularly when these entities have only a dimming of vision as opposed to complete blindness. They may represent a complex differential diagnosis. Age of the patient and sedimentation rate may both be helpful in differentiating retrobulbar neuritis from temporal arteritis. Temporal arteritis is suggested in elderly patients with visual loss and elevated sedimentation rates. Retrobulbar neuritis, however, may be essentially indistinguishable from pharmacologic and toxicologic causes of decreased vision.

Acute changes in the lenses may also cause rapid decrease in vision, although not blindness. Diabetic patients whose blood sugar is significantly elevated may, on an osmotic basis, show marked shifts in the configuration of the lens, resulting in altered visual acuity. Patients with a bilateral decrease in vision and without obvious physical findings should have a blood glucose level obtained along with a sedimentation rate.

The patient with hypertensive encephalopathy may present with decreased vision. These patients generally have other manifestations of their hypertensive problem. Decreased vision should be considered a positive sign of severe involvement of the cerebral vessels and may require a controlled reduction in blood pressure.

Certain common drugs and chemicals have long been recognized as toxins to the visual system (Table 9-11). Lead found in improperly distilled alcohols as well as methanol can seriously affect visual acuity, with minimal findings on funduscopic examination. What is not as well understood is alcohol and tobacco amblyopia. Ethyl alcohol in large doses and large quantities of nicotine in patients unaccustomed to their use have been reported to cause severe decreased vision to the point of total blindness. Alcohol–tobacco amblyopia is usually short-lived and may completely reverse itself in a matter of hours to days. In preadolescents and adolescents presenting with acute visual decrease, a history of tobacco and alcohol use should be discretely obtained.

Acute Double Vision

The complaint of seeing double can be a confusing symptom because the patient may describe decreased or blurred vision as double vision.[17,19] Careful history from the patients about exactly what they are indicating is necessary for proper evaluation. Once it has been determined that the patient is actually seeing split or multiple images, the next step is to separate out monocular from binocular problems (Fig. 9-9).

TABLE 9-11 ——————————————

COMMON DRUGS AND CHEMICALS AFFECTING VISION	
Ethyl alcohol	Chloramphenicol
Methyl alcohol	Sulfanilamides
Quinine and quinidine	Ergot medications
Digitalis	Salicylates
Iodoform	Ethambutol
Methyl chloride	Isoniazid
Methyl bromide	Nicotine

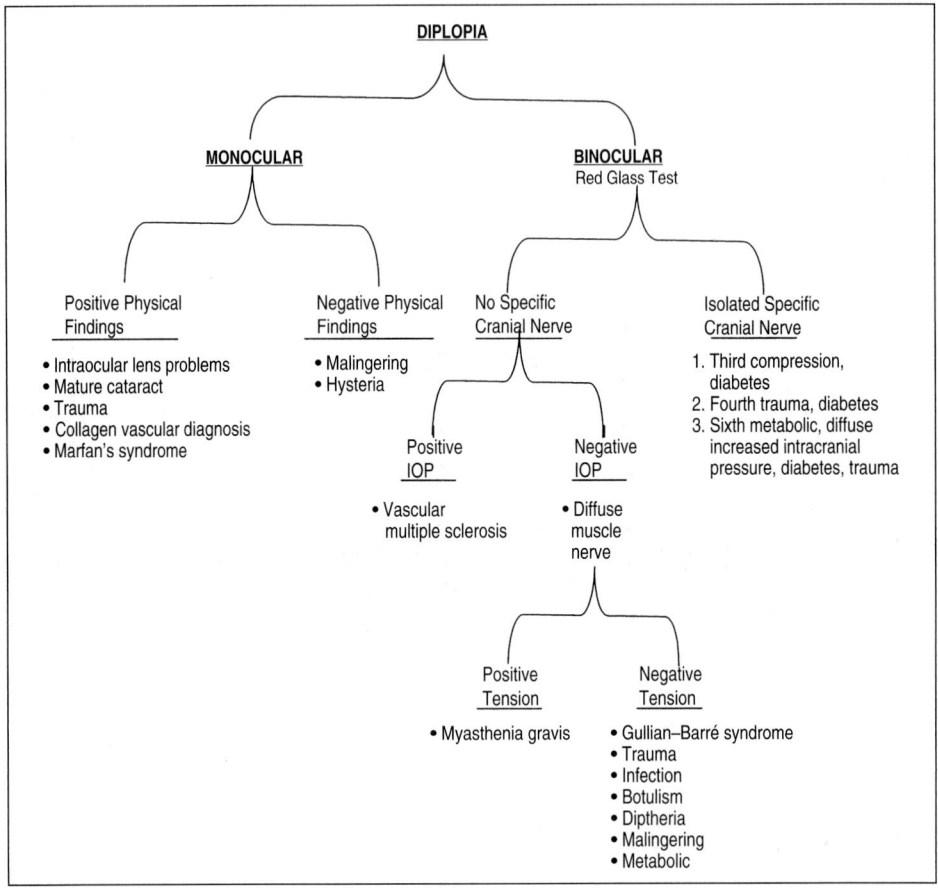

FIGURE 9-9 Evaluation of diplopia. IOP, internuclear ophthalmoplegia.

Monocular Diplopia

Patients with abnormalities of their visual axis including the cornea, lens, and retina may get split images that they interpret as double vision. Testing with the penlight will appear to these patients as two spots or beams of light in the affected eye. All causes of monocular diplopia are in the eye itself, are rare, and may be diagnosable by careful ophthalmologic examination. The ocular lesions that may produce monocular diplopia are varied. With the advent of the implantable intraocular lens, patients may present who have had dislocations or other problems related to these devices. A dislocated or angulated intraocular lens can cause a split image on the retina. Excimer laser surgery has also been associated with monocular diplopia.[20]

Subluxation of the natural lens may also cause abnormal light images. Severe trauma has been reported to dislocate the lens. Patients with collagen vascular diseases such as Marfan's syndrome and homocystinuria develop weak supporting structures for the lens, allowing it to dislocate with little or no trauma.

Maturing cataracts may also form irregular opacities that will split the light image and give the impression of double vision. Note also that a mass behind the retina, although theoretically diagnosable by standard ophthalmologic evaluation, may in its early phases cause mild monocular diplopia by deforming the retina. Such patients should be carefully followed and reevaluated if a retroretinal mass is suspected.

Binocular Diplopia

Binocular diplopia is readily separated from monocular diplopia with a simple cover–uncover test. If the patient sees only one image with each eye independently but has a double image when the eyes are used concomitantly, the patient has a binocular diplopia secondary to abnormalities of alignment of the eyes in various areas of gaze.

The location of the abnormality with limitation of conjugate gaze on command should be thought of in terms of four sites: (1) supranuclear, above the parapontine gaze centers and midbrain, (2) pontine gaze centers, (3) internuclear lesions involving the medial longitudinal fasciculus (MLF), and (4) infranuclear, from the nuclei of the third, fourth, and sixth nerves outward (Tables 9-12 and 9-13).

Supranuclear Causes

Supranuclear causes of gaze palsies (inability to move the eyes conjugately) are due to lesions in central nervous system structures above the brainstem that send signals to the eyes. Such lesions can be anywhere from prefrontal lesions to the motor tracts as they descend through the central core of the brain to the brainstem. These patients maintain

TABLE 9-12

CAUSES OF BINOCULAR DIPLOPIA

1. Orbital trauma: muscle entrapment or hematoma
2. Third (III) nerve palsy
3. Fourth (IV) nerve palsy
4. Sixth (VI) nerve palsy
5. Multiple mixed neuritis—vasculitis, mononeuritis, multiple neuritis, infection (herpes)
6. Myasthenia gravis
7. Tolosa–Hunt syndrome
8. Multiple sclerosis
9. Decompensation of existing phoria or tropia (existing disconjugate gaze)
10. Vascular occlusion—brainstem
11. Wernicke's syndrome
12. Viral Guillain–Barré syndrome
13. Bulbar palsy
14. Diphtheria
15. Botulism
16. Tuberculosis
17. Syphilis

TABLE 9-13 — COMPARISON OF GAZE PALSY FINDINGS AND LOCATIONS

	Strabismus	Diplopia	Nystagmus	Caloric Response	Examples
Supranuclear	None	None	None	Normal deviation; defective; first phalange	Parietal–frontal tumor; hemorrhage; degenerative disease
Pontine gaze center	None	None	None	Paralysis of conjugate eye movement	Infarct in pons
Medial longitudinal fasciculus (internuclear)	On conjugate gaze	Yes	In abducting (good) eye	Adductor weakness	Multiple sclerosis; brainstem infarct; involving medial longitudinal fasciculus
Infranuclear peripheral lesions	Yes	Yes	None	Defect in pull of involved nerve or muscles	Myasthenia gravis; III, IV, VI nerve injuries

conjugate gaze on primary position when looking forward owing to brainstem reflexes. They are not able to move their eyes on command. Because the eyes remain conjugated, the patient relates no diplopia in primary gaze, and on gross inspection, no disconjugate gaze (strabismus) is noted in primary position. Because vestibular nuclei and brainstem centers are all intact, the patient will have normal deviation of the eyes on cold caloric testing. The patient may, however, have problems in the correction phase because of an inability to send information from the cortex. These are extremely rare conditions.

Pontine Gaze Center

Lesions of the pontine gaze center are usually on a vascular basis.[21] In primary position, no disconjugate gaze is noted, and the patient does not complain of diplopia. With voluntary movement of the eyes, the diplopia is elicited. On cold caloric testing, the patient is unable to generate normal conjugate eye movements because the normal flow of information reaching the gaze centers is interrupted.

Internuclear Lesions

Normal control of eye movements is through the MLF in the center of the brainstem. Cortical input passes to the gaze centers, which then send signals to the appropriate sixth nerve nucleus and to the opposite third nerve nucleus through the MLF.[22] Internuclear gaze palsies are the result of either multiple sclerosis or brainstem vascular lesions involving the MLF. Such lesions are referred to as internuclear ophthalmoplegias (IOPs). Relatively minor trauma and the smoking of crack cocaine have also been associated with transient IOP.[6,23] The patient is able to send information to the pontine gaze center and is usually able to abduct the ipsilateral eye. The patient is, however, unable to adduct the contralateral eye, since it requires information being sent from the sixth nucleus to the third nerve nucleus through the MLF. This produces nystagmus in the abducting eye.

Infranuclear Lesions

Infranuclear lesions are those involving nerves III, IV, or VI or the muscles of eye movement that they control. Weakness in either the muscle or a specific nerve lesion can cause strabismus even in primary gaze, and the patient will complain of diplopia. Myasthenia gravis, botulism trauma, and the various diseases that affect the third, fourth, and sixth cranial nerves are examples of infranuclear lesions (see specific nerve lesions).

Paralysis of Upward Gaze

A rarely seen entity is paralysis of upward gaze or Parinaud's syndrome. The lesion in Parinaud's syndrome is generally a vasculitis or mass affecting the region of the pretectal nucleus, thus preventing conjugate upward gaze. This may, on rare occasions, be seen with shunt malfunctions.

Evaluation of Diplopia

An organized evaluation of specific cranial nerves, the connections between the nerves and the muscles that move the eyes, and surrounding structures around the eye are required to analyze diplopia.

Isolated Cranial Nerves

Cranial Nerve III

The muscles innervated by the third nerve move the eye primarily upward and inward. Third cranial nerve lesions present with the involved eye looking laterally and slightly downward. Ptosis may or may not be present depending on the location of the lesion along the nerve.[12] The patient is unable to elevate the involved eye or pull it medially. There is a type of a third cranial nerve lesion that involves only selected motor fibers. This is referred to as a pupil sparing or partial third nerve palsy. A complete third cranial nerve lesion involves motor fibers and the fibers of pupillary constriction. Complete third nerve palsies involving motor and pupillary fibers with a dilation of the pupil that is nonreactive to light should initially be considered to be on a compressive basis (Table 9-14).[12] In the trauma patient in coma, a complete third nerve palsy is usually the result of compression of the third cranial nerve by herniation of the uncus of the temporal lobe. A sudden onset of a complete third cranial nerve lesions in nontraumatic patients should be considered to be the result of compression of the third cranial nerve by an aneurysm of the posterior communicating artery. Sudden onset of complete third nerve palsy, as a result of supratentorial herniation or compression by an aneurysm, represents an emergency. The physician should pay close attention to the patient with an acute headache and complete third nerve palsy. A diagnosis of expanding aneurysm should be entertained until proven otherwise. Incomplete third nerve palsies are those that have motor fibers involved but spare the pupil.

Pupil-sparing third nerve palsies are almost always related to the vascular complications of diabetes mellitus with infarction of the nerve. Pupillary sparing is the result of the pupillary fibers having more collateral blood supply than do the motor fibers, so that with lesions of the vasoneurvorum, the pupillary fibers are less susceptible to small vascular lesions.

Patients who are diabetic and have a new onset of pupil-sparing third nerve palsy can usually be sent home and managed on an outpatient basis if other medical problems are under control.

Cranial Nerve IV

Acute fourth nerve palsies are rare.[4] They may be seen with trauma to the nerve or to the trochlea (tendon pivot point) of the muscle or with vascular involvement of the nerve from

TABLE 9-14

CAUSES OF UNILATERAL THIRD NERVE PALSY

1. Diabetes mellitus, usually incomplete, sparing pupil
2. Aneurysm
3. Other neuropathies
4. Cranial and orbital tumors
5. Migraine
6. Trauma
7. Infection: mononucleosis; syphilis
8. Carotid-cavernous fistula
9. AV malformation

TABLE 9-15
CAUSES OF UNILATERAL SIXTH NERVE PALSY

1. Increased intracranial pressure: trauma, tumor, infection (meningitis)
2. Arteriosclerosis; hypertension
3. Diabetes mellitus
4. Multiple sclerosis
5. Myasthenia gravis, early
6. Gradenigo's syndrome
7. Syphilis
8. Wernicke's syndrome
9. Postlumbar puncture
10. AV malformation

diabetic complications. In very rare cases, hypertension, multiple sclerosis, sickle cell anemia, and systemic lupus have been reported to cause isolated fourth nerve palsies. Fourth nerve palsies may be difficult to recognize if the patient's only complaint is double vision when looking down for reading or walking down stairs. Patients are seen to have their head tilted, with the chin toward the affected side and the ear away from the affected side.

Cranial Nerve VI

The sixth nerve has the longest intracranial course of any of the cranial nerves.[5] Because of its course and position, generalized swelling inside the cranial vault can cause stretching of the nerve, resulting in a sixth nerve palsy. Trauma may affect the nerve directly as it passes through the foramen of the skull. The nerve can be affected indirectly through increased intracranial pressure either focally, such as subdural or epidural pressure, or diffusely with generalized brain swelling. Like the third and fourth cranial nerves, the sixth cranial nerve is also susceptible to vascular insult from complications of diabetes mellitus.

An acute lack of thiamine in the brainstem affects the sixth cranial nerves preferentially. The first sign of an impending Wernicke's syndrome in a nutritionally deficient patient, such as a chronic alcoholic, may be the presence of a sixth nerve palsy. Multiple cranial nerves may subsequently be involved, but the sixth cranial nerves are most commonly affected (Table 9-15).[24]

INTERNUCLEAR OPHTHALMOPLEGIA

For diplopias that do not show a specific cranial nerve pattern, the presence of an IOP may be suspected. An IOP is a lesion of the MLF, which connects the various cranial nerve nuclei in the brainstem that control eye movement. Lesions in this area have a characteristic pattern: (1) inability to adduct the ipsilateral eye on the side of the lesion on contralateral horizontal gaze, (2) normal adduction of the involved eye on convergence testing, and (3) nystagmus in the abducting eye.[22]

The reason for the findings in an IOP is relatively simple if the anatomy of the visual system is considered. When given a command to look laterally, the eye is moved by its ipsilateral sixth nerve nucleus. To move the opposite eye medially at the same time requires that the signal be sent through the brainstem, through the MLF to the opposite third nerve nucleus. A lesion involving MLF fibers will therefore not allow adduction of the eye on the side of involvement on contralateral gaze. With convergence, however, the involved eye will adduct because signals for the convergence reflex come up not from the MLF but from a separate center believed to be part of the nucleus of Perlia. Nystagmus in the abducting eye is the result of the brain getting two images and the brainstem moving to align the eyes. The cortex then sends signals to return the abducting eye in its originally ordered direction.

Whenever an IOP is seen, the differential diagnosis is brief. Vascular lesions of the midbrain, including microhemorrhages or infarcts involving the MLF, may produce an IOP. Severe hypertensive crisis with vascular compromise may also produce such lesions.[7] In rare instances a tumor intrinsic to the midbrain may produce an IOP, but it is extremely rare for this to be the only positive neurologic finding. By far the most common cause of an IOP is multiple sclerosis. In general, young adults with IOPs and without other neurologic findings are manifesting multiple sclerosis. In older adults, an IOP generally indicates vascular disease or a tumor of the brainstem. Other very rare but potentially reversible causes of IOP include minor trauma, Wernicke's syndrome, cocaine use, and systemic lupus.[16]

INFRANUCLEAR DIPLOPIA WITHOUT CRANIAL NERVE INVOLVEMENT

Binocular diplopia without a specific cranial nerve involvement or without evidence of an IOP may represent either involvement of multiple nerves or diffuse neuromuscular disorders. A Tensilon test can be given to separate out diplopias that are caused by myasthenia gravis. A patient who has a marked positive response to this medication is strongly suspected of having myasthenia gravis (see Tensilon test, Chapter 5).

Trauma

Facial trauma may result in blowout fractures of the infraorbital structures, causing entrapment of extraocular muscles. The most common muscle to be involved is the inferior rectus, and the patient has the greatest diplopia when looking up. Patients with blowout fractures generally have a mild to moderate enophthalmos as orbital contents are pushed into the sinus below.

Trauma may also produce diplopia without blowout fracture by causing swelling of the retro-orbital contents or a retro-orbital hematoma. Unlike the blowout fracture patients, these patients tend to have a mild exophthalmus and diffuse limitation of motion and may have decreased vision. A patient with decreased vision and exophthalmus following trauma should be considered to have tension on the optic nerve and may need imaging of the orbital and retro-orbital structures on an acute basis.

Infection

Retro-orbital cellulitis and abscesses may also cause diplopia. Such patients generally have signs of infection and extreme pain on movement of the eyes. These patients are at high risk not only of involving the optic nerve but also of spreading the infection posteriorly to involve the cavernous sinus. Diabetic patients and patients with compromised immune systems may present with indolent infections involving the cavernous sinus and sagittal sinus regions. Nonspecific diplopia and headache in a diabetic patient should trigger the thought of a fungal infection or some other type of orbital infection. Acute CT scanning of the orbital regions can generally delineate the issue and determine the need for surgery.

Diphtheria may present as an acute syndrome that includes diplopia. These patients generally are toxic, with elevated temperature, tachycardia, and oral lesions specifically related to diphtheria.

Botulinum toxin has a predilection for the cranial nerves. The first complaint of a patient with botulism may be diplopia. Although the sixth nerve is most frequently the first involved, by the time the patient presents to a physician, multiple cranial nerves and muscles may be affected, and isolated cranial nerve abnormalities may not be detectable. A specific picture may be difficult to ascertain. Such patients may rapidly go on to other abnormalities of the bulbar musculature and then finally to complete paralysis. The physician needs not only to treat any underlying medical problems but also be prepared to supply airway support.

Guillain–Barré syndrome may also involve the extraocular muscles. These patients generally have diffuse symptomatology and an ascending-type paralysis, but the syndrome may occasionally begin in the cervical and cranial nerve areas (the C. Miller Fisher variant). Again, the patient may move rapidly to requiring airway support.

Metabolic Causes

Metabolic causes of nonspecific diplopia are rare. Although Wernicke's syndrome generally begins with the sixth cranial nerves, it may go on to involve multiple cranial nerve nuclei, thus giving a nonspecific diplopic pattern. Patients considered to be at risk for such nutritional deficiencies, i.e., chronic alcoholics, cancer patients, and the older patients, should be given thiamine if there is any reasonable suspicion.

Psychiatric Causes

The psychiatric patient who presents with diplopia may be extremely difficult to diagnose. The best method to use when this is suspected is to repeat the red glass test several times. It is rare that such an individual can remember exactly what patterns were described in previous examinations. Such patients can represent a difficult diagnostic and therapeutic problem (see Chapter 10).

Summary

The vast majority of visual complaints are nonneurologic and relate only to the eye. The visual system is complex and is intimately related to the nervous system. Separating out structural problems within the eye from neurologic disease requires a directed history and physical examination. The neuroanatomy of vision is, however, both precise and specific, and a precise neurologic diagnosis can be made from visual symptoms in the acute care setting.

REFERENCES

1. Volpe NJ, Gaysas RE. Optic nerve and orbital tumors. *Neurosurg Clin N Am*. 1999;10:699-715.
2. Acheson J. Optic nerve and chiasmal disease. *J Neurol*. 2000;247:587-596.
3. Bense WE, Spalter HF. Vitreous hemorrhage. *Surv Ophthalmol*. 1971;15:297.
4. Bender M, Rudolph S, Stacy C. The neurology of the visual and oculomotor systems. In: Joynt R, Griggs R, eds. *Baker's Clinical Neurology*. Philadelphia: Lippincott Williams & Wilkins; 1998:3-9.
5. Afifi A, Bergman R. *Functional Neuroanatomy: Text and Atlas*. 2nd ed. New York: Lang Medical Books/McGraw-Hill; 2005.
6. Diaz-Calderon E et al. Bilateral internuclear opthalmoplegia after smoking "crack" cocaine. *J Clin Neuroophthalmol*. 1991;11:297-299.
7. Dobbin KR, Saul RF. Transient visual loss after licorice ingestion. *J Neuroophthalmol*. 2000;20:38-41.
8. Miller N, Newman N, eds. *The Essentials: Walsh and Hoyt's Clinical Neuroophthalmology*. Philadelphia: Waverly; 1998.
9. Campbell W. *Pocket Guide and Took Kit to DeJong's Neurological Examination*. Philadelphia: McGraw-Hill, Williams & Wilkins; 2008.
10. Achesan J, Sander M. *Common Problems in Neurophthalmology*. New York: WB Saunders; 1996.
11. Brazis PW. Localization of lesions of the oculomotor nerve: recent concepts. *Mayo Clin Proc*. 1991;66:1029-1035.
12. Brazis PW, Lee AG. Binocular vertical diplopia. *Mayo Clin Proc*. 1998;73:55-66.
13. Jacobon DM. Pupillary responses to dilute pilocarpine in preganglionic third nerve disorders. *Neurology*. 1990;40:804-808.
14. McFadzean R et al. Representation of the visual field in the occupital striate cortex. *Br J Ophthalmol*. 1994;78:185-190.
15. Horton JC, Hoyt WF. Quadrantic visual field defects: a hallmark of lesions in the extra-striate (V2/V3) cortex. *Brain*. 1991;114:1703-1718.
16. Loong SC. The eye in neurology: evaluation of sudden visual loss and diplopia—diagnostic pointers and pitfalls. *Ann Acad Med Singapore*. 2001;30:143-147.
17. Shingleton B, O'Donoghue M. Blurred vision. *N Engl J Med*. 2000;343:556-562.
18. Benavente O et al. Prognosis after transient monocular blindness associated with carotid-artery stenosis. *N Engl J Med*. 2001;345:1084-1090.
19. Richardson LD, Joyce DM. Diplopia in the emergency department. *Emerg Med Clin North Am*. 1997;15:649-664.
20. Hersh PS, Shah SI, Durrie D. Monocular diplopia following excimer laser photorefractive keratectomy after radial keratotomy. *Ophthalmic Surg Lasers*. 1996;27:315-317.
21. Dutt I et al. Unilateral internuclear ophthalmoplegia in systemic lupus erythematous. *J Assoc Physicians India*. 2000;48:1210-1211.
22. Zee DS. Internuclear ophthalmoplegia: pathophysiology and diagnosis. *Baillieres Clin Neurol*. 1992;1:455-470.
23. Chan J. Isolated unilateral post-traumatic internuclear ophthalmoplegia. *J Neuroophthalmol*. 2001;21:212-213.
24. Kumar PD, Nartsupha C, West BC. Unilateral internuclear ophthalmoplegia and recovery with thiamine in Weinicke syndrome. *Am J Med Sci*. 2000;320:278-280.

10
NEUROLOGIC
TRAUMA

Injury to the nervous system is a common cause of death and disability.[1] Injuries to the head often do not occur as an isolated event. Cervical spine injuries are the most significant associated injuries, and extremity injuries are the most common. Associated injuries are at times difficult to detect because of the impaired mental status of the head-injured patient. In this chapter the overall subject of injury to the nervous system is divided into two categories: head injury and spinal cord injury. The focus of the following discussions is on the evaluation and stabilization of patients who have an isolated central nervous system injury, with the understanding that trauma management requires a comprehensive, multisystem approach.

TRAUMATIC BRAIN INJURY

Traumatic brain injury (TBI) is a leading cause of death worldwide, particularly in those younger than 40 years.[2] Head injury and TBI are two distinct entities that are often, but not necessarily, related. A *head injury* is best defined as an injury that is clinically evident upon physical examination and is recognized by the presence of ecchymoses, lacerations, deformities, or the presence of rhinorrhea or otorrhea. *Traumatic brain injury* refers to an injury to the brain itself and can occur without external signs of trauma.

The Glasgow Coma Scale

Historically, the most often used system for grading the severity of a brain injury is the Glasgow Coma Scale (GCS) score. The GCS is based upon three factors: eye opening, verbal function (mental status), and motor function; a modified scale exists for nonverbal children (Table 10-1).[3] Created by Teasdale and Jennett in 1974, the GCS was developed as a standardized clinical scale allowing for reliable interobserver neurologic assessments of TBI patients in coma.[4] The original studies applying the GCS score, as a tool for assessing outcome, required that coma be present for at least 6 hours.[4-6] The scale was not designed to diagnose patients with mild or even moderate TBI nor was it intended to

TABLE 10-1

GLASGOW COMA SCALE FOR ADULTS AND FOR PREVERBAL CHILDREN

Eye opening	
Spontaneous	4
To speech	3
To pain	2
No response	1
Verbal response	
Adults	
Alert and oriented	5
Disoriented	4
Nonsensical speech	3
Moans	2
No response	1
Preverbal Children	
Coos, babbles	5
Irritable cry	4
Cries to pain	3
Moans to pain	2
No response	1
Motor response	
Adults	
Follows commands	6
Localizes pain	5
Withdraws to pain	4
Abnormal flexion	3
Abnormal extension	2
No response	1
Preverbal children	
Moves spontaneously	6
Withdraws to touch	5
Withdraws to pain	4
Abnormal flexion	3
Abnormal extension	2
No response	1
Grading of TBI	
Mild	13–15
Moderate	9–12
Severe	3–8

supplant a neurologic examination. Instead, the GCS was designed to provide an easy-to-use assessment tool for serial evaluations by relatively inexperienced care providers and to facilitate communication between care providers on rotating shifts. A single isolated GCS score is of limited value, is insufficient to determine the degree of brain parenchymal injury after trauma, and does not have prognostic value. On the other hand, serial GCS scores are a valuable clinical tool (when confounding factors such as drugs or alcohol are absent). A low GCS score that remains low, or a high GCS score that decreases, predicts poorer outcomes than high GCS scores that remain high, or a low GCS score that progressively improves. In one of the original multicenter studies validating the score, approximately 13% of patients who ultimately were in coma had a GCS of 15 (note that at the time these studies were done, CT scanning was not available to aid in clinical decision making).[6]

The literature refers to "mild" TBI as those patients with a GCS score greater than 12. Some authors have suggested that patients with a GCS of 13 be excluded from the "mild" category and be placed into the "moderate" risk group because of their high incidence of lesions requiring neurosurgical intervention.[7,8] The key for the clinician is not to overly rely on a GCS score, but instead to use the GCS score in conjunction with a relevant neurologic examination to assess head-injured patients for TBI.

Epidemiology

In the United States, approximately 1.6% of all emergency department (ED) visits are for a head injury. Approximately 90% of these visits are for mild TBI, and 10% for moderate or severe TBI.[9] TBI is the leading cause of death among people younger than 24 years.[10] There are 150,000 deaths due to trauma each year in the United States, of which 50% are due to fatal head injuries. The most common cause of head injuries is motor vehicle accidents in the young and falls in the elderly.[1] Approximately 50% of patients who die from TBI arrive at the hospital alive, a number that can potentially be decreased with early and aggressive interventions.[2]

Pathophysiology

When a head injury occurs there are *primary injuries* directly related to the trauma, e.g., skull fractures or blood vessel and/or brain parenchymal damage. *Secondary injury* refers to damage that results in neuronal death as a consequence of hypoxia, edema, and initiation of inflammatory cascades. Secondary injury greatly impacts outcome and can be minimized by resuscitative efforts.

Parenchymal brain injury results from a sudden deceleration or rotational acceleration that generates shearing forces within the brain. These forces disrupt small blood vessels and axons at gray and white matter interfaces. Injury to these small intraparenchymal vessels results in petechial hemorrhages or focal edema; disruption of extra-axial cerebral convexity "bridging" veins results in subdural hematomas; arterial injury, usually laceration of the middle meningeal artery or its branches within their periosteal course, results in epidural hematomas. Many patients may have a combination of intracranial injuries.

Diffuse Axonal Injury

Diffuse axonal injury (DAI) is a pattern of white matter changes frequently reported in TBI. It results from trauma-related impairment of intra-axonal neurofilament organization, which in turn impairs axonal transport, leading to axonal swelling, Wallerian degeneration, and transection.[11]

Epidural Hematoma

An epidural hematoma results from ongoing arterial bleeding which progressively compresses a portion of the brain resulting in a rapid progression of neurologic symptoms. The classic history is that of an immediate posttraumatic loss of consciousness followed by a "lucid" interval (often lasting hours) during which the patient may either awaken fully or at least show improvement in the level of consciousness, followed by a rapid neurologic deterioration. The treatment for most acute epidural hematomas is immediate surgical evacuation, ideally done in the operating room by a neurosurgeon. Under rare circumstances where a neurosurgeon is not immediately available, an ED burr hole may be lifesaving.

Subdural Hematoma

A subdural hematoma results from the tearing of the veins which bridge from the cerebral cortex toward a major dural venous sinus over a cerebral convexity. The venous bleeding takes place slowly, thus patients frequently present with a less than catastrophic decline in mental status and level of consciousness. However, large lesions can obviously result in profound neurologic damage and require emergent neurosurgical evacuation.

Intracerebral Contusion/Hematoma

An intracerebral contusion is a focal area of damaged parenchyma without significant (i.e., macroscopic) extravasation of blood. Intracerebral hematomas result from shearing forces in the brain. Neurologic deficits result from the combined compressive forces of the hematoma on the brain and the disruption of neural tissue itself. The history in these patients may be similar to that of patients with a subdural hematoma. They will frequently have focal neurologic findings. The decision to evacuate an intracerebral hematoma and the timing of the evacuation is most dependent on the size and location of the bleed, the patient's clinical course, and the patient's intracranial pressure. Hence, the initial baseline evaluation of the patient will be useful in deciding the course of therapy based on subsequent improvement or deterioration.

Cerebral Perfusion Pressure

Cerebral perfusion pressure (CPP) is the physiologic variable that defines the pressure gradient for cerebral blood flow (CBF). The CPP is the difference of the mean arterial pressure minus the intracranial pressure (ICP); thus, monitoring of the ICP is a necessity for CPP assessment. It is generally accepted that CPP is best maintained between 70 and 80 mm Hg. Under normal conditions, the brain is able to tightly control CBF through the process of autoregulation. Autoregulation is often lost in severe brain injury. A low CPP may jeopardize a region of the brain with preexisting or borderline ischemia while a high CPP may result in progressive cerebral edema and neurologic deterioration.

Prehospital Care of the TBI Patient

The overall goals of prehospital management of head-injured patients include rapid recognition and correction of life-threatening conditions, prevention of secondary brain insults, and transportation to the closest appropriate facility (Fig. 10-1).[12] In the case of a moderate

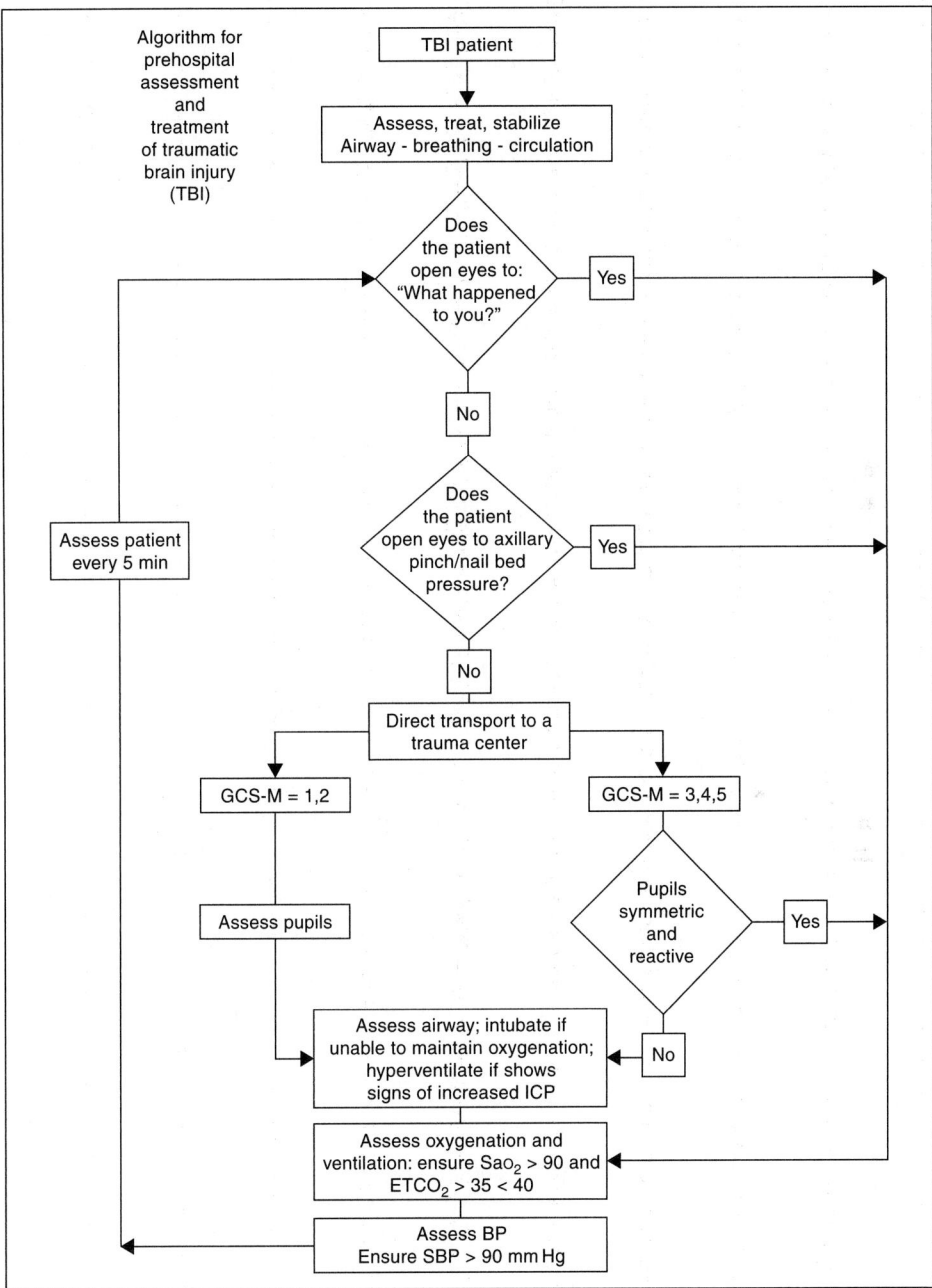

FIGURE 10-1   Prehospital management of patients with traumatic brain injury (TBI).

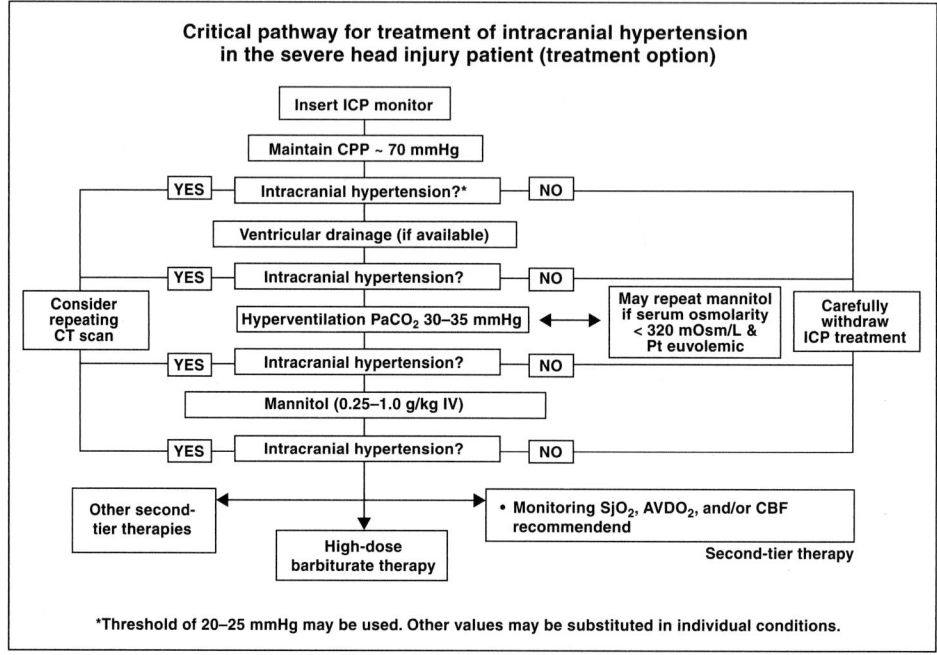

FIGURE 10-2   Hospital management of patients with severe traumatic brain injury. CPP, cerebral perfusion pressure; ICP, intracranial pressure.

or severe TBI patient, transportation ideally should be to a facility with 24-hour availability of neuroimaging and neurosurgical capabilities, including intracranial pressure monitoring and treatment (Fig. 10-2). However, transport decisions are dependent on a number of factors, including the presence of other injuries and the distance to various facilities.

Prehospital protocols begin with stabilizing the "A, B, Cs," including the cervical spine when indicated. Assessment focuses on determining the GCS score, pupillary response, blood pressure, and oxygenation.[12] Mechanism of injury, patient comorbidities, and serial GCS examinations must be used by the prehospital provider to determine the most appropriate target hospital for transport. Patients with a history of a penetrating injury, or the potential for a penetrating injury such as a gunshot to the scalp, deserve special attention and should be transported directly to a trauma center even if the injury appears inconsequential.

Prehospital management of the TBI patient includes assessing for and treating hypoglycemia when present and maintaining oxygen saturation above 90% and blood pressure above 90 mm Hg. Patients in coma who demonstrate signs of increased intracranial pressure are candidates for intubation with hyperventilation (Table 10-2) until the signs of increased intracranial pressure resolve. Intubated patients should be monitored with capnometry and maintained at a PCO_2 between 35 and 40 mm Hg; hypocapnia (PCO_2 <35) in patients who do not have clinical signs of herniation has been associated with worse outcomes in TBI patients.[12] There is no proven role for mannitol in the prehospital arena, especially when transport times are relatively short.[12] Agitated TBI patients must be assessed for confounding factors such as pain, hypoxia, or hypoglycemia; they may be treated with a benzodiazepine or a phenothiazine.

TABLE 10-2

SAMPLE RAPID-SEQUENCE INTUBATION PROTOCOL
FOR THE TBI PATIENT

1. Assess airway for difficulty; ensure ability to bag-valve mask.
2. Preoxygenate with 100% oxygen (do not bag-valve-mask unless necessary).
3. Prepare medications and rescue airway strategies.
4. Premedicate: Lidocaine 1.5 mg/kg and fentanyl 2.0–3.0 μg/kg.
5. Induction: etomidate 0.2 mg/kg.
6. Paralysis: succinylcholine 1.5 mg/kg.
7. Intubate with in-line cervical stabilization.
8. Confirm endotracheal tube placement with capnometry.
9. Consider long-term neuromuscular blockade, sedation, and analgesia.

Emergency Department Evaluation and Management

Evaluation of the head-injured patient requires a careful assessment of historical information that suggests that a brain injury has occurred, and an examination that assesses for focal neurologic deficits, including altered mental status. Table 10-3 lists pearls that may be helpful in evaluating TBI patients.

Initial Stabilization

Resuscitation, including brain-specific interventions, should occur simultaneously with the clinical assessment. As brain injury is a continuum that begins at impact, many secondary insults that exacerbate the initial damage occur during the ensuing hours and days. Identification of the factors predictive of poor outcome may be helpful in directing management and minimizing morbidity and mortality. These factors include hypotension, hypoxemia, hypercarbia, abnormal motor response, impaired or absent eye movements, abnormal pupillary light reflexes, the presence of an intracranial hematoma, or elevation of intracranial pressure over 20 mm Hg.

TABLE 10-3

CLINICAL PEARLS IN THE MANAGEMENT OF
HEAD-INJURED PATIENTS

- Neither loss of consciousness nor amnesia predicts whether or not a head-injured patient has sustained a brain injury.
- Serial Glasgow Coma Scale (GCS) scores, hypoxemia, and hypotension are the best predictors of outcome in traumatic brain injury (TBI) patients in the emergency department.
- A single GCS score determination has no predictive value, and thus the GCS must be repeated serially in select patients.
- Clinical signs of increased intracranial pressure include dilated fixed pupil(s) or extensor posturing and are acutely treated with hyperventilation; once signs of herniation resolve the P_{CO_2} should be maintained at 35–40 mm Hg.
- Patients with moderate or severe TBI should be transported to a hospital with neurosurgical capabilities.

BLOOD PRESSURE AND OXYGENATION Multiple studies have demonstrated the association of hypoxemia and hypotension with poor outcome in TBI patients.[13,14] Consequently, the cornerstone of stabilization is to maintain the oxygen saturation over 90% and the mean systolic blood pressure over 90 mm Hg.

The airway should be secured with rapid sequence intubation (RSI) in TBI patients who fail to ventilate, fail to oxygenate, or fail to protect their airway, or in those patients at risk of losing their airway, especially if they are leaving the ED. Table 10-2 outlines a sample protocol for RSI in TBI patients. Hypotension should be corrected as quickly as possible to bring the mean systolic pressure over 90 mm Hg. Isotonic intravenous crystalloid administration has been the mainstay of initial volume resuscitation.

History

On the initial encounter, it is not possible to determine accurately the degree of brain injury that a head-injured patient has sustained. Neither loss of consciousness nor amnesia has proven to be a reliable discriminator in determining which patients have sustained a TBI.[15] Severe headaches, seizures, vomiting, evidence of trauma above the clavicles, age >64, use of anticoagulants, or antiplatelet medications are concerning and prompt the need for a head CT; the absence of these findings has been found to be highly sensitive in excluding an injury requiring neurosurgical intervention even when loss of consciousness (LOC) has occurred.[15]

Physical Examination

The physical examination begins with a careful set of vital signs and with a general overview of the patient, assessing for evidence of scalp trauma, skull fractures, or signs of a basilar skull fracture ["raccoon eyes," Battle's sign, or the presence of cerebrospinal fluid leakage (otorrhea or rhinorrhea)]. Subtle findings such as an external ear canal laceration or hemotympanum may be critical for directing additional testing. Cushing's sign, i.e., hypertension with bradycardia, is a classic descriptor of severe TBI but unfortunately is a late and unreliable finding. Serial evaluations are useful until the clinician is satisfied that the patient is clinically stable. Finally, no decisions can be made until a focused neurologic examination has been completed.

The neurologic examination is necessary to establish the severity of neurologic injury and to establish the baseline with which subsequent examinations will be compared. The classic sign of an expanding intracranial mass lesion is a unilateral dilated and fixed pupil. This results from uncal herniation from a mass lesion medially displacing the uncus of a temporal lobe, which results in compression of the parasympathetic fibers at the periphery of the ipsilateral third cranial nerve in the suprasellar cistern; this finding is associated with a contralateral hemiparesis (as the ipsilateral cerebral peduncle is compressed). A less common phenomenon, known as Kernohan's notch, refers to a paradoxical motor sign in which there is a dilated and fixed pupil and a hemiparesis or hemiplegia both ipsilateral to the side of the primary lesion. In these cases, the brainstem has been pushed to the side contralateral to the side of the primary injury up against the tentorium resulting in the contralateral cerebral peduncle being compressed (in addition to the ipsilateral third nerve being compressed by the ipsilateral uncal herniation) resulting in hemiparesis and third nerve findings both ipsilateral to the side of the offending lesion.

The presence of focal neurologic findings or an altered mental status is predictive of significant lesions, although, conversely, the absence of such findings does not eliminate the possibility that an injury has occurred. When performing the neurologic examination, particular attention must be paid to cranial nerves III, IV, and VI (see Chapters 3 and 9). Papilledema is a late finding in ICP and thus is not seen in acute head injury. The pupil examination consists of determining pupil size, symmetry, and reactivity to light. Mass effect from edema or an expanding intracranial lesion may result in a unilateral fixed and dilated pupil (see "Kernohan's notch" mentioned earlier). Bilaterally dilated and fixed pupils are consistent with brainstem injury. Hypoxemia, hypotension, and hypothermia are associated with dilated pupil size and abnormal pupil reactivity, making it necessary to resuscitate and stabilize the patient before an accurate pupillary assessment can be performed.[12] Direct trauma to the eye may also result in a dilated pupil, or in an isolated cranial nerve IV or VI deficit that might not be evident until a careful extraocular muscle range-of-motion examination has been performed. An assessment of cognitive function may be helpful in select cases, in that it provides an important baseline in the patient's evaluation. Cognitive function is only superficially assessed in the GCS score through the patient's verbal response. In mild TBI, it has not been shown to be predictive of parenchymal injury demonstrable on head computed tomography (CT).[15]

HERNIATION The signs of cerebral herniation include one or both fixed dilated pupil(s) and extensor posturing (decorticate posturing is not a sign of herniation); in severe TBI patients, a decrease in the GCS score of 2 or more points suggests increasing ICP. Hyperventilation may be considered to be a temporizing measure in acute herniation, while osmotic diuretics (see "Hyperosmolar Therapy") is the mainstay of medical management.

Diagnostic Testing

Laboratory testing is tailored to the individual patient. All patients with altered mental status require an immediate serum glucose determination in order to avoid confusing hypoglycemia with a trauma-related condition. Brain-specific serum markers may have a role in detecting brain injury and in risk stratification for neuroimaging. The most widely studied biomarker is S-100B and the best available evidence suggests that if the serum level of S-100B, determined within 4 hours of injury, is less than 0.1 μg/dL, the risk of an acute traumatic lesion is minimal and a CT does not need to be performed.[15] This recommendation awaits validation before being put into general practice.

A noncontrast head CT is the test of choice for the initial evaluation of the TBI patient. Moderate and severe TBI patients require an imaging study; the only question is the timing of scanning and the possible need for repeat/serial scanning. Brain swelling with associated ICP develops in 10% to 15% of severe TBI patients who have an initial normal head CT, and in 53% to 63% of patients with acute traumatic abnormalities on a hospital admission CT.[2]

In the presence of clinical signs of herniation or progressive neurologic deterioration, the CT scan should be obtained as soon as possible, once the patient has been stabilized. In the absence of clinical signs of herniation or in cases of multiple trauma, CT scanning may be delayed pending the completion of other diagnostic tests though if other portions of the body are being evaluated with CT, the head can also be scanned at that time. Indications for head CT in mild TBI are discussed later in the chapter. There is no evidence that MRI is better than CT in the acute assessment of TBI,[15] though it does have some advantages in identifying brainstem lesions and diffuse axonal injury, and also in identifying nonhemorrhagic lesions in the subacute and chronic stages of care.

Management of Severe TBI

Intracranial Pressure Monitoring

ICP monitoring is used to facilitate maintenance of an adequate cerebral perfusion pressure. The ICP is normally 0 to 10 mm Hg; in general, an ICP of more than 20 mm Hg is an indication to initiate therapy to lower the pressure.[2] In patients with severe TBI, strong consideration should be given to initiation of ICP monitoring. ICP monitoring is indicated in severe TBI patients with CT scan evidence of edema, hemorrhage, hematomas, contusions, or effaced basal cisterns. ICP monitoring is also recommended in severe TBI patients who have a normal head CT but who have at least two of the following three features: age over 40, unilateral or bilateral posturing, and/or a systolic blood pressure of less than 90 mm Hg.[2] When only one of these features is present and the patient has a normal head CT, the risk of developing intracranial hemorrhage is low, and ICP monitoring is probably not indicated.

Hyperventilation

In the past, hyperventilation to maintain a Pco_2 of less than 25 mm Hg was the cornerstone of both acute and chronic management of patients with increased ICP. Indeed, hyperventilation leads to an initial decrease in the ICP by causing an immediate cerebral vasoconstriction with a resultant rise in cerebral vascular resistance and a fall in cerebral blood flow (CBF); however, there is evidence that cerebral anoxia can occur as a result of the cerebral vasoconstriction, resulting in worsening outcomes when hyperventilation is used past the initial resuscitation phase.[2] Hyperventilation therapy, to a Pco_2 of 30 to 35 mm Hg, is recommended only as a temporizing measure in patients with signs of increased ICP and should be discontinued as soon as the signs of increased ICP resolve.

Hyperosmolar Therapy

Mannitol, an osmotic diuretic, can reduce ICP by 25% or more within 5 to 20 minutes of its administration to patients with severe TBI. There is limited evidence to guide the dosing and timing of mannitol.[16] It is generally administered as intermittent boluses of 0.25 to 1 g/kg. Ideally, mannitol is given once ICP monitoring is in place, although therapy should not be delayed in patients showing signs of increased ICP. Also, ICP monitoring can help avoid the deleterious effects of overadministration of mannitol. When mannitol is used, care should be taken to maintain the patient in a euvolemic state by fluid replacement and to keep the serum osmolarity below 320 mOsm to reduce the possibility of renal failure.

Mannitol has two proposed mechanisms of action. One is an immediate but transient plasma-expanding effect, leading to improved cerebral perfusion as the result of reduced hematocrit, reduced blood viscosity, and increased CBF with improved oxygen delivery. The second mechanism is an osmotic effect that is delayed for 15 to 30 minutes while gradients between plasma and cells are established. Smaller and more frequent doses are safe and effective in reducing the ICP while avoiding the risk of osmotic disequilibrium and severe dehydration. After multiple doses or continuous infusions, mannitol may paradoxically elevate ICP by increasing brain swelling, the so-called rebound effect, probably secondary to accumulation of the mannitol in injured tissue.

Hypertonic saline (HTS) (generally 3%, though higher concentrations have been studied) lowers ICP by osmotic mobilization of water across the intact blood–brain barrier, thus reducing cerebral water content.[17] It may improve regional cerebral blood flow by a dehydration effect. HTS therapy causes an increase in intravascular volume leading to an increase in cardiac output. It should be used with caution in patients with cardiac disease. It is unclear if HTS provides an outcome advantage over mannitol and at this time is generally reserved as a secondary intervention when mannitol does not work.[2]

Barbiturates

High-dose barbiturates are recommended in hemodynamically stable severe TBI patients with intracranial hypertension that is refractory to maximal medical and surgical ICP-lowering therapy. However, they have not been shown to affect outcome and are not recommended prophylactically.[2]

Analgesia/Sedation/Neuromuscular Blockade

The severe head-injured patient commonly undergoes episodes of agitation and combativeness, both of which tend to increase ICP and complicate patient care. Therefore, treatment protocols should include the use of short-acting analgesics and sedatives such as fentanyl, midazolam, or propofol.

The use of neuromuscular blockade is also helpful in managing severe TBI patients. Neuromuscular blockade should be considered in any patient whose transportation, management, or diagnostic imaging is complicated by uncontrolled agitation or combativeness. The paralytic agents used should be short acting and discontinued as soon as feasible.

Anticonvulsants

Posttraumatic seizures (PTS) are classified as either early PTS (occurring within 7 days of injury) or late PTS (occurring 7 or more days after the injury). Approximately 15% of severe TBI patients have an early PTS; up to 20% will have a late PTS.[18] Phenytoin decreases the incidence of early PTS to 4% and is recommended in the first week post-TBI. Phenytoin has not been shown to impact on the incidence of late PTS. Consequently, prophylactic phenytoin is not recommended after the first week in patients with severe TBI.[19]

Corticosteroids

Evidence suggests that corticosteroids do not lower ICP or improve outcome in severely head-injured patients and therefore they are not recommended.[2]

Penetrating Trauma

When penetrating trauma occurs and penetrating foreign bodies protrude from the head, they should not be removed in the ED setting. While the foreign body is still lodged in the head, it may be tamponading vessels; release of the tamponade may cause catastrophic bleeding and deterioration in the condition of the patient. Penetrating foreign objects should be removed only in the operating room under controlled conditions.

Mild Traumatic Brain Injury

The question of how best to define a mild TBI is of great importance and has been a source of confusion. A small subset of these patients will harbor a life-threatening injury, while many will suffer neurocognitive sequelae for days to months after the injury (see "Post-concussive Syndrome"). The Centers for Disease Control and Prevention defines mild TBI as the occurrence of injury to the head resulting from blunt trauma or acceleration or deceleration forces with one or more of the following conditions attributable to the head injury during the surveillance period: (1) any period of observed or self-reported transient confusion, disorientation, or impaired consciousness; (2) any period of observed or self-reported dysfunction of memory (amnesia) around the time of injury; (3) observed signs of other neurologic or neuropsychological dysfunction; and (4) any period of observed or self-reported loss of consciousness lasting 30 minutes or less.[20] This definition is extremely broad and explains why there is so much difficulty in interpreting the mild TBI literature.

Skull Films

Skull films continue to be used as the first step in assessing mild TBI in many health care facilities, particularly those in which head CT is not readily available. However, a meta-analysis of the literature has concluded that, although a fracture demonstrated on plain film increases the likelihood of an intracranial lesion, its low sensitivity precludes its use to rule out the diagnosis of an intracranial hemorrhage; thus plain films are of limited clinical value in risk stratification for brain injury.[15] As plain radiographs cannot be used to rule in or rule out an intracranial lesion, they should not be obtained to evaluate trauma to the head with the exception of evaluating possible child abuse patients where they should be included as part of a skeletal survey.

CT in Mild TBI

Approximately 10% of patients with a GCS of 15 will have an acute lesion on noncontrast head CT; less than 1% will have a lesion in need of a neurosurgical intervention.[21] Neither loss of consciousness nor amnesia predicts which patients with mild TBI will have an intracranial injury requiring neurosurgical intervention. The literature does not clearly state which patients with intracranial lesions deteriorate, nor is it clear about the predictive value of the presence of intracranial lesions in predicting the development of postconcussive syndrome.

Well-designed studies and evidence-based practice guidelines recommend that patients with blunt head trauma who experienced loss of consciousness or amnesia, with a GCS score of 15 and a normal neurologic examination, do not need a head CT in the ED if they do not have headache, vomiting, an age over 60, drug or ETOH intoxication, deficits in short-term memory, physical evidence of trauma above the clavicle, or seizure.[15] Patients with any of the above findings, however, and those with a GCS score below 15, should be considered for a head CT, as well as patients on anticoagulants and patients with a history of hemophilia. It is unknown if there is additional risk if a patient is on antiplatelet medications.

Concussion and the Second Impact Syndrome

The *second impact syndrome* refers to the cumulative neuroanatomic damage that occurs when the brain is traumatized a second time before it has fully recovered from the first traumatic event. Controversy regarding the proper sideline evaluation and management of sports-related concussions led to the development of practice guidelines (Table 10-4).[22] However, these practice guidelines are consensus-based and await validation by method-ologically sound studies.

TABLE 10-4

MANAGEMENT RECOMMENDATIONS FOR PATIENTS
WITH CONCUSSION[a]

Grade I: Confusion but no loss of consciousness, no amnesia

Remove from activity (e.g., sporting event) and observe. When patient returns to baseline, have him/her exert him/herself by doing exercises; if patient remains asymptomatic, return to full activity.

Two grade I concussions in one day: no exertional activity for the rest of the day.

Three grade I concussions: no exertional activities that place the patient at risk for head trauma for 3 months.

Grade II: Confusion and amnesia, but no loss of consciousness

Remove from activity that places patient at risk for head trauma for the rest of the day.

Follow-up in 24 hours for reassessment.

No activity that places patient at risk for 1 week.

Two grade II concussions: no activity that places patient at risk for 3 months.

Grade III: Loss of consciousness

Transport to the ED for evaluation and a head CT.

Return to activities 1 month after a 2-week symptom-free interval.

Two grade III concussions: no activity that places patient at risk for head injury for 3 months.

[a]Modified from recommendations made in the Colorado Medical Society Concussion in Sports Guidelines.

Intoxication

In some reports as many as 42% of patients with TBI were "legally" intoxicated at the time they presented to the ED.[23] The difficult task of detecting an intracranial injury is compounded by the danger of attributing observed mental status changes to the alcohol. Although observation is an accepted practice for patients suspected of being intoxicated, the clinician must maintain a high level of suspicion and should combine clinical judgment with neurologic evaluations. There should be a low threshold for obtaining a head CT scan in an intoxicated patient who has signs of head injury.

Postconcussive Symptoms

The postconcussive syndrome (PCS) includes a wide spectrum of symptoms that commonly occur after a TBI. The symptoms are divided into three categories: somatic, cognitive, and affective (Table 10-5). Common symptoms include headache, dizziness/vertigo, difficulty concentrating, and depression. Up to 80% of mild TBI patients report some TBI-related symptoms at 3 months postinjury and up to 15% at 1 year postinjury.[24,25] It appears that well-motivated, young, male patients are at the lowest risk of developing the PCS and that females, those over 55, or patients who experienced prolonged posttraumatic amnesia are at a higher risk of developing PCS. Despite the emerging consensus that somatic and cognitive deficits result from mild TBI, physiogenesis versus psychogenesis of symptoms is debated, especially when symptoms persist for more than 3 months.

TABLE 10-5

SYMPTOMS SEEN IN POSTCONCUSSIVE SYNDROME

Somatic
Headache
Sleep disturbance
Dizziness/vertigo
Nausea
Fatigue
Oversensitivity to noise/light

Cognitive
Attention/concentration problems
Memory problems

Affective
Irritability
Anxiety
Depression
Emotional lability

When managing patients with mild TBI, it is important to take the time to advise them of the potential sequelae of the injury; such advice may significantly assuage their anxiety about permanent damage. A referral to a specialist with expertise in caring for these patients may be helpful for the patient's prognosis. Recovery appears to be linked not only to the underlying lesion but also to psychosocial issues in the patient's life. Consequently, access to multidisciplinary resources may provide the patient with the most comprehensive support services to assist in recovery.

Mild TBI in Infants and Children

Most injuries in infants are from falls, the vast majority of which are from a relatively short height such as from tables, chairs, and sofas. By early childhood the mechanisms of injury parallel those of adults. When the mechanism of injury is unclear or the clinical presentation does not appear to correlate with the reported clinical history, the possibility of child abuse should be considered (see Chapter 2). The current literature on mild TBI in pediatrics, as in adults, does not provide definitive evidence to make clinical decision-making easy. The American Academy of Pediatrics has published recommendations on the management of minor closed head injury in children older than 2 years[26] (Table 10-6). In essence, management is based on a careful neurologic examination, and decisions must take into account the environment to which the child is returning. Infants are much more difficult to assess clinically, in that their presentations are typically subtle and potentially misleading. Infants require careful observation; for patients with a history of a fall from less than 3 ft, observation alone is sufficient if the neurologic examination is normal and there is no evidence of scalp trauma.[27] Falls from more than 3 ft or an abnormal neurologic examination should prompt consideration for a CT scan.

TABLE 10-6

SUMMARY OF RECOMMENDATIONS BY THE AMERICAN ACADEMY OF PEDIATRICS FOR THE MANAGEMENT OF MINOR CLOSED HEAD INJURY IN CHILDREN 2 YEARS OR OLDER

- The use of head CT, skull radiograph, or MRI is not recommended for the initial evaluation and management of the child with minor closed head injury and no loss of consciousness.
- The use of skull radiographs or MRI in the initial management of children with minor closed head injury and loss of consciousness is not recommended.
- Skull radiographs have only a limited role in the management of the child with loss of consciousness: CT scanning is the imaging modality of choice.
- The risk–benefit ratio for the evaluation and management modalities of CT scanning or observation is unknown. For children who are neurologically normal after minor closed head injury with loss of consciousness, cranial CT scanning along with observation is an acceptable management option.
- Patients may be discharged from the hospital for observation by a reliable observer if the postinjury CT scan is interpreted as normal.

Disposition in TBI

Patients with severe or moderate TBI are usually admitted to the hospital. Patients with mild TBI and a positive CT scan for acute injury also require neurosurgical consultation, if available, and possibly admission for observation. Considerations for admission to the hospital or to an observation unit when the CT is normal include an abnormal mental status or neurologic examination, intractable vomiting, drug or alcohol intoxication, or suspicion of child abuse or domestic violence; consideration for admission should also be given to elderly patients on anticoagulants who do not have a competent observer at home.

Neuroimaging has resulted in a decline in the number of mild TBI patients admitted to the hospital for observation without a reported increase in adverse outcomes.[1] Although the safety of discharge after a normal CT has been established, patients with TBI may not remember their discharge instructions emphasizing the need not only to give patients written instructions, but also to provide a family member or friend with important information that will impact the patient during the recovery period. Table 10-7 provides the framework for discharge instructions.

Spinal Cord Injury

An essential part of early care of a traumatic event includes the assessment and management of the patient with the potential for injury to the vertebral column and spinal cord. Spinal cord injury can be devastating, with long-term disability, yet may be preventable if proper stabilization and early interventions are initiated. This section focuses on the acute management of the patient with potential vertebral column and/or spinal cord injury. The emphasis is on diagnostic approaches and initial management.

TABLE 10-7

SAMPLE DISCHARGE INSTRUCTIONS FOR MILD TBI PATIENTS

1. Thank you for coming to the emergency department. You have been evaluated for an injury to your head and for the possibility of an injury to your brain.
   ❑ You had a CT scan of your brain and no injury was identified.
   ❑ You did not have a CT of your brain because it was determined that it was not needed.
2. Very rarely after a head injury serious complications develop. You should return immediately to the emergency department if any of the following develop:
   ➤ Vomiting more than once
   ➤ Worsening or severe headache
   ➤ Progressive tiredness and unable to stay awake during times you would normally be awake
   ➤ Seizure
   ➤ Difficulty walking or difficulty with your vision
   ➤ Any new symptom that concerns you
3. It has been determined that it is safe for you to go home; however, it is very important to understand that many people often experience a variety of symptoms during the days and weeks after a head injury. These "postconcussive symptoms" may include headache, nausea, difficulty concentrating or remembering, tiredness, difficulty sleeping, emotional lability, or irritability. Generally these symptoms gradually go away with rest and time.
4. Tips for feeling better:
   ➤ Rest, get plenty of sleep, and gradually increase activity as able
   ➤ Avoid doing too much too fast
   ➤ Avoid alcohol
   ➤ Discuss return to sports with your trainer/team physician/primary care provider
5. Until you are back to feeling 100%, you should not drive; you should avoid physically and mentally stressful situations. It is reasonable for you to take time off from school or work until you feel able to fully do your work.
6. If you are not back to feeling normal within 5 to 10 days, follow up with your primary care provider or with a health care provider who has experience with treating head injury.
7. More information about head injury can be found at
   www.cdc.gov
   www.braintrauma.org
   www.biausa.org

Epidemiology

The National Spinal Cord Injury Database (NSCID) has been used to compile epidemiologic data on spinal cord injury patients in the United States since 1973; the current database contains more than 21,000 cases.[28] Data from the NSCID estimate 12,000 new cases of spinal cord injury each year. Four times as many vertebral column fractures occur without neurologic sequelae. Most patients with spinal cord injury are victims of vehicular trauma, followed by acts of violence, falls, and recreational sporting activities.

The incidence of cervical spine fracture in most series of blunt trauma patients is between 1% and 6%; fractures of the thoracolumbar spine occur in 2% to 3%. Roughly 65% of vertebral injuries involve the cervical spine, 20% the thoracic spine, and 15% the lumbar spine.[29] The most common site of fracture in the cervical spine is C2 (including the odontoid), which accounts for roughly 24% of fractures. The upper cervical spine (C1 through C3) is more likely to sustain injury in children (younger than 12 years) and in the elderly (older than 50 years), whereas the lower cervical spine (C6 through T1) is more often injured in young adults (12–50 years). Approximately 40% of cervical injuries in patients older than 50 years will involve the atlantoaxial complex.[30] If a patient has one spinal column injury, there is an increased risk of a second spinal injury being present.

Anatomy and Pathophysiology

The support structures of the spine are composed of 33 individual units grouped into five general divisions according to location and anatomic characteristics. Typically, there are 7 cervical vertebrae, 12 thoracic vertebrae, 5 lumbar vertebrae, 5 sacral vertebrae, and 3 to 5 coccygeal vertebrae. Separating each cervical vertebral body (except at the C1 through C2 level), each thoracic and lumbar vertebral body, and variably separating each sacral vertebral body are somewhat compressible intervertebral discs that form slightly movable articulations. The intercentral ligaments connecting vertebral bodies consist of these intervertebral discs in addition to the anterior and posterior longitudinal ligaments. Posterior vertebral arch osseous elements are attached to those at contiguous levels by additional cephalocaudad-oriented ligaments including the ligamenta flava, interspinous ligaments, joint–capsular ligaments, and the supraspinatus ligament.

In the transverse section, the spinal cord consists of (1) a butterfly-shaped central gray substance composed of collections of cell bodies and their processes and (2) a surrounding mantle of white matter composed of bundles of myelinated fibers that are divided into either ascending or descending tracts (see Fig. 10-3).

Ascending Tracts

The posterior columns of the spinal cord include the medially located fasciculus gracilis and the laterally located fasciculus cuneatus that together convey impulses cephalad and which are concerned with touch-pressure and kinesthesia (i.e., vibratory and position sense). As they ascend in the posterior columns, the fibers of these tracts shift medially and posteriorly creating a somatotopic organization of the fibers. Fibers ascend to the junction of the spinal cord and medulla and then to the respective nucleus gracilis and cuneatus in the ipsilateral medulla where they terminate on relay nuclei whose secondary fibers cross the midline to ascend in the contralateral medial lemniscus to the thalamus.

The lateral spinothalamic tract transmits impulses cephalad through the spinal cord, which are concerned with pain and thermal sensation. The spinothalamic fibers cross to

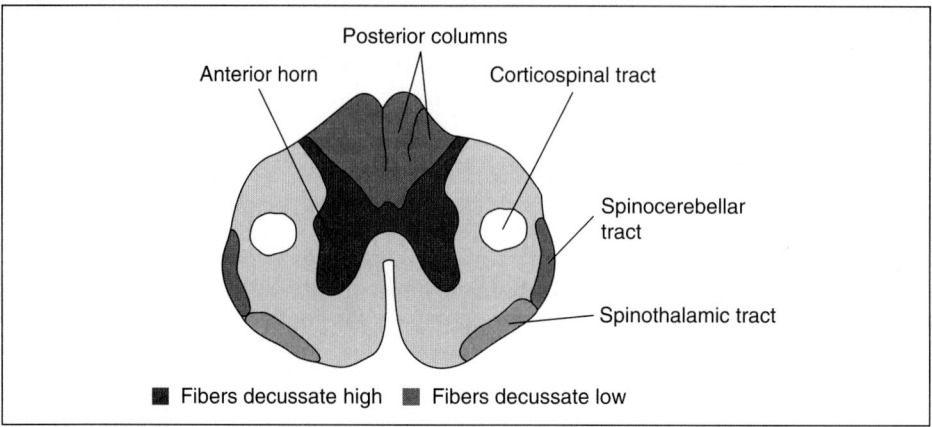

FIGURE 10-3   Transverse section of the spinal cord.

the opposite side of the spinal cord in the anterior white commissure within one or two spinal segments of their origin. This tract is also somatotopically organized, with the sacral and lumbar segments located laterally, and the thoracic and cervical segments located more medially.

Descending Tracts

Descending tracts are concerned with motor function and visceral innervation. The fibers of the corticospinal tracts originate in the cerebral cortex. In the lower medulla, at the pyramidal decussation, the corticospinal tracts undergo incomplete decussations dividing into three tracts: (1) the large lateral corticospinal tract (all fibers cross), (2) the small anterior corticospinal tract (fibers are uncrossed), and (3) the small anterolateral corticospinal tract (fibers are uncrossed).

Spinal fractures and dislocations carry a 14% incidence of spinal cord injury. Dysfunction of the spinal cord can result from mechanical impingement on the cord by bone, disc material, or hematoma. In the cervical region, the incidence of neurologic deficit with fracture is 39%. If there has not been anatomic transection of the spinal cord, a contusion of the cord can result in a progressive sequence of changes that begin initially as small hemorrhages centrally within the cord. These can evolve over minutes to hours with variable progressive hemorrhage, edema, and coagulation necrosis.

Initial Stabilization

Most patients with spinal cord injury will manifest impairment at the time of injury. However, manipulation may worsen an injury or cause injury in a patient without an initial cord injury who has an unstable spinal fracture; thus extreme care must be taken to protect and stabilize the spine until the true extent of a spinal injury is known. Maximum spinal immobilization is provided by a rigid cervical collar (which incorporates the upper thorax), sand bags or taped blocks, and a long spine board (padded or unpadded). Provisions for vigorous suctioning to prevent aspiration of blood and secretions should also be made readily available.

In most victims of major trauma requiring urgent airway management, intubation will be done *before* a full assessment of the cervical spine is possible. Rapid sequence intubation (RSI) protocols incorporating in-line cervical spine stabilization are recommended. There is no evidence that endotracheal intubation with in-line stabilization significantly increases the risk of neurologic injury in patients with unstable cervical spine fractures.[31] Some situations will require alternative airway management techniques such as fiberoptic laryngoscopy, lighted stylets, or an intubating laryngeal mask.

History

When obtaining the history of a cervical spine injury, an attempt should be made to delineate the mechanism of injury (flexion, extension, direct blow, rotation, etc.), magnitude of the forces involved (height of fall, speed of accident), timing of the onset of symptoms, and the time course of symptoms since the injury. The presence of spine pain, radicular pain, dysesthesias, and other neurologic symptoms (numbness, weakness) should be elicited and particular attention directed to whether neurologic deficits were complete or incomplete. Care must be taken to ensure that other injuries (e.g., chest, abdomen, pelvis, extremities) do not distract from detecting and fully evaluating a spinal injury.

If the history is unreliable because of intoxication or head injury, the lack of reported spine pain should be ignored, and one should treat an injury as spinal until disproved or until the history can be trusted. A history of osteoporosis, ankylosing spondylitis, idiopathic skeletal hyperostosis, rheumatoid arthritis, or previous spinal fusion raises the level of concern that a spinal injury could have occurred, even if an injury appears to be minor, as these patients are at increased risk of spinal fractures.

Physical Examination

A systematic neurologic examination is important in the initial evaluation of the patient with a possible spinal injury. Serial examinations are of equal importance in order to identify and document evolving neurologic pathology. Guidelines for motor and sensory evaluations have been established by the American Spinal Injury Association (ASIA; Table 10-8). In the awake, interactive patient, sensation is assessed by dermatome to localize the most cephalad extent of the spinal cord injury; on the anterior chest, dermatome levels abruptly change from C4 through T2 just above the nipple line. A spinal cord level can also be assessed by checking deep tendon reflexes (DTRs; Table 10-9). Pain sensation can be used to test contralateral spinothalamic tract function. Motor function, indicative of ipsilateral corticospinal tract integrity, is assessed on a 0 to 5 scale (see Chapter 3 for information on the neurologic exam). Dorsal column testing, which includes light touch, should not be neglected, as it will differentiate between a complete lesion and an anterior cord syndrome (see "Anterior Cord Syndrome"). The dorsal columns are best examined by assessing proprioception or vibration in the distal extremities. Special attention should be paid to rectal tone, sacral sensation, and bladder function to avoid missing injuries affecting the conus medullaris (terminal portion of the spinal cord at the thoracolumbar junction) and cauda equina, as well as documenting a complete versus incomplete spinal cord injury.

Spinal shock is a state of complete areflexia below the level of an acute, severe transverse spinal cord lesion. All spinal function and reflexes are lost for up to 6 weeks. In men, reversal of spinal shock is heralded by the return of the bulbocavernosus reflex. This reflex

TABLE 10-8

AMERICAN SPINAL INJURY ASSOCIATION
IMPAIRMENT CRITERIA

Grade A: Complete motor and sensory loss below level of lesion
Grade B: Complete motor loss with some sensory sparing below level of lesion
with sacral sparing
Grade C: Motor function intact including key muscles below the lesion level with
muscle grade less than 3
Grade D: Motor function intact including key muscles below the lesion level with
muscle grade greater than or equal to 3
Grade E: Motor and sensory function normal

is easily tested by pinching the glans penis or foreskin, which should elicit a contraction of
the bulbocavernosus muscle at the base of the penis and contraction of the rectal sphincter.

Cervical Spine Injury Patterns

While a full discussion of injuries of the cervical spine is beyond the scope of this text,
cervical spine injuries can be categorized according to four basic mechanisms of injury
and resultant radiographic alterations: flexion, extension, axial load, and rotational.

It should be remembered that the cervical spine can be thought of as being composed of two columns—namely an "anterior column" that includes the anterior longitudinal ligament, the vertebral bodies, and the posterior longitudinal ligament; and a "posterior column" that includes all structures located posterior to the posterior longitudinal
ligament including the osseous and ligamentous structures of the neural arch and the
intracanalicular structures including the spinal cord.

TABLE 10-9

ASSESSMENT OF DEEP TENDON REFLEXES IN RELATION
TO SPINAL CORD LEVEL

Upper extremities/torso
Pectoral C4–C5
Biceps C5–C6
Triceps C7 (C8)
Brachioradialis C5–C6
Upper abdomen T6–T9
Lower abdomen T10–T12

Lower extremities
Patellar L2–L4
Achilles S1–S2
Hamstrings L5–S1
Cremasteric L1–L2
Bulbocavernosus S3–S4
Anal wink S3–S5

Flexion

Flexion injuries cause compression of the anterior spinal column structures and distraction of the posterior column structures. This results in varying degrees of crush injury of the anterior aspect of the vertebral body, as well as variable degrees of ligamentous disruption and distraction of posterior column structures ("crushed in the front and wide in the back"). Simple wedge fractures, flexion "teardrop" fractures, unilateral facet dislocations, and bilateral facet dislocations represent a progression of severity (and instability) of flexion injuries.

Extension

Extension injuries cause distraction of the anterior column structures and compression of the posterior column structures. There is variable disruption and widening of the anterior column ligaments, as well as varying degrees of crush injury of the posterior column elements ("wide in the front and crushed in the back"). Extension injuries include the hangman's fracture and extension "teardrop" fractures.

Axial Load

Axial load injuries cause compression of both anterior and posterior column structures. These are the result of forces from above (skull) or below (pelvis) that are applied to the vertebral column in neutral position at the time of impact. Adjacent vertebral bodies are forced against each other with overwhelming force. The resultant force vectors cause the vertebral body to shatter outward, resulting in a *burst* fracture. A burst fracture is generally a stable fracture because the nearby ligamentous structures of the vertebral column remain intact. An exception is a burst fracture of the C1 vertebra (Jefferson's fracture), which is unstable and, like many spinal fractures, requires neurosurgical consultation.

Rotation

Rotational injuries occur when one of the facet joints (which are paired posterior column intervertebral articulations) acts as a fulcrum, and abnormal rotation with some degree of flexion causes the contralateral facet joint to dislocate. For any given two contiguous vertebra, such facetal dislocation is manifest by the inferior articulating facet of the more cephalad vertebra "jumping" superior to and then anterior to, the superior articulating facet of the more inferiorly located vertebra. Thus, the articulating facet of the upper vertebra (inferior) comes to rest in the intervertebral foramen region anterior to the articulating facet of the lower vertebra (superior). This injury, when unilateral, results in a "locked-in" position and is considered a stable injury (even though the posterior ligaments are somewhat disrupted). An anteroposterior radiograph will show that the usually midline spinous process above the level of the injury will be angled away from the midline in the direction of the rotational injury. On the lateral radiograph, a subluxation of the vertebra above the facet dislocation can be seen. These injuries can be subtle on plain radiographs, but are easily delineated on CT. Note should be made that when the above-described injury occurs bilaterally resulting in bilateral "jumped" facets, the spinal injury is often unstable.

Spinal Imaging

As discussed in Chapter 2, for evaluation of the cervical spine, some patients require no imaging, some may be evaluated with limited plain radiography, and some require CT.

Most patients with a fracture identified on plain x-ray will subsequently undergo CT scanning to further characterize the fracture and to search for additional occult fractures. Patients with spinal trauma and neurologic symptoms consistent with spinal canal injury will almost always also undergo MRI regardless of whether a fracture is identified on plain radiographs or CT. Patients with spinal fractures, but no neurologic findings do not necessarily have to undergo MRI, but many do so to search for associated spinal canal hematomas, injured ligaments, or herniated discs before spinal surgery is performed.

Spine Radiography

As with all tests, a positive finding on a plain radiograph has meaning, but a negative result does not disprove injury. There can be significant ligamentous instability or spinal cord injury without radiographic findings. In addition, patients with one spinous fracture frequently have another spine fracture. The National Emergency X-Radiography Utilization Study (NEXUS) was a prospective, multicenter, observational study that included 34,069 patients with potential cervical spine injury.[32] It identified negative predictors of cervical spine injury (Table 10-10). In a follow-up study of 818 patients, 5.5% of patients with a cervical fracture had a distracting injury and 3% had altered alertness or intoxication as the only criteria that predicted their cervical spine injury.[33] Similar studies have been conducted for thoracic and lumbar imaging, although they are not as large as NEXUS.[34] Based on these studies, it is reasonable to use criteria similar to those established by NEXUS for imaging the thoracolumbar spine.

Three-View Versus Five-View Versus Seven-View Cervical Radiography

A single cross-table lateral view of the cervical spine has a sensitivity between 57% and 85% for identifying a fracture. Addition of the anteroposterior and open-mouth odontoid views to the cross-table lateral view increases the sensitivity to 99%.[35] Consequently, a minimum of three radiographic views should be obtained. Adding two oblique views provides improved visualization of posterior column structures (pedicles, articular pillars, neural foramina, and lamina). These views are also useful in visualizing the cervicothoracic junction and may be used instead of the "swimmer's" view. They are indicated in patients with a poor-quality three-view series of radiographs or in patients suspected of having a pedicle fracture (Table 10-11).

Lateral flexion and extension radiographs complete a seven-view cervical spine series. They assess for ligamentous injury and can be considered in patients who have

TABLE 10-10

INDICATIONS FOR CERVICAL RADIOGRAPHY FOLLOWING BLUNT TRAUMA[a]

1. Neck pain
2. Midline cervical tenderness
3. Altered mental status including any evidence of intoxication
4. Focal neurologic deficits or complaints
5. Distracting painful injury

[a]Based on the NEXUS data; cervical radiography is not indicated in the absence of all five criteria.

TABLE 10-11 ———————————————————————

INTERPRETATION OF CERVICAL SPINE RADIOGRAPHS

Lateral view
Alignment: anterior, middle, and posterior arcs
Bones: uniformity and height of vertebrae and spinous processes
Cartilage: intervertebral disc space height and length
Soft tissue: prevertebral soft tissue width

Anteroposterior view
Alignment of spinous processes
Distance between spinous processes
Uniformity and height of vertebrae

Open–mouth odontoid view
Spacing of dens and lateral masses
Lateral alignment of C1 and C2
Uniformity of bones

neck pain but are neurologically intact. Timing of these views is controversial, but in general they are usually obtained 2 to 3 days to weeks after an injury as initial muscular spasm can give a false negative study.[36]

Computed Tomography and Magnetic Resonance Imaging

Multidetector CT scanning is the best modality for identifying fractures of the spine (see Chapter 2). CT is much better than MRI for identifying osseous lesions, and therefore spinal fractures cannot be ruled out on an MRI scan; however, MRI is far superior to CT for detecting soft tissue and spinal cord lesions (see "MRI"). It is recognized that CT is increasingly being used as the initial screen in trauma patients due to its ready availability, ease of use, and cost-effectiveness.[37] With modern scanners, the entire cervical spine can be scanned at 1- to 2-mm intervals with creation of multiplanar 2-dimensional and 3-dimensional reformatted images in a matter of seconds. However, except in major trauma patients, at some institutions, CT is still sometimes reserved for patients with questionable lesions on plain film radiographs or in patients with persisting pain despite "normal" plain films.

MRI

MRI plays an important role in the evaluation of suspected spinal cord injury (see Chapter 2). It has replaced myelography for evaluation of these patients, except in those patients with contraindications to MRI or indwelling foreign material that, while still MR compatible, might result in artifacts, which could obscure areas of clinical interest. The advantages of MRI include its lack of ionizing radiation, its noninvasiveness (e.g., as opposed to myelography), its multiplanar imaging capabilities, its lack of need to introduce a contrast agent, and, most importantly, its superior "contrast resolution" which results in superior delineation of soft tissues (e.g., disc material, ligamentous structures, pathology such as hematomas, etc., as well as the spinal cord itself). Current indications for emergent MRI evaluation in the setting of acute spinal trauma include complete or incomplete neurologic deficits or ongoing deterioration of neurologic function. Relative indications for emergent MRI include assessing for associated incidental spinal canal hematomas or herniated discs in neurologically intact patients with spinal fractures who are about to undergo spinal surgery and in some patients with suspicion of ligamentous injury despite negative flexion/extension films.

Spinal Cord Lesions

Complete Cord Lesions

Complete transection of the spinal cord is most commonly caused by trauma (other rarer causes include spinal cord infarction, hemorrhage, and acute compressive disc herniation). Below the level of the lesion there is loss of motor, sensory, and autonomic (including sphincter) function. All reflex function below the level of the lesion is acutely lost secondary to spinal shock (see "Physical Examination"). Lesions in the cervical region can interrupt all sympathetic fibers before they exit the spine in the thoracic region (T1 through T10 levels). This results in functional sympathectomy, with a decrease in systemic and pulmonary vascular resistance. Because of the loss of this sympathetic tone, there is a relative increase in vagal tone to the heart with concomitant decrease in cardiac contractility and cardiac output. This results in a syndrome of bradycardia with hypotension. Loss of sympathetic tone is accompanied by gastric atony, bowel and bladder dysfunction, and impairment in temperature regulation. Lesions involving the C3 through C5 levels result in loss of phrenic nerve function, diaphragmatic paralysis, and respiratory compromise.

Acute lesions below the cervical region usually do not affect sympathetic tone in such a dramatic fashion, but all motor, sensory, and reflex functions also will be lost below the level of the lesion.

Complete motor–sensory deficit signifies a poor prognosis, especially if it persists for 24 hours post injury; the presence of neurologic sparing represents an incomplete injury with a better long-term prognosis. The perianal region is most commonly spared in both sensory and reflex testing. A complete lesion that persists for 24 hours has only extremely rarely been associated with useful motor recovery. Complete spinal lesions cannot be diagnosed until spinal shock has worn off (reflexes are regained), which is usually within 24 hours of injury.

In caring for patients with complete spinal cord lesions, a careful examination must be performed to ensure that associated hypotension is not due to internal bleeding or drugs before it is attributed to the spinal injury. Once spinal shock is diagnosed, treatment is with fluids and vasopressors. These patients also require meticulous supportive care in order to avoid injury such as aspiration and pressure sores.

Incomplete Spinal Cord Injuries

BROWN-SEQUARD SYNDROME   True hemisection of the spinal cord is a rare occurrence; if found, it is usually associated with penetrating trauma. The syndrome, in its pure form, is characterized by ipsilateral loss of motor function and proprioception with contralateral loss of pain and temperature sensation. As the fibers in the lateral spinothalamic tract move up and down one or two segments before crossing to the contralateral side, analgesia may be noted one or two segments above the lesion. There may be an ipsilateral loss of pinprick sensation at the level of the lesion because the nerves that carry this information have not yet crossed to the contralateral–lateral spinothalamic tract. In reality, a "partial Brown–Sequard syndrome" is more often seen with varying degrees of paresis and analgesia.

ANTERIOR CORD SYNDROME   Anterior cord lesions are characterized by loss of motor function and pinprick sensation below the level of the lesion. The posterior columns are preserved; therefore, light touch, position, and vibratory senses remain intact. This lesion is typically seen following hyperflexion injuries with acutely dislocated vertebral body fragments or acutely herniated disc material compressing the anterior spinal artery and spinal cord.

CENTRAL CORD SYNDROME   The central cord syndrome is the most prevalent of the partial cord syndromes. It is characterized by bilateral motor paresis that is greater in the upper extremities than in the lower extremities. The paresis is often denser more distally in the extremities than proximally. There is variable sensory impairment and bladder dysfunction. This syndrome is commonly associated with hyperextension neck injuries in elderly patients with preexisting cervical spondylosis. A good mnemonic for this syndrome is MUD: *M*otor > sensory, *U*pper > lower, and *D*istal > proximal.

Anatomically, the central cord syndrome can be explained by the somatotopic organization of the long tracts of the spinal cord. As the deeper (i.e., most central) portions of the posterior columns, the corticospinal tracts, and the lateral spinothalamic tracts contain fibers from the upper extremities, the degree and extent of neurologic deficits, while dependent on the size of these central lesions, have a greater tendency to involve the upper extremities.

CONUS MEDULLARIS SYNDROME   The conus medullaris is the terminal portion of the spinal cord usually located at approximately the thoracolumbar junction or upper lumbar spinal canal in adults. Isolated lesions of the conus medullaris are rare but they produce a typical syndrome. Disturbances of urination, specifically a denervated autonomic bladder, are common. Primary sphincteric involvement as well as loss of sexual function are prominent features. Sensory abnormalities may involve only the lower sacral and coccygeal segments or may present as complete saddle anesthesia. These often present as a mixture of upper and lower motor neuron deficits involving the gluteal musculature and, depending on the extent of the lesion, the lower extremities. The bulbocavernosus reflex is absent.

Spinal Injury in Children

Cervical spine injuries are infrequent in children, and those that do occur frequently involve the occipitoatlantoaxial segment (the craniovertebral junction region). This is the result of a proportionally heavier head, a higher fulcrum of flexion, greater ligamentous laxity (allowing for more mobility at C1 through C2), the presence of unfused physes, and the presence of horizontally inclined articular facets that facilitate sliding in younger children.

There are also a number of anatomic characteristics unique to the pediatric cervical spine that may mimic injury, but should not be confused with a significant injury. These include pseudosubluxation at either the C2 vertebra over the C3 vertebra or C3 over C4, some degree of anterior wedging of vertebral bodies, secondary ossification centers that may mimic posttraumatic avulsions, variable interspinous distances, widening of the atlantoaxial interval ("predental") space (up to 5 mm), and apparent lateral displacement of the lateral masses of C1 on C2.

There were 3,065 patients in the NEXUS database who were younger than 18 years, of which 30 had sustained a cervical spine injury. Only 4 of the 30 injured children were younger than 9 years and none were younger than 2 years. The decision rule correctly identified all pediatric cervical spine injury victims; however, the small number of infants and toddlers in the study precludes definitive recommendations.

Spinal Cord Injury Without Radiographic Abnormality

Spinal cord injury without radiographic abnormality or SCIWORA is a syndrome of neurologic injury without evidence of osseous injury or significant spinal malalignment on plain radiographs or CT. It occurs in the pediatric population, making up 4% to 67% of all pediatric spinal injuries; it results from highly elastic ligaments and increased spinal mobility.[38] SCIWORA usually occurs in adults as the result of preexisting spondylitic changes of the cervical spine, resulting in reduced diameters of the cervical spinal canal. There were 27 cases of SCIWORA in the NEXUS database; all were in adults, none were in children.[32]

The presentation of SCIWORA ranges from complete paralysis to subjective complaints of numbness. Patients with SCIWORA have positive MRI findings ranging from spinal cord hemorrhage or edema to intervertebral disc herniation and spinal cord transection. MRI findings appear to correlate with outcome: patients with transient symptoms and a normal MRI have an excellent prognosis, those with cord edema but no hemorrhage do variably well, and those with major cord damage (e.g., cord transection or hemorrhage) have an extremely poor prognosis.

Spinal Cord Injury Management

Early treatment for any spinal cord injury, incomplete or presumed complete, must address vertebral column alignment and stability and decompression of the spinal cord or nerve roots. Alignment and stability are initially attempted in the cervical region by head-traction devices. When this cannot be accomplished in a timely manner by closed techniques, operative reduction with internal fixation is considered.[39] In the thoracic region, malalignment is uncommon because of the stabilizing properties of the ribs. Thoracic injury sufficient to cause spinal malalignment/dislocation usually results in concomitant massive injury to other intrathoracic structures. Thoracic immobilization is usually accomplished by bed rest. Lumbar immobilization is similarly accomplished, but occasionally operative reduction may also be necessary.

Intuitively, it would seem reasonable to decompress a compromised spinal cord or nerve root surgically. However, there is no conclusive evidence that early surgery to remove bone and disc fragments provides improved outcomes over conservative management. Management of these patients remains controversial and is dependent on the local neurosurgical practice.[39]

There is evidence that management of acute spinal trauma results in better outcomes and a lower incidence of paralysis when the patient is managed in a trauma center with high volumes of spinal cord injuries.[40] Neurosurgical intervention in acute spinal trauma varies from center to center and is dependent on the prevailing experience of the treating physician.

Pharmacotherapy for Acute Spinal Cord Injury

A number of agents have been studied in an attempt to improve neurologic outcome following spinal cord injury, including naloxone, glucocorticoids, nimodipine, tirilazad mesylate, and GM-1 ganglioside. The National Acute Spinal Cord Injury Studies (NASCIS) suggested an outcome benefit of high-dose methylprednisolone therapy when given within 8 hours of spinal cord injury.[41] The recommendation was the result of a secondary analysis of the data and the overall methodology of the trials has received considerable criticism.[42] A randomized trial in France using an identical treatment protocol failed to show a benefit of corticosteroid therapy.[43] The American Academy of Neurologic Surgeons performed a critical analysis of the trials on steroids in spinal trauma and questioned the benefit of treatment.[44] Currently, corticosteroids in spinal trauma are a treatment option and the negligible potential benefit must be carefully weighed against the potential for harm, i.e., increased risk of infection.

SUMMARY

The possibility of a spinal injury should be considered in all trauma patients. Patients with moderate or severe TBI, altered mental status, or multiple trauma and fractures elsewhere should be carefully assessed for a spine or spinal cord injury. Initial evaluation is directed at stabilizing the patient, establishing baseline neurologic function, and determining the appropriate degree of acute imaging evaluation necessary with respect to the spinal injury. Particular attention to perianal sensation and reflexes may detect signs of function in a patient who would otherwise be classified as having a complete cord lesion. Early specific therapy is directed at immobilization and reduction of dislocations; the use of corticosteroids remains controversial but generally is not recommended. Prevention of the complications of paralysis should start at the time of initial diagnosis, utilizing a multidisciplinary team approach.

REFERENCES

1. Thurman D, Guerrero J. Trends in hospitalization associated with traumatic brain injury. *JAMA*. 1999;282:954-957.
2. Brain Trauma Foundation. Guidelines for the Management of Severe Head Injury. 3rd ed. *J Neurotrauma*. 2007;24:S1-S82.
3. Chameides, L, Hazinski M, eds. *Textbook of Pediatric Advanced Life Support*. Vol 8. Dallas, TX: American Heart Association; 1994:3.
4. Teasdale G, Jennett B. Assessment of coma and impaired consciousness; a practical scale. *Lancet*. 1974;4:81-83.
5. Teasdale G, Jennett B. Assessment and prognosis of coma after head injury. *Acta Neurochir*. 1976;34:45-55.
6. Jennett B et al. Severe head injuries in three countries. *J Neurol Neurosurg Psychiatry*. 1977;40:291-298.
7. Stein SC, Ross SE. Mild head injury: a plea for routine early CT scanning. *J Trauma*. 1992;33:11.

8. Williams D, Levin M, Howard E. Mild head injury classification. *Neurosurgery*. 1990;27:422.

9. Jager T, Weiss H, Coben J, et al. Traumatic brain injuries evaluated in U.S. emergency departments, 1992–1994. *Acad Emerg Med*. 2000;7:134-140.

10. White BC, Krause GS. Brain injury and repair mechanisms: the potential for pharmacologic therapy in closed head trauma. *Ann Emerg Med*. 1993;22:970.

11. Povlishock J. Pathobiology of traumatically induced axonal injury in animals and man. *Ann Emerg Med*. 1992;22:980-986.

12. Brain Trauma Foundation. Guidelines for prehospital management of severe traumatic brain injury. *Prehosp Emerg Care*. 2007;12(suppl):S1-S50.

13. Chesnut R et al. The role of secondary brain injury in determining outcome from severe head injury. *J Trauma*. 1993;34:216-222.

14. Kokoska E et al. Early hypotension worsens neurological outcome in pediatric patients with moderately severe head trauma. *J Pediatr Surg*. 1998;33:333-338.

15. Jagoda A, Bazarian J, Bruns J, et al. Clinical policy: neuroimaging and decision making in adult mild traumatic brain injury in the acute setting. *Ann Emerg Med*. 2008;52:714-748.

16. Wakai A, Morley E, Zahtabchi S. Mannitol for traumatic brain injury: searching for the evidence. *Ann Emerg Med*. 2008;52:298-300.

18. Quereshi AI, Suarez JI. Use of hypertonic saline solutions in treatment of cerebral edema and intracranial hypertension. *Crit Care Med*. 2000;28(9):3301-3313.

19. Temkin N et al. A randomized, double-blind study of phenytoin for the prevention of posttraumatic seizures. *N Engl J Med*. 1990;323:497-502.

20. Chang BS, Lowenstein DH. Practice parameter: antiepileptic drug prophylaxis in severe traumatic brain injury: report of the Quality Standards Subcommittee of the American Academy of Neurology. *Neurology*. 2003;60:10-16.

21. Centers for Disease Control and Prevention, National Center for Injury Prevention and Control. Report to Congress on mild traumatic brain injury in the United States: steps to prevent a serious public health problem. Atlanta, GA: Centers for Disease Control and Prevention; 2003:1-47.

22. Colorado Medical Society Sports Medicine Society. *Guidelines for the Management of Concussion in Sports*. Denver, CO: Colorado Medical Society, 1991.

23. Dikmen S, Machamer J, Konovan D, et al. Alcohol use before and after traumatic head injury. *Ann Emerg Med*. 1995;26:167-176.

24. Alves W, Macciocchi S, Barth J. Postconcussive symptoms after uncomplicated mild head injury. *J Head Trauma Rehab*. 1993;8:48-54.

25. Rutherford WH, Merret JD, McDonald JR. Symptoms at one year following concussion from minor head injuries. *Injury*. 1978;10:225.

26. American Academy of Pediatrics. The management of minor closed head injury in children. *Pediatrics*. 1999;104:1407-1415.

27. Gruskin K, Schutzman S. Head trauma in children younger than 2 years: are there predictors for complications? *Arch Pediatr Adolesc Med*. 1999;153:15-20.

28. Spinal Cord Injury Information Network. Spinal Cord Injury: facts and figures at a glance. June 2006. www.spinalcord.uab.edu. Accessed November 23, 2009.

29. Burney RE et al. Incidence, characteristics and outcome of spinal cord injury at trauma centers in North America. *Arch Surg*. 1993;128:596-599.

30. Goldberg W et al. Distribution and patterns of blunt traumatic cervical spine injury. *Ann Emerg Med*. 2001;38:17-21.

31. Manoach S, Paladino L. Manual in-line stabilization for acute airway management of suspected cervical spine injury: historical review and current questions. *Ann Emerg Med*. 2007;50:236-245.

32. Hoffman JR et al. Validity of a set of clinical criteria to rule out injury to the cervical spine in patients with blunt trauma. *N Engl J Med*. 2000;343:94-99.

33. Panacek EA et al. Test performance of the individual NEXUS low-risk clinical screening criteria for cervical spine injury. *Ann Emerg Med*. 2001;38:22-25.

34. Terrigino CA et al. Selective indications for thoracic and lumbar radiography in blunt trauma. *Ann Emerg Med*. 1995;26:126-129.

35. MacDonald RL, Schwartz ML, Mirich D, et al. Diagnosis of cervical spine injury in motor vehicle crash victims: How many x-rays are enough? *J Trauma*. 1990;30:392-397.

36. Pollack CV et al. Use of flexion–extension radiographs of the cervical spine in blunt trauma. *Ann Emerg Med*. 2001;38:8-11.

37. Schenarts PJ, Diaz J, Kaiser C, et al. Prospective comparison of admission CT scan and plain films in the upper cervical spine in trauma patients with altered mental status. *J Trauma*. 2001;51(4):663-668.

38. Gupta SK et al. Spinal cord injury without radiographic abnormality in adults. *Spinal Cord*. 1999;37:726-729.

39. McDonald J. Spinal-cord injury. *Lancet*. 2002;359:417-425.

40. Macias C, Rosengart M, Puyana J, et al. The effects of trauma center care, admission volume, and surgical volume on paralysis after traumatic spinal cord injury. *Ann Surg*. 2009;249:10-17.

41. Bracken MB et al. A randomized, controlled trial of methylprednisolone or naloxone in the treatment of acute spinal cord injury. *N Engl J Med*. 1990;322:1405.

42. Hurlbert RJ. Methylprednisolone for acute spinal cord injury: an inappropriate standard of care. *J Neurosurg*. 2000;93:1-7.

43. Pointillant V et al. Pharmacological therapy of spinal cord injury during the acute phase. *Spinal Cord*. 2000;38:71-76.

44. American Association of Neurological Surgeons and the Congress of Neurological Surgeons. Pharmacological therapy after acute cervical spinal cord injury. *Neurosurgery*. 2002;50(suppl 3): S63-S72.

PSYCHOGENIC NEUROLOGIC SYNDROMES

The evaluation of patients with presumed psychogenic neurologic symptoms presents a great challenge to the skills of any physician. Because disease affecting the nervous system can manifest in a multitude of ways, differentiation of true organic from functional neurologic manifestations can, at times, be extremely difficult. Psychogenic neurologic syndromes are not uncommon, and there may be a psychogenic origin to some aspect of patients presenting symptoms.[1] The term *psychogenic neurologic syndrome* is used to describe a collection of psychologic disorders presenting with neurologic signs and symptoms that have no identifiable organic etiology within the nervous system. They have also been termed pseudoneurologic syndromes[2] or "functional" disorders.

For the purposes of this chapter, some basic definitions are needed.[3] The term malingering is used to describe a willful, deliberate imitation or exaggeration of illness that is intended to deceive others for a consciously desired end. Malingering is divided into three types. The first is pure malingering, in which there is not even a presumed organic basis for the symptoms and signs. The second is partial malingering or exaggeration. In this condition, which is a much more common presentation to physicians, there is an expansion of true disability or symptoms that would ordinarily be attributed to a documented organic problem. The third type of malingering, false imputation, occurs when a patient may indeed have a real disease; however, the symptoms described are not those that could reasonably be attributed to that disease entity. While there is a rich and extensive literature on malingering in many settings and for many conditions, most involve the use of testing not available in the acute care setting. However, many of the lessons learned in clinical practice will be emphasized here. It is useful to know, however, that sophisticated testing designed to evaluate for suspected malingering exist.

By contrast, the term *hysteria* has been used to imply that a patient is not conscious of the unreality of their symptoms. This determination can be difficult. The range of possible symptoms is as broad as all of neurology. Although the term *hysteria* is no longer used in a number of official diagnostic classifications, it is in common use in practice and in medical

TABLE 11-1

MEDICAL CONDITIONS WITH FEATURES SUGGESTING CONVERSION DISORDER

Guillain–Barre syndrome
Multiple sclerosis
Nonconvulsive status epilepticus
Pure sensory stroke
Ciguatera poisoning
Hypoglycemia
Electrolyte disorders
Brain/spinal abscess
Dystonic-type medication reaction

literature.[4] To the extent that the term does not convey the psychiatric nature of the illness, it should be avoided and the term conversion disorder be used. Signs and symptoms of conversion disorder have been labeled as hysteria in the past.[5] Only those syndromes common to the emergency department (ED) or acute outpatient settings are addressed herein. One should be careful in applying the label of conversion disorder, as patients initially so labeled are not uncommonly later diagnosed with an organic illness.[6] Table 11-1 lists some medical conditions that can easily be mistaken for conversion disorder. When a language or cultural barrier exists, be especially careful. Table 11-2 lists key aspects of the *Diagnostic*

TABLE 11-2

DIAGNOSTIC CRITERIA FOR 300.11 CONVERSION DISORDER

A. One or more symptoms or deficits affecting voluntary motor or sensory function that suggest a neurologic or other medical condition.
B. Psychological factors are judged to be associated with the symptom or deficit because the initiation or exacerbation of the symptom or deficit is preceded by conflicts or other stressors.
C. The symptom or deficit is not intentionally produced or feigned (as in factitious disorder or malingering).
D. The symptom or deficit cannot, after appropriate investigation, be fully explained by a general medical condition, or by the direct effects of a substance, or as a culturally sanctioned behavior or experience.
E. The symptom or deficit causes clinically significant distress or impairment in social, occupational, or other important areas of functioning or warrants medical evaluation.
F. The symptom or deficit is not limited to pain or sexual dysfunction, does not occur exclusively during the course of somatization disorder, and is not better accounted for by another mental disorder.

Specify type of symptom or deficit:
  With motor symptom or deficit
  With sensory symptom or deficit
  With seizures or convulsions with mixed presentation

and Statistical Manual, 4th edition (*DSM-IV*), criteria for the diagnosis of conversion disorder.[7] It is helpful not to be biased by the preliminary perceptions of others, as such bias can result in a "chain of presumption" that the problem is not an organic one.[8]

In this chapter, emphasis is placed on a mode of examination and a style of practice that will allow one to gather the information necessary to render an appropriate diagnosis while at the same time establishing a trusting therapeutic relationship with the patient. It may be appropriate in selected circumstances to obtain a formal psychiatry[9] or neurology referral.[10]

It cannot be overemphasized that the role of any physician faced with patients presenting with possible psychogenic complaints should be that of making the differentiation between two varieties of illness. One must view the differentiation between two legitimate illnesses (psychogenic and organic) in somewhat the same manner as a physician would approach the differentiation between appendicitis and gastroenteritis. The physician's attitude should be that of a caring problem-solver. The communication of this attitude will go far in establishing an appropriate relationship with the patient and significant others.

GENERAL APPROACH

Physicians must communicate to patients, through actions and words, that they are the patients' advocate. A physician's attitude must be one of trying to do the best that can be done for the patient. As in other parts of medicine, this will be accomplished by firmly establishing a diagnosis while at the same time developing a trusting relationship.

Open-ended questions can be the most productive. Specifics will be elicited, and they are covered under specific subject headings later in this chapter. Frequently, when patients are allowed to respond to an open-ended question, they reveal data that would not otherwise have been elicited. Asking what the circumstances were and what was going on in the patient's life at the time the symptoms occurred will allow patients the option of expressing what is uppermost in their minds, thereby furnishing facts that might have gone unsuspected by the physician. An independent history taken from family members or friends may be extremely helpful.

A functional neurologic diagnosis should be based on the demonstration of positive signs. The patient must demonstrate neurologic signs and symptoms that are inconsistent with the functioning of the nervous system[2] thereby allowing examiners to best differentiate organic from nonorganic illness. This presupposes a relatively detailed knowledge of the anatomical, physiological, and pathologic manifestations of dysfunction in the nervous system. It also presupposes that patients lack the sophisticated knowledge of the nervous system that physicians possess. At times such might not be the case, because some patients can be extremely sophisticated in their knowledge. Early in the encounter with the patient, the examiner must assess this level of sophistication in order to pursue an appropriate line of questioning and examination.

The positive signs that are inconsistent with the functions of the nervous system will be the academic substance of this chapter. The method of obtaining these signs has more to do with the art of medicine.

Because knowledge of anatomic and physiologic mechanisms in neurologic illness is incomplete and current methods of objective verification have limitations, a general attitude of caution is preferable in diagnostic evaluation. Often, patients with neurologically unexplained disorders have a history of other medically unexplained disorders.[11]

For the examiner to convince the patient and everyone involved that a careful opinion has been rendered, a focused history and a detailed, relevant, professional neurologic examination are important. It is only when the patient is taken seriously that all concerned will recognize that the physician is carefully pursuing the problem.

The physician must constantly ascertain the level of certainty of the information obtained. For example, the sensory examination is primarily subjective. There are limitations to asking nonmedical firsthand observers to describe what may be a relatively sophisticated neurologic event. At times, however, firsthand observers and witnesses, such as emergency medical technicians, paramedics, and bystanders, may render information that is much more important than is any neurologic test. Communication with relatives, other physicians, and others may provide a great deal of useful information, as can a review of past records.

The neurologic examination should be conducted with attention to certain details. The reasons for this are many. For most patients the neurologic examination is something outside their usual experience. It is common for them to realize that injured extremities will be palpated and chests will be auscultated. However, the neurologic examination is something different. The tapping of reflexes, observation of coordinated motor acts, and ophthalmologic examinations are unusual experiences. It is a legitimate use of this aspect of the neurologic examination to communicate to the patient that the examiner does truly possess a sophisticated knowledge of the nervous system, which will in turn lead to trust and confidence in the examining physician. Although the subject matter of this chapter is that of psychogenic neurologic syndromes, one must always be alert to exclude organic, but unrelated, medical conditions. When an organic medical condition is discovered, the patient may simply drop all the functional complaints, having adopted a genuine focus of medical attention.

The best attitude for the physician to adopt is one of intellectual humility. The most experienced and concerned physician will at times label a syndrome as functional only to find it attributed to an organic problem at a later date. Diseases of the nervous system and their presentations are so variable that 100% accuracy is impossible.

Remember the words of William Beaumont, "Even if the story we are told is a tangle of impossibility, copied from the repertoire of the father of lies, and worthy of the mother of invention, it may have a genuine pathological basis."[12]

The examiner should be aware of the limitations of the clinical neurologic examination. Testing of coordination, motor function, and strength is done on a somewhat subjective basis. These functions are not usually tested in a repetitive, strictly reproducible and quantifiable fashion. Confrontation visual field testing, for example, is crude by comparison with that obtained by a tangent-screen apparatus. The sensory examination is likewise a highly subjective examination, and all examinations are performed at one moment in time in the course of a patient's illness.

Most experienced examiners have encountered patients with large nervous system lesions who had a normal examination relative to the functional area of the nervous system involved.[13] This is not to say that the neurologic examination is a poor starting point for neurologic evaluation. There is nothing more informative, cost-effective, or valuable

TABLE 11-3

CLUES TO PSYCHOGENIC ORIGIN

Indifferent attitude
Bizarre symptoms
Fluctuating, suggestible, or alternating deficits
Past history of psychogenic symptoms
Having a role model for symptoms
Temporal psychological proximity for stressor

to the evaluation than a carefully obtained history and properly performed neurologic examination.

One final point relative to the neurologic examination is worth emphasis. In general, patients who are malingering will not be interested in or will agree to only a few examinations. They are consciously trying to imitate a neurologic deficit, which involves intense concentration for reproducibility. Therefore, if one gets a sense from a patient that he or she does not wish to be examined, this may be the first indication of malingering. This is in contrast to patients with a conversion disorder, who, because they lack knowledge of the unreality of their symptoms, are not aware that they may sometimes present with conflicting and shifting neurologic deficits (Table 11-3).

PSYCHOGENIC NUMBNESS

Numbness is a difficult neurologic symptom to evaluate. It is subjective and frequently vague. Each patient has his or her own idea of what it means. By numbness, most physicians mean an area of altered sensation. Examiners clearly separate the sensory functions from the motor functions. Patients, however, frequently do not separate these two functions. Examiners must determine early on in the interaction that they and the patient have the same perception of altered sensation and not some other symptom.

Patients with numbness on an organic basis are usually specific about the sensory modality involved and the location, as opposed to patients with psychogenic complaints, in whom numbness may be vague or shifting, or not clearly defined in the patient's mind. One must establish whether the patient feels the area of numbness is that of complete anesthesia, or of analgesia (meaning lack of painful sensation), or some other alteration of sensory modality. Precise definition of the involved area is essential. There are several classic psychogenic locations of numbness (Table 11-4).

While taking the history, one should note the time course of the symptom and what actions were taken by the patient. An indifferent attitude to the sudden onset of large areas of numbness, possibly associated with other neurologic symptoms, can be seen in functional patients. The mode of onset and particularly a history of trauma should be elicited. It is during this time that one asks about the circumstances under which the event took place, thereby allowing the patient a means of expressing feelings related to an event that may have caused psychological trauma. Asking how a problem has affected the patient will give further clues to a psychogenic complaint. Patients may say that it kept them from caring for a child or performing a specific task. Without asking such

TABLE 11-4

SIGNS OF PSYCHOGENIC NUMBNESS

Split vibratory senses
Touch response when not touched
Motion but not position sense
Pin withdrawal
Glove-and-stocking anesthesia stopping at joint lines
Hemigenitalia–hemirectum anesthesia
Crossed interlocked finger test

specific questions, physicians might be unaware of the significance of a psychogenic complaint. Asking relatives or others similar questions is a valuable tool, because relatives might be able to relate how this deficit has impaired the patient's ability to interact with others.

A key to the neurologic examination is observation. One first notes the affect of the patient. What is the attitude expressed toward what could potentially be a significant neurologic illness? As mentioned before, an indifferent attitude, seen frequently in conversion disorder, can be a clue.

The neurologic examination, excluding the sensory examination, should be performed first so as to isolate the complaint and allow one to examine the sensory system indirectly without drawing attention to the examination. The examiner realizes that motor and sensory examinations are linked as a functional unit and in areas such as reflex arcs. The examiner, but not the patient, realizes that many sensory functions have been found to be normal prior to a more formal sensory examination. Certain classic neurologic findings, which one can begin to elicit and document, are inconsistent with the normal functioning of the nervous system. Although split vibratory sensory loss, with the lack of reporting of vibration on one side of a bilateral structure such as the cranium, has been classically associated with psychogenic illness, infrequently patients with organic disease have reported this phenomenon.[13]

Extremely unsophisticated patients can be examined with a technique in which they are asked to close their eyes and respond when they feel they have been touched with a "yes" and a "no" when they feel they have not been touched. The examiner then proceeds to touch various parts of the body. Patients with a psychogenic complaint may promptly report "no" immediately after an area has been touched, indicating that they had some sensation there but are not yet willing to say they felt it. This obviously suggests that one is dealing with a very unsophisticated patient, so the test must be done rather quickly and not repeated very often, for even the most unsophisticated patient will realize its contradictory nature.

An additional test can be done when testing position sense. Classically, when position sense is tested, the proximal interphalangeal joint of the finger is fixed and then the examiner either elevates or depresses the distal interphalangeal joint of the finger. With their eyes closed, patients are instructed to respond with an "up," a "down," or an "I don't know" with respect to the movement of the distal phalanx. If they respond promptly "I don't know" to every position change of the distal phalanx, they are at least reporting that they have intact motion sense and touch.[14] Motion and position sense are very closely aligned in the nervous system, so the patients have demonstrated that they do have motion sense. However, be aware that one can have loss of position sense with other sensations, e.g., pain, being intact on an organic basis.

Withdrawal to a pinprick is another test. The patient's withdrawal from a brief pinprick at least demonstrates that the reflex arc is intact. If there is associated verbalization of pain, then that sensation has at least reached consciousness. Some altered sensation may be present, but at least one has documented the presence of some sensation; at this point the patient may realize that sensation has been demonstrated and reverse the complaint. Isolated sensory symptoms, either loss of sensation or spontaneous pain, may, however, occur from thalamic stroke.[15]

One other classic pattern of sensory loss is that of the glove-and-stocking distribution. Although glove-and-stocking distribution sensory loss is commonly seen with peripheral neuropathies, these are not of acute onset, and they do not stop abruptly at joint lines, as they often do with psychogenic complaints. There is no anatomic sensory boundary at the elbow, wrist, or shoulder. Acute vascular insufficiency to an extremity could give this pattern, but it should be obvious clinically.

Physicians should tailor their sensory examination to what they predict will be the most productive modalities to test, since it is impossible to test all of them all the time. It is sometimes useful to do sensory testing on the interlocked crossed fingers[16] (Fig. 11-1). The midline sensory supply of the trunk can be tested. There is some crossover to either side of the midline, and patients with organic lesions will usually have some preservation of sensation over the midline and then gradual diminution after that. Sensory loss directly at the midline is uncommon in organic lesions.

PSYCHOGENIC WEAKNESS

A psychogenic complaint of weakness is common. The examiner should be careful to differentiate between weakness and numbness and should be aware of the patient's meaning. Although the physician may initially think of weakness in terms of specific anatomic locations or nerve distributions, patients may have a concept of weakness as a generalized loss of energy or neurasthenia. They may feel there is a lack of energy throughout the body.

The history from a patient complaining of weakness should be obtained in a way similar to that described for numbness. The physician should first attempt to find out what the patient means with respect to the weakness (i.e., was it complete or partial, what its relative time course was, and what functions were lost and what functions were preserved). Frequently patients with weakness on a psychogenic basis are unable to perform certain acts (for instance, picking up a pen and writing one's name or picking up a child to care for them), whereas other motor actions that require use of the same muscles are preserved. Questioning the patient concerning trauma and especially emotional trauma can be productive.

Observation of the patient is again the key to the neurologic examination. Watching the patient undress, sign the chart, move about the room, or gesture during the examination can be superior to the formal muscle strength testing that is a usual part of the neurologic examination, because the patient is somewhat distracted by questions and routines.

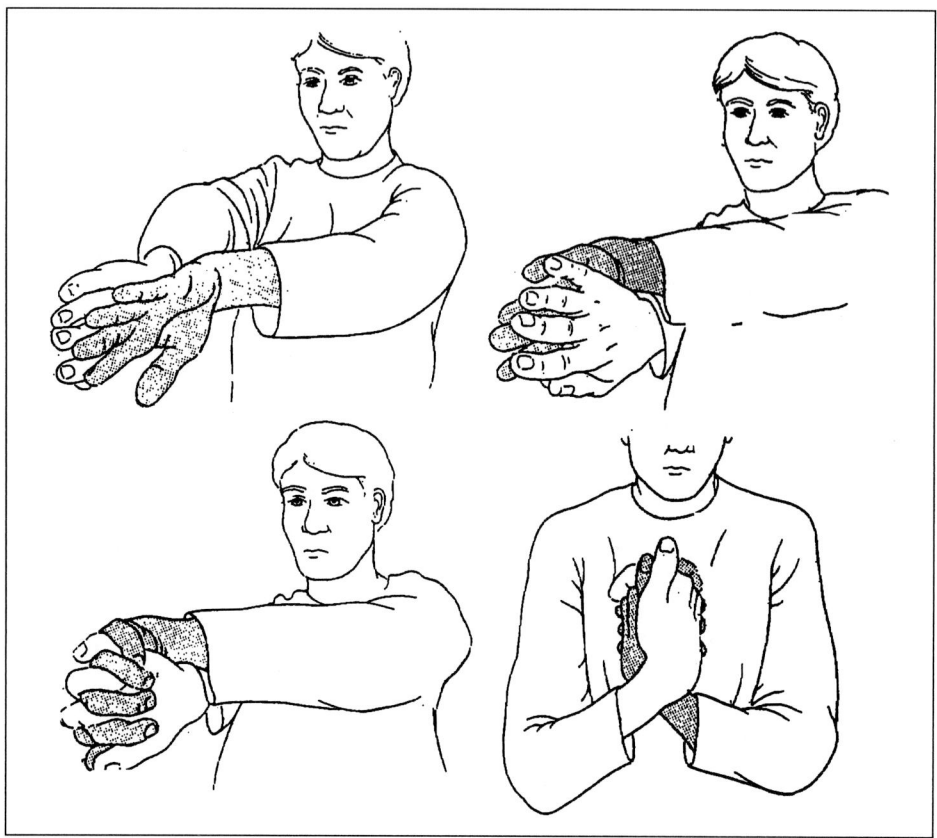

FIGURE 11-1   Interlocked crossed fingers.

A classic sign of psychogenic weakness is that of giveway weakness (Table 11-5). It is difficult to imitate the true mild decrease in muscle strength that accompanies a true organic deficit. The patient may try to simulate something less than full strength. When formal muscle strength resistance testing is performed, one feels a cogwheel or ratchet-type loss of strength. If examiners vary resistance continually over a wide range, they will find at times that their most powerful effort cannot overcome the patient's muscle; at

TABLE 11-5

SIGNS OF PSYCHOGENIC WEAKNESS

Weakness of motion but not specific muscles
Giveway weakness
Abduction test
Hoover's sign
Astasia–abasia
Falling toward safety
Active contraction of antagonist

other times, a very weak effort can overcome it. This is what is meant by giveway weakness. One commonly sees a giveway weakness in a painful limb as an organic cause. Frequently, when the extremity is dropped, such as back down to the patient's lap or examining table, it falls at less than the speed that would be dictated by gravity alone. It may sometimes fall into a very natural position into the lap.

There are means of testing cooperation and effort and not specifically the degree of power in the muscle. The first is the abduction test. To perform the test as diagrammed (Fig. 11-2), patients are asked to abduct their legs while lying supine. This is a bilaterally innervated function, and if they are truly trying to move the supposed weak leg, the examiner will feel the supposed normal leg making a counterbalancing effort. This is also

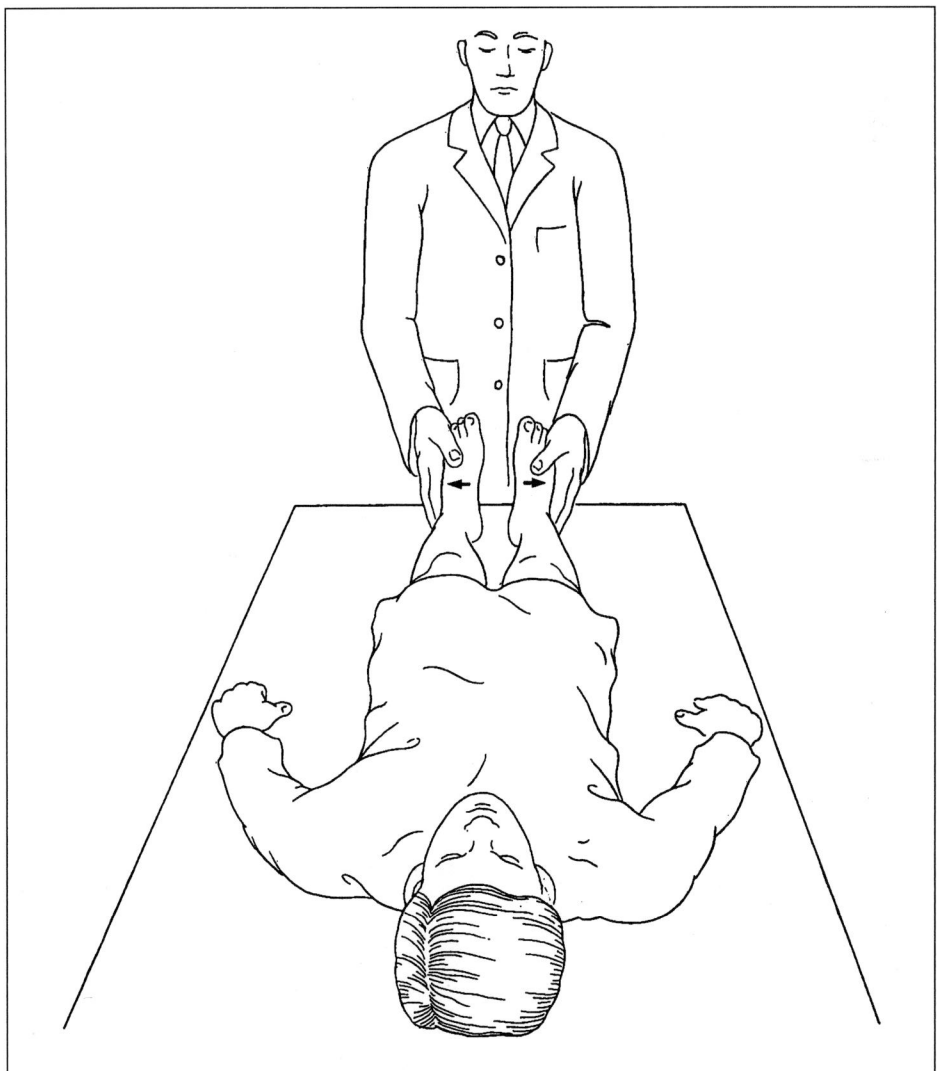

FIGURE 11-2 Abduction test. Patients abduct their legs while lying supine.

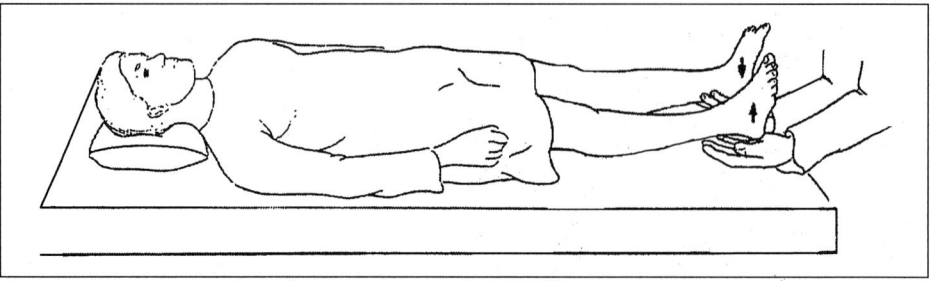

FIGURE 11-3   Hoover's sign. Examiner's hands are placed beneath the heels of the patient.

the basis of Hoover's sign. In this test, the examiner's hands are placed beneath the heels of the patient, as in Figure 11-3, and the patient is asked to raise the supposedly weak leg. The examiner should feel increased pressure under the good leg as the patient presses down to counterbalance an effort to raise the supposed weak leg. Failure to feel this is a sign that the patient is not making a conscious effort. It must be emphasized that the most these tests reveal is that the patient is not cooperating with the examination. Whether the patient is truly weak in addition to this cannot be determined by these tests.

Other motor signs are occasionally seen in the patient who complains of weakness and/or difficulty with coordination. This is referred to as astasia–abasia: the patient's loss of coordination is accompanied by a wild flinging motion of the arms and possibly the legs. The patient tries to walk or stand on one foot with large flinging motions of the arms but does not fall. This actually demonstrates superior balance, muscle strength, and coordination, as opposed to the poor results the patient may have wished to demonstrate. Psychogenic gait problems are characterized by exaggerated efforts, extreme slowness, variability, and unusual or uneconomic postures.[17]

Frequently a patient with a psychogenic weakness will fall only to the side of the examiner or a supportive relative or friend. Falling only toward the stretcher or toward the door of the examination room is also seen. When placed in the middle of the room, such patients seem to walk well until they approach a "safe" object, and then they fall and grasp the object. The fall may be theatrical.

Another sign seen in patients with supposed weakness in one leg is that of actually dragging a foot as if it were made of lead. It is as though the patient were pressing the foot very tightly to the floor.

Testing the action of the sternocleidomastoid muscle in turning the chin to the opposite side has somewhat limited applicability. A patient with a hysterical paralysis involving the right side of the body may not realize that the right sternocleidomastoid turns the head to the left. Motion in that direction may be strong, and motion in the other direction may be paradoxically weak.

An important sign that can be demonstrated when doing individual muscle strength testing is that the patient is actively contracting the antagonistic muscle to the action being requested. By palpating the antagonistic muscle, the examiner can demonstrate good strength in the opposing muscle. If one then asks for the antagonistic action to be performed, the patient may contract the muscle that was supposedly weak.

The examiner must obviously be selective in choosing which one of these signs to try to elicit. The signs should be elicited once or at most twice and not repeated, because their usefulness tends to decline with time as the patient becomes more familiar with the tests. The tests should be performed with an attitude that they are routine, not to somehow trick the patient, but simply to reveal the nature of the problem.

DISORDERS OF CONSCIOUSNESS

Coma and alterations of consciousness are common as psychogenic problems (Table 11-6). The disorders are often an embellishment on a mild organic deficit, or they may occur in the setting of other, serious diseases. For example, mild alcohol or other drug intoxication may be embellished to the point of coma when in reality it may produce only minimal lethargy. There is no other area in which firsthand observers are as helpful in obtaining a history, especially if the patient has awakened upon arrival in the ED. One may need to search for a history of diabetes, drug ingestion, seizure disorder, and trauma (both physical and emotional in the appropriate setting). There is also no other time when one can lose rapport faster with the patient than when conducting the coma examination unless meticulous care is exercised. The patient and significant others must place trust in the examiner as a caring physician in order to arrive at a reasonable disposition. Efforts to "awaken" the patient that involve painful stimuli or other degrading or humiliating procedures serve only to weaken whatever limited therapeutic relationship existed at the start. As always, part of the initial observation of the patient is to ensure the patient's airway and circulation are adequate prior to other examinations.

Several important clues to disorders of consciousness can alert the examiner to a psychogenic possibility. Patients may be in a trancelike state in which their eyes are open. They seem to be unresponsive and may have alternating laughing and crying spells. They may have unresponsiveness but purposeful movements. If one suspects embellishment on a true deficit and feel that laboratory analyses may be in order (toxicologic screens, glucose, or other laboratory work), it is expeditious to obtain these tests very early in the evaluation, because later the patient may not be cooperative. It cannot be emphasized strongly enough that using painful stimuli and other provocative procedures, such as ammonia capsules, Foley catheters, needle punctures, etc., to awaken the patient with psychogenic unresponsiveness is unproductive and jeopardizes the caring relationship that the physician should wish to establish. Noxious procedures may turn a patient who was benignly "comatose" into a belligerent and physically aggressive person. It may also be interpreted by the family as lack of respect and sensitivity toward the patient.

TABLE 11-6

SIGNS OF PSYCHOGENIC COMA

Trancelike states
Normal postures and tone
Voluntary eyelid closure
Bell's phenomenon
Normal involuntary movements
Fixed downward gaze on opening the eyes

Simple observation over time may be very productive as the patient may tire of the effort required to maintain the deception.

In many patients, unresponsiveness on a psychogenic basis can be established by pulling open the eyelids and observing the eyes. Once the patient has made eye contact with the physician, they may begin to respond and talk. Sometimes only the sclera is seen, thus demonstrating Bell's phenomenon. This voluntary eyelid resistance to lid opening causes the eyes to turn up in the head, and one can then see only the sclera. This signifies voluntary eyelid closure on the part of the patient. If this has not occurred, the physician can examine the pupils and check extraocular movements. It is frequently with this maneuver alone that patients can no longer maintain unresponsiveness; once they establish eye contact, they will proceed to become "responsive." Patients may always look to the side away from the examiner. This has been described as the eye's consistently being "deviated" toward the side of the bed.[14] Also, the slow, very gradual, and often incomplete eyelid closure that occurs in truly comatose patients when the lids are released from the open position cannot be simulated.

Observation alone may alert the physician that the patient may not be truly unconscious. Patients may have purposeful motor movements when being transferred from stretcher to bed or X-ray table. They may grasp at personal objects. They may cross their legs, set their hands behind their head, or assume other normal voluntary postures. If the examiner feels certain that there has been no trauma to the cervical spine, sitting patients up may cause them to become responsive. Dropping the hand onto the face is a relatively poor test. Patients may in fact allow the hand to strike the face. A better test is to see that they actually have voluntary limb resistance, or that the hand, when dropped, falls too slowly. Although intact slow- and fast-phase nystagmus on ice water caloric testing indicates that the patient is physiologically awake, it is usually uncomfortable and unnecessary.

Simply talking to patients in a normal conversational tone and establishing oneself as a physician is important. Asking them to cooperate so that you might help them establishes the fact that you are on the side of the patient and that you understand they are not unconscious. Moreover, it illustrates that you know they are troubled and that you are there to try to help with whatever kind of problem they have, regardless of its nature. Minimally provocative tests, such as nasal tickle, will provoke patients to use their extremities in a coordinated and purposeful way and to open their eyes. Once eye contact has been made, patients can be further examined. Frequently a brief discussion with patients whose eyes are closed about the fact that the physician is aware they may be having some problems is useful. This can be followed by a brief period of observation, which will allow patients the dignity of reversing their "coma." Allowing patients their dignity while performing these maneuvers strengthens the therapeutic alliance with the physician.

If there is sufficient doubt about whether the embellishment on a mild deficit may be organic or not, one should manage patients as if they have disorders of consciousness. As mentioned above, laboratory specimens can be obtained early in the evaluation of the patient and then held should the examiner find it necessary to analyze them. Performing a general physical examination sufficient to exclude a true unrelated medical problem such as the result of trauma is important.

Even in the best of hands of the most caring physician, some patients deprived of their "comatose" state may become uncooperative and leave the ED without the physician's having had the opportunity to establish the fact that such patients had no physical evidence of a serious condition.

PSEUDOSEIZURES

Patients who present with pseudoseizures have varying levels of sophistication and knowledge of what constitutes a true seizure. Frequently pseudoseizures, also termed nonepileptic seizures or psychogenic nonepileptic seizures,[18] are an embellishment on a true seizure disorder, which makes evaluation even more difficult. Ten to fifty percent of patients with pseudoseizures have an underlying seizure disorder.[19] The neurologic literature is clear on the point that many varieties of abnormal behavior can be attributed to a seizure disorder. Conversely, there are almost no manifestations of true epilepsy that cannot be simulated in conversion disorder or malingering. There are certainly patients, usually with an underlying seizure disorder, who present with pseudoseizures that are difficult even for the most experienced examiner to differentiate. Simultaneous video and EEG recording, while not available in the usual outpatient or ER setting, can at times be useful in differentiating psychogenic from organic seizures in problematic cases. The majority of pseudoseizures, however, are very unsophisticated and are easy for an examiner with sufficient experience in observing true seizure disorders to differentiate.

It is important for the physician to observe the episode. Without direct observation, it is difficult to make the differentiation. If one must resort to the report of a firsthand observer, there are several areas to be questioned. The nature of the shaking movements is the most important. The position of the eyes in the head and other associated events such as verbalizations are also important subjects to cover. It may be difficult for observers to either describe or imitate the motions of a seizure. Frequently there is embarrassment at trying to imitate what seems to be a bizarre act, but given some encouragement and possibly a brief demonstration of what the physician is looking for will allow the observer to differentiate the nature of the shaking movements. The true tonic–clonic movements seen with a major motor seizure are frequently not very well imitated. The nature of the shaking movement may be such that there is a wild flinging of the arms; frequently there are purposeful movements and goal-oriented behavior. However, in nonconvulsive status epilepticus (see Chapter 12), unusual and seemingly purposeful movements may occur. Partially treated organic seizure disorders, on the other hand, may be somewhat "abortive." Assaultive behavior is not representative of a seizure disorder, nor is such activity as grabbing the physician or other medical personnel. Asynchronous movements of the extremities and pelvic thrusting are unusual, but not unheard of especially in frontal lobe partial seizures,[20] in organic seizures, as is weeping[21] (Table 11-7).

Shaking movements in pseudoseizures are at times tremulous, similar to those of impending DTs or those with a fever. During a pseudoseizure patients will frequently look directly at the observer or examiner. At other times they will speak on request during the "seizure" event. Although it is true that focal motor seizures can present without loss of consciousness and without impairment of mentation or speech, it is not possible for a generalized tonic–clonic seizure to have preservation of speech. It is somewhat difficult to describe the exact nature of a pseudoseizure, but one is usually aware of a

TABLE 11-7

SIGNS OF PSEUDOSEIZURES

Purposeful movements
Flinging movements
Harmful movements
Theatrical movements
Preservation of voluntary speech

theatrical quality to the spell. It usually happens only when there are observers present. A pseudoseizure frequently may involve something that will look potentially harmful to the patient, such as slamming the arm against the wall. It frequently happens at the time of emotional upset, and questioning observers about this can be revealing. Also, patients may not be aware that consciousness is usually impaired during a seizure. Simply talking to them, telling them that the seizure will soon abate, or asking them to perform coordinated motor action during a seizure reveals the true nature of the spell. Patients with pseudoseizures may very rarely bite their tongue or become incontinent of urine.[22] Accidental injuries do not rule out pseudoseizures. Such injuries or urinary incontinence can be caused by patients with true organic seizure disorders who know that after a true seizure they sometimes have a small bite mark on their tongue or have been incontinent of urine. Incontinence of stool is extremely unusual in pseudoseizures. Cyanosis is obviously a strong sign of organic seizure, but brief breath-holding spells may be found with pseudoseizures.

As with the other disorders previously described, one should consider a true, unrelated emergent medical condition. Although simultaneous electroencephalography (EEG) and video recording is outside consideration in the initial evaluation of these patients, it may be helpful in difficult cases of suspected pseudoseizures.[23] If the patient is on anticonvulsants, it may be necessary to check the anticonvulsant level and to discuss care and follow-up with the patient's personal physician.

PSYCHOGENIC VISUAL COMPLAINTS

Psychogenic visual complaints are unusual as an isolated event. The physician should establish whether the patient means that the visual loss is complete or partial and whether it involves one or both eyes, because the examination will be different depending on such initial history (Chapter 9). Malingered blindness is usually unilateral, and hysterical blindness is usually bilateral (Table 11-8).

Psychogenic visual complaints are frequently embellished on a partial deficit. The patient may have decreased vision owing to some organic problem and then "lose" vision completely. The best and easiest test is again observation. Patients who are truly blind in both eyes will protect themselves from harm. They will not walk purposely into doors, will not walk quickly about a room, and will act as any other person would when awakened from sleep in a dark room, i.e., take a wide-based stance with hands out protecting themselves from harm and seek other sensory input to get about in their environment. They will look directly at someone when talking to them, using the tracking

TABLE 11-8

SIGNS OF PSYCHOGENIC BLINDNESS

Intact optokinetic nystagmus
Threat response
Looking away from examiner
Lack of concern to protect self from harm
Inability to write name legibly
Inability to touch finger to finger

function of the auditory system, which is so good that a truly blind patient can almost look one in the eye. A truly blind person can look at his or her own hand. The classic finding of someone feigning blindness is that of walking into objects to cause oneself minimal harm.

There are patients with denial of blindness on an organic basis, the so-called Anton's syndrome, who may initially present like those with a psychogenic syndrome. This is a cortical blindness. If a patient is complaining of a partial deficit, the tests cannot be used as well. However, noticing whether the patient gazes in the direction of the examiner can still be used as a sign. Threat response, elicited by moving the examiner's hand toward the eye, can be used to demonstrate some intact vision.[22] However, one should be careful that they are not eliciting a corneal reflex by a gust of air on the patient's cornea. Optokinetic nystagmus testing is more sophisticated but can be extremely useful (Chapter 9). To perform the test, a striped object or revolving drum is placed in front of the patients' eyes; if they have intact vision, their eyes will demonstrate nystagmoid jerks as their eyes transiently track the moving object. This cannot be faked and essentially cannot be suppressed except by a very select group of individuals, such as ballerinas and ice skaters, who perform rotatory movements and can at the same time suppress optokinetic nystagmus.

Other highly sophisticated tests can be done for the hysterical or malingering patient's visual complaints; these are beyond the scope of a preliminary examination. It is, however, useful to know that these can be done in the eventual evaluation of these patients. For example, different-colored lenses can be placed over both eyes, and reading material is presented in two different colors. The patient is then asked to take a test based on the facts presented. There are other similarly sophisticated tests with prisms to isolate the images of the two eyes, in addition to EEG tests of visual-evoked response.

The examination should include the pupils and the position and motion of the eyes. It is unusual for a truly blind eye to have a direct response to light; however, one can have a cortical lesion and be blind on a cortical basis with preservation of pupillary reflexes (see Chapter 9). Pupillary responses may be altered by instillation of drops in malingerers. Drug-induced mydriasis is virtually the only cause for a dilated pupil not to respond to pilocarpine. Patients with psychogenic loss of visual acuity may be able to read only the top line on the Snellen chart regardless of how far they stand from it.

Psychogenic diplopia may present as monocular diplopia, which is found only in extremely unusual organic lesions,[6] such as dislocation of the lens, either artificially implanted or natural.

Psychogenic hearing loss

Psychogenic hearing loss is an uncommon problem in an acute care setting. It may be part of a "pansensory" or "hemisensory" loss. These occur when patients have loss of feeling, smell, vision, taste, hearing, and movement on one side of the body. This obviously cannot happen on an organic basis. Psychogenic hearing loss is a common malingerer's problem and has been common in both military and civilian circumstances. Again, there are highly sophisticated tests to determine the extent of hearing loss, which would not be performed as part of an initial evaluation but several general principles can be applied to the examination. Truly deaf people try to develop some sensory input from their environment. They will attend to the examiner's face and lips.

Whether they can lip-read or not, they will try to get sensory input. Patients who cannot hear, and who stare in another direction and appear to be ignoring someone, are not trying to get that sensory input. Unilateral hearing loss usually results in turning of the good ear toward the examiner. This is such a natural phenomenon that the lack of it may be a clue that there is no hearing loss. Patients with true long-standing hearing loss may raise their voice.

There are sophisticated tests in which the two ears are isolated with stereophonic headphones, information is presented to either or both ears, and the patient is then asked to take a test based on that information. It is sufficient to know that the tests exist and can be performed, if needed, in the eventual full evaluation of the patient.

Smell and taste

Aberrations of, or loss of smell and taste are extremely uncommon as an isolated psychogenic complaint. Irritating substances, such as ammonia or acetic acid, do not test smell but are perceived by the fifth cranial nerve because they are an irritant in the nose. Complete lack of taste requires bilateral seventh, ninth, and tenth nerve deficits, which is clearly a devastating neurologic insult. The most common cause of decreased taste is decreased smell, because most of our perception of taste is associated with smell. This will not be dealt with further because of the rarity of its presentation.

Speech

Disorders of speech are common in psychogenic syndromes, particularly in conversion disorders. As mentioned in the motor system examination discussion, patients may have a concept of the nervous system malfunction that simulates a lack of energy, or neurasthenia. They feel that they cannot speak in a full voice, but only whisper. There is no neurologic deficit that results in patients' whispering; it actually involves no less energy to whisper than it does to speak.

Hysterical patients may move their mouth normally, but no sound will come out or they may only whisper. Sometimes it can be mentioned to the patient that the physician perceives that they have some difficulty with speaking and that perhaps if they talked in whispers he or she might be able to help them further. The examiner can then obtain an entire history in whispers. Sometimes there will be no speech, or there will be a very abrupt onset and termination of the ability to speak. Occasionally there is stuttering, which again does not have an organic neurologic deficit as its cause.[24] The speech may be very slow or garbled or sound like baby talk. Although it is sometimes difficult to differentiate these disorders of speech from true dysphasia or aphasia, for the most part it is not a difficult differentiation. The patient with a true aphasia will usually try to speak.

Disposition

Once a diagnosis of a psychogenic complaint has been made, which may be easy, the most difficult part of the encounter with the patient begins: the disposition. It must be emphasized that the diagnosis must be based on positive findings that are inconsistent with known knowledge of the nervous system. One must have established a relationship of trust and caring with the patient and their family so that opinions, once rendered, will be taken seriously. The opinion that will be rendered is frequently unpopular with both the patient and the family.

One can separate the disposition into several categories based on the reason for the psychogenic complaint. Obvious malingerers can sometimes be allowed to simply reverse their story without losing face. A brief mention of some contradictory facts or a demonstration during the examination to such patients of a contradictory fact will allow them to realize that the complaint is on a nonorganic basis. The examiner usually need not confront such patients. Simply suggesting the fact that the symptom will be resolved very quickly or that it will not be a problem will allow patients to reverse their story and preserve their dignity. Sometimes a brief period of observation is all that is required, with the encouraging report of the physician that all seems to be well, thus allowing patients to then reverse the problem on their own terms. If this is insufficient, it is not inappropriate to seek an opinion from another physician. It is important to let patients know that all the records obtained during any encounter will be available to anyone who will see them so that they are given the feeling that nothing about the encounter, no matter how contradictory, will ever be lost to anyone who is looking into the problem. This alone may discourage the patient from pursuing a malingered complaint. Frequently one must simply explain what has been observed, without drawing a conclusion. It may be helpful to state that as a careful physician and a concerned examiner, you have examined the patient and to the best of your ability cannot document a problem that might cause a complaint. If the physician has established rapport with a patient and has done a careful examination, then the truth of the matter (that he or she is unable to document a problem) is all that can be said. It is obviously clear to both the physician and the patient that this does not mean it is impossible for the problem to exist. A problem may exist that the physician is simply unable to uncover with an honest attempt. Such problems are frequently difficult to deal with in disposition, and it is not uncommon that a second examination by a different examiner, or referral to a specialist, or referral for further diagnostic testing must be obtained before a diagnosis is accepted or an organic one made.

Embellishment on a true deficit is one of the most common settings seen and the most difficult one in which to establish a diagnosis. Patients are seeking to have a disease, and once they are given one they may let go of all the parts that do not fit that disease. Sometimes a brief discussion of what can be explained on the basis of their illness and what cannot be explained will encourage them to simply drop the embellished symptoms and pursue the true organic parts of their illness. Treat what can be treated and call to the attention of the patient what specific symptoms will be treated. Mention should be made of the fact that there are components to the complaint that cannot fit known knowledge of the nervous system. Again, seeking consultation, arranging for follow-up, and letting patients know that all records will be available to other examining physicians are important parts of the disposition. The obviously nonorganic patient is sometimes the easiest to diagnose. The diagnosis of functional neurologic complaint can be made at times within seconds. However, the disposition becomes extremely difficult. Patients may agree to a combined workup that is both neurologic and psychiatric. It is rare that patients with acute conversion disorder will have their disposition settled and their problem sufficiently evaluated on one brief outpatient basis. Hospitalization is sometimes necessary in some settings to arrive at an equitable disposition for such patients. Patients who are in coma on a psychogenic basis and allow various humiliating procedures to be performed upon them truly have a serious illness. The illness may not be an organic one as we currently understand it, but it is serious and it probably will not be resolved by allowing them to leave the healthcare system.

TREATMENT

Treatment of psychogenic neurologic disorders is beyond the scope of this text. It is rare that a psychogenic neurologic disorder is the sole manifestation of a patient's problems. It may be appropriate to refer a patient to certain resources to deal with other problems, i.e., social, psychiatric, substance abuse, etc. These resources vary with location and medical setting but may include psychiatrists, psychologists, social workers, and counselors, in addition to the patients' physicians. Even though the psychogenic syndrome seen may be only one facet of the patients' spectrum of problems, they may be most amenable to intervention following an acute episode, so that efforts to direct them to therapy may be rewarding. A precise psychiatric diagnosis is rarely made in the acute care setting and is rarely necessary.

SUMMARY

Psychogenic complaints need a systematic evaluation. They are frequently embellishments on true, established organic problems. The examiner must approach the patient with humility and must never lose the rapport and trust of the patient while performing the examination and gathering data. The most important part of the examination is that of skilled observation.

REFERENCES

1. Lempert T et al. Psychogenic disorders in neurology: frequency and clinical spectrum. *Acta Neurol Scand*. 1990;82:335-340.
2. Shaibani A, Sabbagh MN. Pseudoneurologic syndromes: recognition and diagnosis. *Am Fam Physician*. 1998;57:2485-2494.

3. DeJong RN. *The Neurologic Examination*. 3rd ed. New York: Harper & Row; 1970.

4. Mai FM. "Hysteria" in clinical neurology. *Can J Neurol Sci*. 1995;22:101-110.

5. American Psychiatric Association. *Diagnostic and Statistical Manual of Mental Disorders*. 4th ed. Washington, DC: American Psychiatric Association; 1994:452-457.

6. Moene FC et al. Organic syndromes diagnosed as conversion disorder: identification and frequency in a study of 85 patients. *J Psychosom Res*. 2000;49:7-12.

7. Schuepbach WM, Adler RH, Sabbioni ME. Accuracy of the clinical diagnosis of 'psychogenic disorders' in the presence of physical symptoms suggesting a general medical conditions: a 5-year follow-up in 162 patients. *Psychother Psychosom*. 2002;71(1):11-17.

8. Glick TH. Suspected conversion disorder: foreseeable risks and avoidable errors. *Acad Emerg Med*. 2000;7:1272.

9. Smith HE, Rynning RE, et al. Evaluation of neurologic deficit without apparent cause: the importance of a multidisciplinary approach. *J Spinal Cord Med*. 2007;30(5):509-517.

10. Dula D, DeNaples L. Emergency department presentation of patients with conversion disorder. *Acad Emerg Med*. 1995;2:120-123.

11. Schrag A, Brown RJ, Trimble MR. Reliability of self-reported diagnoses in patients with neurologically unexplained symptoms. *J Neurol Neurosurg Psychiatry*. 2004;75(4):608-611.

12. Beaumont WM. Malingering in relation to sight. In: Jones, Llewellyn, eds. *Malingering or the Simulation of Disease*. London: Heinemann; 1917.

13. Gould R et al. The validity of hysterical signs and symptoms. *J Nerv Ment Dis*. 1986;174:593.

14. Magee KR. Hysterical hemiplegia and hemianesthesia. *Postgrad Med*. 1962;31:339.

15. Paciaroni M, Bogousslavsky J. Pure sensory syndromes in thalamic stroke. *Eur Neurol*. 1998;39:211-217.

16. Bowlus WE, Currier RD. A test for hysterical hemianalgesia. *N Engl J Med*. 1963;269:1253.

17. Hayes MW et al. A video review of the diagnosis of psychogenic gait: appendix and commentary. *Mov Disord*. 1999;14:914-921.

18. Rosenbaum M. Psychogenic seizures—why women? *Psychosomatics*. 2000;41:147-149.

19. Benbadis SR, Agrawal V, Tatum WO IV. How many patients with psychogenic non-epileptic seizures also have epilepsy? *Neurology*. 2001;57:915-917.

20. Saygi S, Katz A, Marks D, et al. Frontal lobe partial seizures and psychogenic seizures: comparison of clinical and ictal characteristics. *Neurology*. 1992;42:1274-1277.

21. Walczak TS, Bogolioubov A. Weeping during psychogenic nonepileptic seizures. *Epilepsia*. 1996;37:208-210.

22. Peguero E et al. Self-injury and incontinence in psychogenic seizures. *Epilepsia*. 1995;36:586-591.

23. Krumholz A. Nonepileptic seizures: diagnosis and management. *Neurology*. 1999;53(5)(suppl 2):S76-S83.

24. Mahr G, Leith W. Psychogenic stuttering of adult onset. *J Speech Hear Res*. 1992;35:283-286.

CHAPTER

12
SEIZURES

A seizure is frequently the presenting symptom that precipitates a patient's entrance into the medical care system. The key in emergency management of seizures is identifying reversible etiologies. This chapter deals with the evaluation and stabilization of the seizure patient in the acute care setting. The focus is on a differential diagnostic approach as well as clinical decision making. Status epilepticus and febrile seizures are discussed in detail.

Ictus refers to the period during which a seizure occurs. An *aura* is not just a "premonition" that a seizure is going to occur but is actually a partial seizure; thus its manifestation depends on the area in the brain that is affected. A focal seizure can remain focal or spread into a generalized event; a corollary to this is that patients with a primary generalized seizure disorder do not have an aura (see discussion below). *The postictal period* is the time after a seizure ends but before the patient returns to baseline. *Epilepsy* is a condition of recurrent unprovoked seizures. Despite historical definitions that used a time frame of 30 minutes, *Status epilepticus* is often practically defined as a seizure that lasts more than 5 to 10 minutes, or recurrent seizures without a return to baseline mental status between events.[1]

CLASSIFICATION AND ETIOLOGIES

A seizure can be the result of an acute process, in which case it is referred to as an *acute symptomatic seizure;* it can result from a past intracranial insult such as stroke, trauma, or anoxia, in which case it is referred to as a *remote symptomatic seizure;* or it can be *idiopathic,* i.e., no etiology identified. A seizure's manifestation depends on the area of the brain that is discharging and whether or not the abnormal discharges are focal or generalized throughout the cerebral cortex. Consequently, the clinical spectrum of seizures includes focal or generalized motor activity, altered mental status, sensory or psychic

TABLE 12-1

CLASSIFICATION OF SEIZURES

Partial seizures
Simple partial (without alteration of consciousness)
   Motor
   Somatosensory
   Autonomic
   Psychic
Complex partial
   With focal onset prior to alteration in consciousness
   Without focal onset prior to alteration in consciousness

Generalized seizures
Primary generalized nonconvulsive
   Absence
Primary generalized convulsive
   Tonic–clonic
   Clonic
   Tonic
   Myoclonic
   Atonic
Secondary generalized
   Convulsive
   Nonconvulsive

Status epilepticus
Convulsive generalized
   Primary generalized
   Secondary generalized
Convulsive focal
Nonconvulsive
   Primary generalized (absence)
   Partial with or without secondary generalization (complex partial)

experiences, and/or autonomic disturbances. The classification of seizure types is presented in Table 12-1. In essence, generalized seizures are always associated with altered mental status.

Acute symptomatic seizures are associated with acute or progressive neurologic insult or physiologic stressors. Clinicians are challenged with identifying those patients with potentially reversible etiologies (Table 12-2). Hypoglycemia is the most common metabolic cause of seizures, while hyponatremia and hypocalcemia are rare.[1-3] The metabolic encephalopathies such as nonketotic hyperglycemia and uremia can cause both focal and generalized seizures. Alcohol is the most common toxin associated with seizures followed by tricyclics, cocaine, amphetamines, antihistamines, theophylline, and isoniazid.[4] Drug withdrawal, including noncompliance with anticonvulsant medications in a patient with a known seizure disorder, is a leading cause of recurrent seizures.[5]

TABLE 12-2 ————————————————————————

ETIOLOGIES OF SECONDARY SEIZURES

Tumors
Vascular event
    Subarachnoid hemorrhage
    Subdural hemorrhage
    Epidural hemorrhage
    Stroke
    Vasculitis
Infection
    Meningitis
    Encephalitis
    Abscess
Metabolic
    Hypoglycemia[a]
    Hyponatremia[b]
    Hypomagnesemia[c]
    Hypocalcemia
Toxic (consider the following in overdose):
    Cocaine and sympathomimetics
    Tricyclic antidepressants
    Anticholinergics
    Theophylline
    Isoniazid
Eclampsia

[a] The most common metabolic cause of seizures.
[b] A rare cause of seizures except in infants <6 months of age.
[c] Rarely an isolated cause of seizures; possibly facilitates seizures, especially in malnourished patients, e.g., alcoholics.

Infections can result in physiologic stress and lower the seizure threshold. Acute central nervous system (CNS) infections are responsible for 4% to 12% of acute isolated seizures and up to 28% of cases of refractory status epilepticus. Aside from those seizures caused directly by HIV, toxoplasmosis and cryptococcal meningitis make up the majority of infection-related seizures in AIDS patients.[6]

EPIDEMIOLOGY

Seizures account for an estimated 1% of emergency department (ED) visits.[7] The prevalence of active epilepsy is approximately 6 per 1000, and approximately 25% to 55% of patients with epilepsy continue to have recurrent seizures despite therapy.[8] Under the best of circumstances, excluding noncompliance and other variables, it is estimated that 5% to 10% of patients will have intractable epilepsy despite optimal medical management. The cumulative prevalence of all epilepsy is estimated to be 1.2% of the population through age 24, increasing to 4.4% by age 85.[9]

There is a projected annual incidence of status epilepticus of 50 per 100,000 population, with an overall mortality of 22% (3% in children and 26% in adults).[10] More than half of the patients presenting to the ED in status epilepticus have no prior seizure history. Mortality in patients with status epilepticus is linked to the duration of the seizures and the underlying etiology.

PATHOPHYSIOLOGY

Seizures result from either recurrent excitatory connections in the cerebral cortex or a loss of synchronization between aggregates of neurons. The excitability can be due to positive feedback loops or lack of inhibitory pathways. At the neuronal level, hyperexcitability can occur from hypoxic or hypoglycemic impairment of the Na–K pump. Glutamic acid is an excitatory transmitter and γ-aminobutyric acid (GABA) an inhibitory transmitter; disturbances in the balance between these two transmitters result in seizures. For example, vitamin B_6 is necessary for the syntheses of GABA, and deficiency may result in seizures; this explains the intractable seizures related to isoniazid overdose, which depletes vitamin B_6. The mechanism of action of anticonvulsants is primarily through selective blockade of high-frequency action potentials or potentiation of the inhibitory effect of GABA.

There are a number of pathophysiologic consequences of a seizure. There is often a period of transient apnea and hypoxia during a convulsion. Early in a motor seizure, there is an increase in blood pressure, followed later by a fall in the blood pressure. Serum lactate and serum glucose levels increase, and there is often an increase in the white blood cell count (but with no increase in bands). Body temperature is frequently elevated, with up to 43% of patients who have a generalized convulsion experiencing a rise in temperature above 100°F.[11,12] Acidosis due to elevated lactate occurs within 60 seconds of a convulsive event but should normalize within 1 hour after ictus. A transient cerebrospinal fluid (CSF) pleocytosis of up to 20 white blood cells (WBC)/mm³ has been reported to occur in 2% to 23% of patients with seizures.

If the seizure lasts for more than 30 minutes, the body's homeostatic regulating mechanisms begin to deteriorate. Cerebral blood flow autoregulation may be lost and, combined with alterations in blood pressure, cerebral perfusion may be compromised. The addition of increased neuronal metabolism to this picture may result in significant neuronal damage. Even if systemic factors such as acidosis and hypoxia are controlled, prolonged status epilepticus results in neuronal damage secondary to the release of neurotoxic excitatory amino acids and influx of calcium into cells.

DIFFERENTIAL DIAGNOSIS

A number of conditions can mimic or be misinterpreted as seizures. These include convulsive syncope, with or without cardiac dysrhythmias; decerebrate posturing; psychogenic events; and migraine headaches. Careful consideration of these mimickers is clearly important since misdiagnosis may have significant impact on patient management. Neither tetanus nor strychnine poisoning results in altered mental status, thus they are rarely confused with a seizure.

Syncope

As per the observational studies in blood donors, up to 40% of patients who have syncope will have some component of motor activity, most commonly involving tonic extension of the trunk or myoclonic jerks of the extremities.[13] This will usually occur if the patient is kept in a sitting position. These events are termed convulsive syncope and are not usually associated with tonic–clonic movements, tongue biting, cyanosis, incontinence, or postictal amnesia.

Cardiac Dysrhythmias

Cardiac dysrhythmias can cause hypotension with CNS hypoperfusion, resulting in symptoms that can be confused with convulsive or nonconvulsive seizures.[14] A careful history will often identify preceding cardiac symptoms such as palpitations, lightheadedness, or diaphoresis (see Chapter 13). Review of the ECG may be diagnostic as in the case of patients with long QTc syndrome: in one case series, 5 of 10 patients who had long QTc syndrome were initially misdiagnosed as having epilepsy resulting in a significant delay in making the final correct diagnosis.[15] The diagnosis frequently requires careful coordination with the patient's primary care physician for Holter monitoring, continuous cardiac loop monitoring, and head-up tilt table testing.

Decerebrate Posturing

Decerebrate posturing has been mistaken for tonic seizures, resulting in misdiagnosis and delay in providing potentially life-saving interventions for increased intracranial pressure.[16] It should be remembered that tonic seizures are rare in adults, and when they do occur they are usually of short duration with upper extremity abduction. Decerebrate posturing results in both upper and lower extremity extension.

Migraines

Migraines are typically diagnosed by characteristic symptom patterns associated with a unilateral throbbing headache. However, rare migraine variants have been associated with transient loss of consciousness or confusion as the primary complaint, making it difficult to distinguish this form of migraine from complex partial seizures, postictal vascular headaches, drop attacks, or transient ischemic attacks.

Psychogenic Seizures

See Chapter 11.

Dystonia

Dystonia is muscle rigidity with or without autonomic instability. Seizures can be excluded since there is no alteration of mental status or postictal confusion.

ANTIEPILEPTIC DRUGS

The "traditional" antiepileptic drugs (AEDs: phenytoin, phenobarbital, carbamazepine, valproic acid, and ethosuximide) suppress the repetitive, high-frequency neuronal firing characteristic of seizure activity through one of three general mechanisms: (1) blockade of voltage-dependent sodium channels, e.g., phenytoin; (2) potentiation of GABA-mediated postsynaptic inhibition, e.g., phenobarbital; and (3) blockade of calcium channels, e.g., ethosuximide. Traditionally, the first-line treatment for partial seizures, with or without secondary generalization, has been carbamazepine, valproic acid, phenytoin, and phenobarbital (listed in order of preference; valproic acid is contraindicated in pregnancy). For primary generalized convulsive epilepsy, valproic acid and phenytoin are recommended, whereas ethosuximide is used for absence seizures.

Over the past decade, new AEDs have been introduced that have greatly expanded the drug armamentarium available for treating epilepsy (Table 12-3). Most of the new AEDs are FDA approved only as adjunctive therapy since the FDA requires that new drugs demonstrate superiority not just equivalence. A practice parameter from the American Academy of Neurology lists gabapentin, lamotrigine, topiramate, and oxcarbazepine as potential first-line drugs for new onset partial/mixed seizure disorders and identifies lamotrigine as a potential first-line agent for absence.[17] In general, the decision to initiate a new AED or to add an AED to a therapeutic regimen is best done in consultation with the clinician who will be providing long-term management of the patient's seizure disorder.

PREHOSPITAL MANAGEMENT/INITIAL STABILIZATION

Prehospital management of the convulsing patient centers on securing the airway, maintaining oxygenation, obtaining intravenous access, and protecting the patient from injury. Fortunately most seizures are of short duration and in most cases little else needs to be done. The use of a padded tongue blade is contraindicated since it may induce emesis or break a tooth; a nasal trumpet may be helpful. Patients having seizures require an immediate blood sugar determination or, if not available, dextrose can be given empirically. If the seizure continues for more than several minutes, lorazepam 2 mg IV every minute up to a maximum of 10 mg can be administered; diazepam 5 mg IV every minute up to a total of 20 mg can also be used, but its shorter duration of action makes it less desirable than lorazepam.[18] Intramuscular midazolam and rectal diazepam are alternatives when intravenous access is not available.

Patients who have had a first-time seizure should be transported to the ED via an advanced life support unit, when available. Patients who have a known seizure disorder, who experience a "typical" event, and who are asymptomatic do not necessarily require transport to the hospital if they have capacity and are familiar with their disorder. These patients should be advised to contact their primary care provider as soon as possible. All other asymptomatic patients who have had a seizure should be transported to an ED for evaluation.

EMERGENCY DEPARTMENT EVALUATION

In approaching the seizure patient, the physician is often constrained by the paucity and questionable reliability of historical information, and by the limited resources available

TABLE 12-3   ANTIEPILEPTIC DRUGS

Drug	Trade Name	Route	Seizure Type	Loading Dose (mg/kg)	Daily Dose (mg) in Adults	Therapeutic Range (μg/mL)
Phenytoin	Dilantin	PO, IV	P, GC	20	300–400	10–20
Fosphenytoin	Cerebrex	IV, IM	P, GC	20		10–20
Carbamazepine[a]	Tegretol	PO	P, GC	—	800–1,600	6–12
Valproate[b]	Depakene	PO	All	—	1,000–3,000	50–120
Divalproex sodium	Depakote	PO	All	—	1,000–4,800	50–120
	Depacon	IV	All	10–20		50–120
Phenobarbital		PO, IV, IM	P, GC	10–20	90–150	15–35
Primidone	Mysoline	PO	P, GC	—	750–1,250	6–12
Clonazepam	Klonopin	PO	A, M	—	1.5–20	0.02–0.08
Ethosuximide[c]	Zarontin	PO	A	—	750–1,250	40–100
Levetiracetam	Keppra	PO, IV	P, GC	—	10–20	500–2000
Lamotrigine	Lamictal	PO	All	—	200–600	—
Gabapentin[d]	Neurontin	PO	P, GC	—	1,200–4,800	—
Topiramate	Topamax	PO	P, GC	—	200–600	—
Tiagabine		PO	P, GC	—	32–48	—
Diazepam[e]	Diastat	Rectal	All	0.2–0.5	—	—
Zonisamide		PO	P	—	100–200	—

Abbreviations: P, partial seizure; GC, generalized convulsive seizure; A, absence seizure; M, myoclonic seizure.
[a] Drug of choice for partial seizures, with or without secondary generalization.
[b] Drug of choice for primary generalized tonic–clonic seizures.
[c] Drug of choice for absence seizures.
[d] Only anticonvulsant that is renally metabolized; recommended in patients with multiple medical problems.
[e] Used primarily in children to control clusters of breakthrough seizures.

to some patients in obtaining the follow-up care that their condition might require. Consequently, multiple factors must be carefully weighed when deciding on the best approach to the diagnostic testing and therapeutic interventions initiated in the ED.

History

The history begins with a careful description of the event and its surrounding circumstances, with documentation of the preliminary symptoms, progression of the clinical pattern, the duration of the event including the postictal period, and the presence of incontinence or biting of the tongue (Table 12-4). Efforts should be made to obtain a clear description of the event(s) from witnesses. In patients with known epilepsy, any changes in the character of the seizure such as frequency or clinical features should be investigated. Noncompliance with anticonvulsants is the most common cause of recurrent seizures in this group of patients. The use of anticonvulsants and other medications should be ascertained, if possible. Initiation of new medications may have altered the bioavailability of the AEDs a patient with epilepsy may be using. Seizure disorders may be exacerbated by a number of stressors, such as fatigue, pregnancy, or systemic infection. Identification of the stressors may explain an event and become the focus of management.

Physical Examination

Seizure activity tends to prompt aggressive interventions, but it is critical to stress the importance of taking the time to carefully observe the patient and perform a physical exam. Obtain an accurate set of vital signs including a rectal temperature. Assess the mental status, skin color, and pupil position and reactivity. If the patient is actively convulsing, describe the motor activity. Look for "automatisms," which are repetitive actions such as lip smacking, swallowing, chewing, or fumbling. Automatisms are frequently seen in complex partial seizures and may be the only indicator that there is ongoing seizure activity.

Seizures resulting from drug overdose may be suggested by the presence of a toxic syndrome, as is seen in anticholinergic, sympathomimetic, or tricyclic ingestions. Hypertension with bradycardia may indicate an intracranial catastrophe, whereas fever may be the manifestation of a central nervous system (CNS) infection (although seizures may independently result in elevated temperatures from muscular hyperactivity or central deregulation). Irregular heart rate or carotid bruits may suggest a stroke as the seizure etiology, a common cause of new-onset seizures in the elderly.

Evaluate the patient for both soft tissue and skeletal trauma, especially head trauma and tongue lacerations. Seizure activity has been reported to directly cause both dislocations and fractures. However, seizure-induced fractures are rare, occurring in less than 1% of events; they most commonly involve the humerus, thoracic spine, and femur.[19]

Perform a complete neurologic examination identifying focal deficits that may represent an old lesion, new intracranial pathology, or reversible postictal neurologic compromise (Todd's paralysis). In cases of a new Todd's paralysis, consider the presence of a new structural lesion. Other physical findings suggesting that a seizure has occurred include hyperreflexia and extensor plantar responses, both of which should resolve during the immediate postictal period.

TABLE 12-4 ─────────────────────────────────
ELEMENTS OF HISTORY OF EVENTS AND PHYSICAL EXAMINATION

History
Description of the event including
   Initial symptoms
   Sensory or autonomic symptoms
   Motor activity: focal versus generalized
   Altered consciousness or awareness
   Timing of event (wakefulness vs. asleep)
   Duration
   Postictal period
   Incontinence
Provoking conditions
   Pregnancy
   Sleep, e.g., deprivation
   Systemic infection
   Drugs or medications
   Environment
Current medications
Past history of similar events
Past medical history including
   Malignancy
   Immunocompromise
   Vascular disease
   Trauma
   Febrile seizures
Family history

Physical examination
Vital signs
Evidence of head trauma
Eye examination including
   Pupil reactivity and size
   Fundi
   Deviation
   Nystagmus
Mouth examination for evidence of intraoral trauma
Neck/spine for meningismus/tenderness
Extremity examination for evidence of trauma
Neurologic examination
   Level of consciousness/mental status
   Abnormal movements/eye deviation
   Automatisms
   Cranial nerves
   Focal weakness
   Hyperreflexia/upgoing toes
Skin for evidence of trauma or intravenous drug use

TABLE 12-5 ⎯⎯⎯⎯⎯⎯⎯⎯⎯⎯⎯⎯⎯⎯⎯⎯⎯⎯⎯

DIFFERENTIAL DIAGNOSIS OF ALTERED MENTAL STATUS IN
THE PATIENT WHO HAS SEIZED

Postictal state
Nonconvulsive status or subtle convulsive status
Hypoglycemia
CNS infection
CNS vascular event
Drug toxicity
Psychiatric disorder

Document the patient's mental status, with the assistance of persons familiar with the patient. Postictal confusion usually resolves over several hours, and the failure of gradual improvement to occur should prompt a search for other causes (Table 12-5). In particular, nonconvulsive status epilepticus can present with subtle behavioral changes that may be discounted unless the clinician maintains a high index of suspicion (see "Nonconvulsive Status Epilepticus" section later in the chapter).

Laboratory Studies

For patients presenting after a first-time seizure who are alert, oriented, and have no clinical findings, appropriate laboratory studies include a serum glucose level, electrolytes, and a pregnancy test in women of child-bearing age[20,21] (Fig. 12-1). A drug-of-abuse screen should be considered. Other tests are of very low yield in this group of patients.[22] Patients who are on dialysis, malnourished, or taking diuretics or who have underlying significant medical disorders usually require more extensive testing including a complete blood count (CBC), blood urea nitrogen (BUN), creatinine, calcium, phosphate, and magnesium, as well as a urinalysis.

Rhabdomyolysis is a rare consequence of a seizure and is diagnosed if the urine tests positive for blood in the absence of red blood cells on the microscopic exam. Serum creatine phosphokinase (CPK) levels are not useful in differentiating seizures from other causes of loss of consciousness.

Patients with a known seizure disorder who have a "typical" event but who are asymptomatic, alert, and oriented in the ED need only a serum anticonvulsant level (if they are taking their medication) unless they have other underlying disease such as diabetes that could result in a metabolic derangement. It is important to consider potential precipitants such as infections or new medications that might have contributed to the event.

Patients in convulsive status epilepticus, as well as patients who are not actively convulsing but who are persistently postictal, require comprehensive diagnostic testing, which may include serum glucose, electrolytes, urea nitrogen, creatinine, magnesium, phosphate, calcium, CBC, pregnancy test in women of child-bearing age, AED levels, liver function tests, and a drug-of-abuse screen. An arterial blood gas analysis (ABG) obtained in a convulsing patient will show an anion gap metabolic acidosis that is usually secondary to lactic acidosis. The anion gap acidosis should resolve within 1 hour after the seizure ends; persistence of seizure after 1 hour suggests the presence of one of the other causes of an anion gap acidosis.

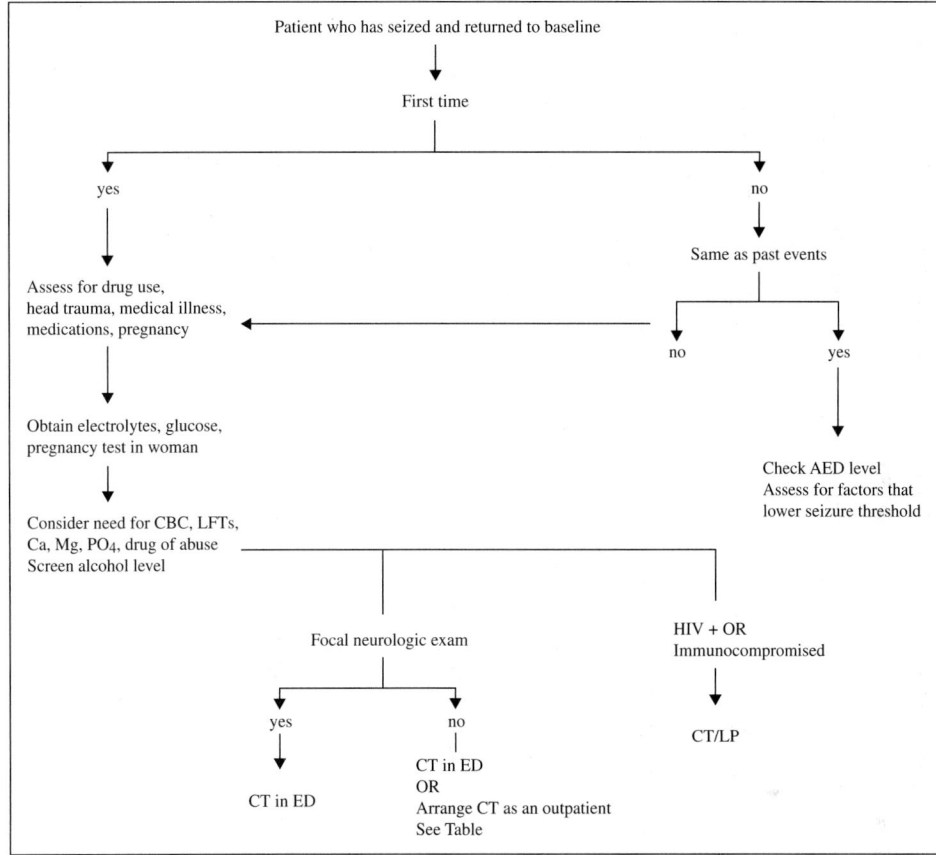

FIGURE 12-1 Approach to a patient who has seized and returned to baseline. AED, antiepileptic drug; CBC, complete blood count; CT, computed tomography; LFT, liver function test; LP, lumbar puncture.

Lumbar Puncture

A lumbar puncture is considered in patients who are in status epilepticus of undetermined etiology, who have an unresolving postictal state, fever, headache, meningeal signs, or positive HIV history, or who are otherwise immunocompromised. There is no evidence to support the performance of a lumbar puncture as part of the diagnostic evaluation in the ED on patients who are alert, oriented, asymptomatic, and not immunocompromised, even if the seizure was a first-time event.[23]

Neuroimaging

Up to 40% of adult patients with a first-time seizure have an abnormal head CT.[2,21] An estimated 20% of patients with a first-time seizure and an abnormal CT have a normal neurologic examination. A head CT in adults should be performed in the ED whenever a seizure patient has a suspected acute intracranial process, a history of acute head trauma, malignancy, immunocompromise, fever, persistent headache, anticoagulation, or a new focal neurologic examination.[24] In those cases where the patient has a normal neurologic examination, has returned to a normal baseline, and has no concerning comorbidities, a neuroimaging study can be deferred if the patient has access to timely follow-up.[24]

Electroencephalography

An electroencephalogram (EEG) in the ED may be useful for those patients with persisting altered mental status in whom subtle convulsive or nonconvulsive status epilepticus is suspected (see below). An EEG may also be useful when a patient's motor activity has been suppressed by either paralysis or barbiturate coma and there is a need to assess ongoing seizure activity.

MANAGEMENT OF CONVULSIVE STATUS EPILEPTICUS

Management of status epilepticus must take into consideration potentially treatable etiologies (Table 12-2), since it will be difficult to control the seizures unless the precipitating causes are addressed. Therefore a comprehensive approach must be taken that concomitantly ensures oxygenation and intravenous access, obtains diagnostic studies, and initiates pharmacologic interventions (Fig. 12-2).

Oxygenation is monitored with pulse oximetry. If at any time breathing appears compromised, rapid-sequence intubation is recommended. Long-acting paralyzing agents are relatively contraindicated until bedside EEG monitoring becomes available, since they mask clinical findings that guide pharmacologic interventions. Intravenous access is best secured with a nondextrose solution since dextrose will precipitate phenytoin if administered concurrently (dextrose solutions are safe with fosphenytoin). A rapid bedside serum glucose determination should be obtained and dextrose given if the level is less than 80 mg/dL; if a rapid dextrose determination is unavailable, administer 50 mL of 50% dextrose intravenously in adults, or 2 mL/kg of 25% dextrose in children. Thiamine, 100 mg, is recommended with dextrose boluses in patients who appear malnourished or abuse alcohol. If a CNS infection is suspected, early consideration must be given to empiric antibiotic treatment, since head CT and lumbar puncture will most likely be delayed pending patient stabilization. Likewise, early administration of activated charcoal, 1 g/kg, is recommended in cases of suspected overdose.

Benzodiazepines are the first-line drugs in managing status epilepticus and have been shown to be equal to phenobarbital alone and superior to phenytoin alone.[25] Diazepam, 0.2 mg/kg at 5 mg/min, and lorazepam, 0.1 mg/kg at 2 mg/min, are equally effective in terminating seizures; lorazepam has the advantage of a much smaller volume of distribution, with anticonvulsant benefit lasting up to 12 hours versus 20 minutes for diazepam. In patients with no intravenous access, intramuscular or intranasal midazolam is an excellent alternative since it is water-soluble, nonirritating, and rapidly absorbed.

When diazepam is used as the initial AED, intravenous phenytoin loading, 18 to 20 mg/kg, should also be started; 18 mg/kg is the dose found to give serum drug levels that remained above 10 mg/dL for 24 hours. The dose of phenytoin can be increased up to a total of 30 mg/kg if the seizures do not stop after the initial load.[26] Phenytoin loading can result in infusion site irritation, hypotension, confusion, and ataxia; it will rarely result in progressive distal limb edema discolorations and ischemia. Infusions are best administered through a large vein to minimize sclerosis from the alkaline pH. The

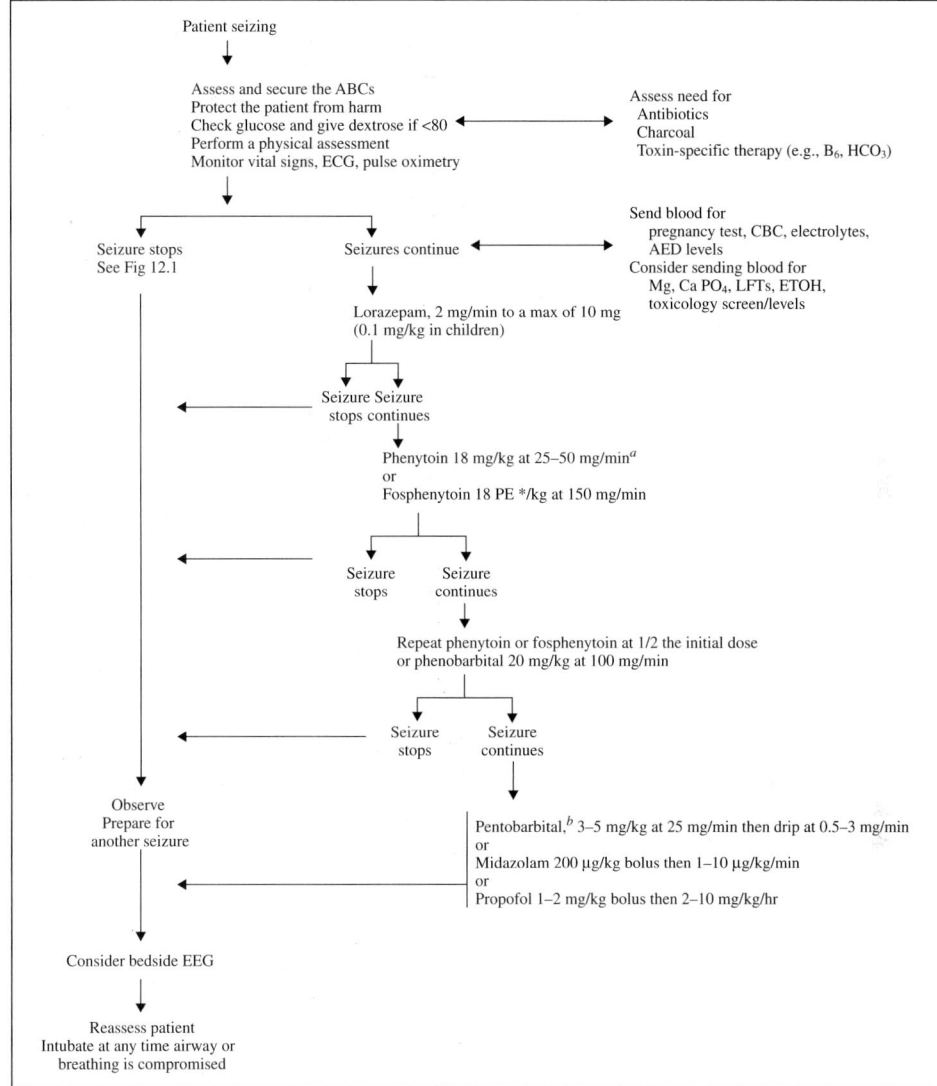

FIGURE 12-2 Approach to a patient who is undergoing a seizure. [a]Slower rates for patients with cardiovascular disease; infusion should be through a large-bore intravenous drip. [b]Watch for hypotension and treat initially with fluids; give dopamine if needed. AED, antiepileptic drug; CBC, complete blood count; LFT, liver function test; ECG, electrocardiogram; EEG, electroencephalogram; PE, phenytoin equivalent.

infusion rate should be no faster than 25 mg/min in patients with cardiac disease, to minimize cardiovascular complications, and 50 mg/min in other patients.[27]

Fosphenytoin, a phosphate ester of phenytoin, has a safety profile that makes it preferable to phenytoin: it is water-soluble and nonirritating and thus can be given intramuscularly with 100% bioavailability. It has fewer cardiotoxic effects than phenytoin, although hypotension can occur. The loading dose is 18 to 20 phenytoin equivalent units (PE)/kg. In emergencies, when given intravenously, the recommended infusion rate is 150 mg/min.

An alternative to phenytoin, particularly in patients who have seized secondary to subtherapeutic valproic acid levels, is intravenous valproic acid. A loading dose is 20 mg/kg, which can be infused at 150 mg/min. Phenobarbital, 20 mg/kg at 100 mg/min, has been used as a first-line drug in status epilepticus, although it is generally reserved for patients who continue to seize despite benzodiazepine and phenytoin loading or who are seizing from drug withdrawal. Resuscitation interventions should be continually reassessed to ensure that the patient is properly oxygenated and is not hypoglycemic, that intravenous lines are functioning, and that phenytoin was not administered in a dextrose solution.

After phenobarbital, there are three options for cases of refractory status epilepticus, i.e., cases that do not respond to first- and second-line AEDs: pentobarbital, propofol, and a benzodiazepine infusion.[28] Pentobarbital, 5 mg/kg, followed by an infusion of 0.5 to 3 mg/kg/h, is effective in suppressing electrical discharges. Pentobarbital can compromise cardiovascular status, and its use necessitates EEG monitoring since motor activity will be suppressed. Pentobarbital-induced hypotension is initially managed with fluid boluses followed by dopamine in resistant cases. Levetiracetam, 500 to 4000 mg, has been recommended as a third-line drug; however, there are no good studies beyond case reports to support its use at this time. Other drugs that have been used include lidocaine, propofol, etomidate, and paraldehyde.[29]

NONCONVULSIVE STATUS EPILEPTICUS

Nonconvulsive status epilepticus (NCS), like convulsive status epilepticus, is a state of continuous or intermittent seizure activity lasting for more than 30 minutes without a return to baseline function. The hallmark of NCS is altered mental status, which can range from subtle behavioral changes to paranoia to coma. Therefore, unless it is suspected, the diagnosis can be easily missed. The literature reports many patients presenting with altered mental status who were initially labeled as psychiatric and only at a later time in their evaluation was the correct diagnosis identified, either by EEG or by onset of a convulsive component to the status.[30] Nonconvulsive status can be either a primary generalized process, in which case it is absence status, or secondarily generalized process, i.e., complex partial status. NCS can occur on a continuum with convulsive seizures. Although the distinction is not clear in the literature, NCS in general should be distinguished from subtle generalized convulsive status epilepticus. This is the end stage of generalized convulsive status when the patient is in continuous coma with only subtle motor convulsions; unlike NCS, this entity has a very poor prognosis. Up to 15% of patients with a prolonged postictal period after convulsive status epilepticus are in NCS.[31]

When NCS is suspected, an EEG should be obtained. NCS is highly responsive to the benzodiazepines, either diazepam or lorazepam; thus, some clinicians recommend a trial of a benzodiazepine when EEG monitoring is not available; this is generally best done in coordinatation with the neurologist who will be assuming the patient's care.

ALCOHOL-RELATED SEIZURES

The risk of an unprovoked seizure is increased with increased alcohol intake, but, interestingly, studies have questioned the existence of "alcohol withdrawal seizures" as a distinct entity.[32] The increased risk is multifactorial and possibly linked to increased comorbidities in alcoholics including incidence of head trauma. The alcoholic who has had a seizure must be approached with caution in order to avoid bias influencing clinical decision making. In a study of 259 patients with suspected alcohol withdrawal seizure, 58% had an abnormal CT; 16 of these patients (6%) had a clinically significant lesion.[33] Phenytoin does not have a role in managing withdrawal seizures or controlling recurrent alcohol-related seizures.[34] Lorazepam, 2 mg IV, is effective in decreasing recurrent seizures related to alcohol use and decreases the need for hospitalization in these patients.[35]

SUBTHERAPEUTIC AED LEVELS IN THE ED

Many patients with a history of seizures present to the ED with low serum AED levels. Serum levels can be brought up to therapeutic range by oral, intramuscular, or intravenous supplementation depending on the urgency of the situation and the AED. When oral loading is used for phenytoin, 19 mg/kg in men and 23 mg/kg in women provide therapeutic serum levels of AED within 4 hours in the majority of patients. Single dose loading has been shown to be safe, although patients should be watched for ataxia and dizziness.[36,37] Intramuscular fosphenytoin, intravenous phenytoin, or fosphenytoin is other option. Valproic acid and carbamazepine cannot be orally loaded with a single dose. Intravenous valproic acid is available and provides physicians with an alternative when rapid therapeutic levels are needed.

SEIZURES IN PREGNANCY

Faced with a pregnant patient having a seizure, physicians must determine whether the seizure is associated with an existing disorder, is of new onset, or is due to eclampsia. Patients whose gestation has progressed beyond 20 weeks should be checked for hypertension, proteinuria, and edema. Patients with seizures due to eclampsia are treated with magnesium sulfate, which has been shown to be superior to phenytoin and diazepam in eclamptic seizures.[38] Once eclampsia has been ruled out, precipitating etiologies such as sleep deprivation, infections, and drug toxicities should be considered. In patients with a history of seizures, compliance with therapy should be explored. Pregnancy changes the "free" AED level of those AEDs that are protein bound. "Free AED levels" are required to accurately assess the true serum drug level. Fetal monitoring is a consideration in patients in the second half of pregnancy, and an obstetrics consultation should be obtained.

PEDIATRIC SEIZURES

Absence Seizures

Primary generalized nonconvulsive seizures, also called petit mal or absence seizures, are typically characterized by a sudden onset of unresponsiveness that is not preceded by an aura or succeeded by a postictal period. Absence seizures account for approximately 15% of all cases of childhood epilepsy. They are seen primarily in the young, usually beginning between the ages of 5 and 10 years, and are rare after the midteens. The average duration of an absence event is 10 seconds, but they may occur many times each day. They are easily misinterpreted by parents, teachers, and others as inattentiveness or "daydreaming." Atypical absence seizures (possibly complex partial seizures with rapid generalization) are events that last longer, have more complex automatisms or associated motor activity, and often have a postictal period.

Patients are generally not aware that the seizure has occurred. The treatment of choice is ethosuximide unless the child also has motor seizures, in which case valproic acid is recommended. Lamotrigine has recently been recommended as an option.[17]

Febrile Seizures

A febrile seizure occurs between 6 months and 5 years of age, is associated with fever, and has no identifiable underlying cause.[39] Simple febrile seizures are generalized tonic–clonic events with no focality, last less than 15 minutes, and have a short postictal period. Complex febrile seizures last longer than 15 minutes or occur in a series, or have a focal onset or a prolonged postictal period. Two to four percent of all children will have a simple febrile seizure. Children who have had a febrile seizure have a 25% to 50% chance of having a second event associated with a fever, usually within a year. Children at highest risk for recurrence are those with a first-degree relative who has had a febrile seizure, those who had a complex first febrile seizure, or those who were younger than 1 year when the first event occurred.

Simple febrile seizures are a benign process; when they occur in children older than 18 months who have not been on antibiotics, they do not require any diagnostic workup, even for a first-time event.[40] Management focuses on a careful history and physical examination and on parental education. Diagnostic studies are guided by general fever protocols. In patients between 6 and 12 months, the physical examination is unreliable for meningitis, and lumbar puncture is recommended; between the ages of 12 and 18 months, clinical signs of meningitis may be subtle, and consideration should be given to obtaining CSF for analysis. Electrolytes, calcium, phosphorus, magnesium, blood sugar, CBC, or neuroimaging is not routinely necessary in patients with simple febrile seizures. Because simple febrile seizures are a benign entity, AEDs as a preventive therapy are unwarranted.[40]

Complex febrile seizures necessitate a complete diagnostic workup looking for underlying precipitating etiologies. Ten to fifty percent of cases of status epilepticus in children are associated with febrile seizures, and status epilepticus in this group is a consistent predictor of increased risk for subsequent seizures.

DISPOSITION

Patients who were in status epilepticus or who have persisting altered mental status or a new neurologic deficit require a period of observation. Initiation of AED therapy in the ED in patients with new-onset seizures is best coordinated with the patient's primary care provider. In general, this decision can only be made on the basis of the underlying cause of the seizure, which requires the results of laboratory testing, a neuroimaging study, and an EEG. All these data are rarely available prior to ED discharge. Consequently, decision making (whether to admit to the hospital and whether to initiate AED therapy) must be based on the predicted risk for seizure recurrence, with the understanding that even if an AED is initiated, seizure recurrence may not be changed.[9]

The chances of a patient having a recurrent event after one unprovoked seizure vary depending on patient's age and the underlying etiology of the seizure. Seizure etiology and EEG findings are the best predictors of recurrence. Patients who have structural lesions on CT or patients with focal seizures that secondarily generalize have a risk of recurrence of up to 65%; this is the group of patients that will probably benefit from initiation of AED therapy. Patients with a new-onset seizure who have returned to baseline and who have a normal neurologic examination, a normal head CT, and normal electrolytes and glucose can be safely sent home on no therapy. Follow-up with a primary care provider or neurologist, as well as the importance of not driving or engaging in other activities that may be dangerous if the seizure recurs, should be discussed with the patient.

Summary

The approach to the seizure patient begins with a careful assessment of the event with consideration given to the various disorders that can mimic epileptic seizure activity. History, physical examination, and diagnostic tests are obtained to elucidate the seizure's etiology and to guide management. When possible, care should be coordinated with the patient's primary care physician or neurologist. Disposition from the ED must take into consideration the patient's social situation, resources, and compliance. All patients who have had a seizure must be advised not to drive and to avoid placing themselves or others in potentially dangerous situations. All states have laws regulating driving and epilepsy, although few states actually have mandatory reporting requirements.

References

1. Lowenstein DH, Bleck T, MacDonald RL. It's time to revise the definition of status epilepticus. *Epilepsia*. 1999;40:120-122.
2. Henneman P, DeRoos F, Lewis R. Determining the need for admission in patients with new-onset seizures. *Ann Emerg Med*. 1994;24:1108-1114.
3. Sempere A et al. First seizure in adults: a prospective study from the ED. *Acta Neurol Scand*. 1992;86:134-138.
4. DeLorenzo R et al. Seizures associated with poisoning and drug overdose. *Am J Emerg Med*. 1993;11:565-568.
5. DeLorenzo R et al. A prospective, population-based epidemiologic study of status epilepticus in Richmond, Virginia. *Neurology*. 1996;46:1029-1035.
6. Wong M, Suite N, Labar D. Seizures in human immunodeficiency virus infections. *Arch Neurol*. 1990;47:640-642.
7. Krumholz A et al. Seizures and seizure care in an emergency department. *Epilepsia*. 1989;30: 175-181.
8. Hauser W. The natural history of drug resistant epilepsy: epidemiologic considerations. *Epilepsia*. 1992(suppl 5):25-28.

9. Hauser W et al. Seizure recurrence after a first unprovoked seizure: an extended followup. *Neurology*. 1990;40:1163-1170.

10. Wachtel T, Steele G, Day J. Natural history of fever following seizure. *Arch Intern Med*. 1987;147:1153-1155.

11. Aminoff M, Simon R. Status epilepticus: causes, clinical features and consequences in 98 patients. *Am J Med*. 1980;69:657-666.

12. Aminoff M et al. Cerebrospinal fluid analysis in children with seizures. *Pediatr Emerg Care*. 1995;11:226-229.

13. Lin J. Convulsive syncope in blood donors. *Ann Neurol*. 1982;11:525-528.

14. Linzer M et al. Cardiovascular causes of loss of consciousness in patients with presumed epilepsy: a cause of increased sudden death rate in people with epilepsy. *Am J Med*. 1994;96:146-154.

15. MacCormick J, McAlister H, Crawford J, et al. Misdiagnosis of long QT syndrome in epilepsy at first presentation. *Ann Emerg Med*. 2009;54:26-32.

16. Haines S. Decerebrate posturing misinterpreted as seizure activity. *Am J Emerg Med*. 1988;6:173-177.

17. French J, Kanner A, Bautista J, et al. Efficacy and tolerability of the new antiepileptic drugs: treatment of new onset epilepsy. Report of the Therapeutics and Technology Assessment Subcommittee and Quality Standards Subcommittee of the American Academy of Neurology and the American Epilepsy Society. *Neurology*. 2004;62:1252-1260.

18. Alldredge BK, Gelb AM, Isaacs SM, et al. A comparison of lorazepam, diazepam, and placebo for the treatment of out-of-hospital status epilepticus. *N Engl J Med*. 2001;30;345:631-637.

19. Lawn N, Bamlet W, Radhakrishnan K, et al. Injuries due to seizures in persons with epilepsy. *Neurology*. 2004;63:1565-1570.

20. American Academy of Neurology. Practice parameter: evaluating a first nonfebrile seizure in children. *Neurology*. 2000;55:616-623.

21. American College of Emergency Physicians. Clinical policy: critical issues in the evaluation and management of adult patients presenting to the emergency department with seizures. *Ann Emerg Med*. 2004;43:605-625.

22. American Academy of Neurology. Practice parameter: evaluating an apparent unprovoked first seizure in adults (an evidence based review). *Neurology*. 2007;69:1996-2007.

23. Green S et al. Can seizures be the sole manifestation of meningitis in febrile children? *Pediatrics*. 1993;92:527-534.

24. American Academy of Neurology. Reassessment: neuroimaging in the emergency patient presenting with seizure (an evidence based review). *Neurology*. 2007;69:1772-1780.

25. Treiman D et al. A comparison of four treatments for generalized convulsive status epilepticus. *N Engl J Med*. 1998;339:792-798.

26. Lowenstein D, Alldredge B. Status epilepticus. *N Engl J Med*. 1998;338:970-976.

27. Donovan P. Phenytoin administration by constant intravenous infusion: Selective rates of administration. *Ann Emerg Med*. 1991;20:139-142.

28. Ziai W, Kaplan P. Seizures and status epilepticus in the intensive care unit. *Semin Neurol*. 2008;28:668-681.

29. Jagoda A, Riggio S. Refractory status epilepticus. *Ann Emerg Med*. 1993;22:1337-1348.

30. Tomson T, Lindbom U, Nilsson B. Nonconvulsive status epilepticus in adults: thirty two consecutive patients from a general hospital population. *Epilepsia*. 1992;33:829-835.

31. Delorenzo R et al. Persistent nonconvulsive status epilepticus after the control of convulsive status epilepticus. *Epilepsia*. 1998;39:833-840.

32. Ng S, Hauser A, Brust J, Susser M. Alcohol consumption and withdrawal in new onset seizures. *N Engl J Med*. 1988;319:666-673.

33. Earnest M et al. Intracranial lesions shown by CT scans in 259 cases of first alcohol related seizures. *Neurology*. 1988;38:1561-1565.

34. Rathlev N et al. The lack of efficacy of phenytoin in the prevention of recurrent alcohol related seizures. *Ann Emerg Med*. 1994;23:513-518.

35. D'Orofrio G et al. Lorazepam for the prevention of recurrent seizures related to alcohol. *N Engl J Med*. 1999;340:915-919.

36. Ratanakorn D et al. Single oral loading dose of phenytoin: a pharmacokinetics study. *J Neurol Sci*. 1997;147:89-92.

37. van der Meyden CH et al. Acute oral loading of carbamazepine-CR and phenytoin in a double-blind randomized study of patients at risk of seizures. *Epilepsia*. 1994;35:189-194.

38. Lucas MJ, Leveno KJ, Cunningham FG. A comparison of magnesium sulfate with phenytoin for the prevention of eclampsia. *N Engl J Med*. 1995;333:201-205.

39. American Academy of Pediatrics. Practice parameter: the neurodiagnostic evaluation of the child with a first simple febrile seizure. *Pediatrics*. 1996;97:769-775.

40. American Academy of Pediatrics. Practice parameter: long term treatment of the child with a simple febrile seizure. *Pediatrics*. 1999;103:1307-1309.

Syncope is the sudden loss of consciousness and postural tone with spontaneous rapid return to normal without medical intervention. Syncope is a symptom not a disease *per se*; it is the final common pathway for a number of underlying conditions the majority of which are benign. However, a concerning minority of patients with syncope have an underlying life-threatening process, thus explaining why syncope is often referred to as a "low risk/high stakes" symptom. Most cases of syncope are due to a reduction in cerebral blood flow, or a transient episode of absent cerebral blood flow. Syncope, like coma, is characterized by lack of self-awareness, yet, unlike coma, it is very brief. Presyncope, near-syncope, or faintness is the sensation of severe light-headedness or impending loss of consciousness that may precede frank syncope or occur without syncope. These symptoms occur along a continuum of severity. Their respective causes are generally the same as syncope, with the major difference being the magnitude of the physiologic derangements. Although syncope has a very narrow definition, other conditions may simulate syncope or cause transiently altered consciousness.

OBJECTIVES

The primary emergency department (ED) objective in evaluation of the syncopal patient is to determine whether the event is the manifestation of a life-threatening condition. Syncope is a common problem and represents up to 2% of emergency department visits.[1] In general, the older the patient and the more comorbidities, the greater the likelihood that an adverse event, including death, will follow; conversely, the younger the patient, the less likelihood of an adverse event. That said, there are many exceptions thus driving initiatives to develop prediction models designed to identify high-risk and low-risk patients with syncope.[1,2]

The transient and episodic nature of syncopal episodes can result in making a firm diagnosis, a challenge. In evaluating the patient who has recovered from a syncopal episode, the conditions prevailing at the time of the event are, almost by definition, no longer present. Even if a current abnormality can be found, establishing cause and effect can be difficult. Causes for syncope range from benign to life-threatening, and a specific etiology cannot be found in up to 50% of cases despite numerous investigations.[3,4]

Syncope is a common symptom, with a prevalence of 15% in the pediatric population and 19% in the adult population.[5] It accounts for up to 3% of hospital admissions with health care expenditures of over $2 billion annually.[6] Emergency department overcrowding and the shortage of inpatient hospital beds makes the systematic evaluation of patients with syncope more important than ever in order to properly use limited resources and minimize risk of missing life-threatening disorders.

PATHOPHYSIOLOGY

In order for consciousness to be lost, the factors that sustain consciousness must be transiently, but reversibly, interrupted. Loss of consciousness, as can be seen from the chapter on coma (Chapter 4), involves loss of normal, organized electrical activity of both cerebral hemispheres or brainstem centers, or acute loss of substrates, primarily glucose and oxygen, which are necessary for cerebral metabolism. Such losses usually occur because of inadequate cerebral perfusion. Cerebral blood flow of approximately 55 mL/100 g brain tissue/min is necessary for an adequate supply of oxygen and glucose; if it falls to the 20 mL/100 g brain tissue/min level, then syncope occurs. The brain does not store energy resources and is dependent on a continuous supply of substrate. Isolated deficiencies of glucose or possibly oxygen rarely occur and, if they did occur, would have to reverse rapidly to mimic a syncopal event. The process of cerebral hypoperfusion must be rapidly reversible, or death would ensue. The two prerequisites of rapidity of onset and rapid reversibility limit the number of etiologies to be considered.

Although much individual variation exists in the magnitude of decrease in cerebral blood flow that can cause syncope, systolic pressures below 70 mm Hg or mean arterial pressure as low as 40 mm Hg may result in syncope, depending on the individual's general state of health, existence of impaired cerebral circulation, intrinsic capabilities for blood flow compensation, and prior blood pressure levels. Several pathophysiologic changes can combine in a given patient to produce syncope, even when none of these changes by themselves is of sufficient magnitude to cause a syncopal event. Regardless of the exact mechanisms involved, virtually all syncopal episodes occur in the upright posture and are generally mitigated or terminated with supine positioning.

Response to Change from Supine to Upright Position

When a person changes from the supine to an upright position, there is a shift of approximately 300 to 800 mL of blood to the lower extremities. This results in less return of venous blood to the heart, less ventricular filling, decreased cardiac output, and reduced arterial pressure. Such a drop in pressure stimulates baroreceptors in the carotid sinus and aortic arch to reduce inhibitory control of the medulla's vasomotor center. This results in enhanced sympathetic tone and diminished parasympathetic

TABLE 13-1

CAUSES OF SYNCOPE[a, 9]

Unknown	37%
Vasodepressor	28%[b]
Cardiac	10%
Orthostatic	9%
Medication	7%
Seizure	5%
Stroke/TIA	4%

[a] Based on a cohort of 822 patients.
[b] Includes cough syncope, micturition syncope, and situational syncope.

tone. Catecholamines, vasopressin, and other neurohumoral substances are released resulting in an increase in systemic vascular resistance, myocardial contractility, and heart rate, resulting in restoration of blood pressure or blunting of the decrease in blood pressure. Interruption of any part of this regulatory pathway can impair the body's ability to maintain normal arterial pressure and cerebral perfusion and thus cause or contribute to syncope.

CLASSIFICATION

There are a number of ways to classify syncope, some of which are listed in Tables 13-1 and 13-2. Grouping disorders that result in similar pathophysiologic changes is a common method of categorization, though frequently syncope results from a combination of etiologies, e.g., medications plus a vasovagal stimulus. Considerable overlap exists in mixed organ system and pathophysiologic classification schemes. Frequently, several factors, none of which would cause syncope individually, combine to transiently impair cerebral blood flow to the point of loss of consciousness. Compensatory mechanisms then reverse one or more factors, and cerebral blood flow and consciousness are restored. It is uncommon that the blood flow solely to parts of the brainstem critical for maintenance of consciousness occurs in a rapidly reversible fashion without affecting other brainstem structures. It is likewise uncommon that the availability of the substrates oxygen and/or glucose is transiently diminished to the point of loss of consciousness.

GENERAL APPROACH TO THE SYNCOPAL PATIENT

The history and physical examination are key in the evaluation of the patient with syncope; they provide the information needed to determine which diagnostic tests, if any, are needed; and they provide the information needed to risk-stratify patients into going home or being admitted to the hospital. Key information focuses on identifying possible etiologies (see "Syncope Syndromes").

Cardiac arrhythmia is one of the most concerning categories for the etiology of syncope. Typically the prodromal symptoms are brief (less than 5 seconds) or absent. An

TABLE 13-2

PHYSIOLOGIC CAUSES OF SYNCOPE

Generalized Low Cardiac Output

Pump failure
Acute MI
Cardiac tamponade
Aortic dissection

Decreased venous return
Hypovolemia
Orthostatic hypotension
Drug-induced
Autonomic neuropathies

Cardiac arrhythmia
Bradyarrhythmia
  Carotid sinus sensitivity
  Sick sinus syndrome
  Second- and third-degree AV blocks
  Pacemaker malfunction
Tachyarrhythmia
  Supraventricular tachycardia
  Ventricular tachycardia
  Runaway pacemaker
  Torsades de pointes
  Long QT syndromes with resultant arrhythmia

Obstruction to flow
Left ventricular outflow obstruction
  Aortic stenosis
  Hypertrophic cardiomyopathy
  Left atrial myxoma
  Mitral stenosis
Right ventricular outflow obstruction
  Pulmonic valvular stenosis
  Pulmonary embolism
  Pulmonary hypertension
  Right atrial myxoma

Combinations
Vasovagal (neurally mediated, neurocardiogenic, vasodepressor)
Pulmonary embolus
Situational (micturition, defecation, cough, swallow)

arrhythmia may occur in isolation (ventricular tachycardia) or in combination with other factors (vasovagal). An arrhythmia may result from a variety of etiologies including underlying conduction disorders (e.g., accessory pathway or nodal disease), structural causes (e.g., valve disease, tamponade), or medications (e.g., inducers of prolonged QTc). Syncope that occurs when the patient is sitting or lying down is most likely to be due to a cardiac etiology (versus syncope that occurs after standing which suggests orthostatic hypotension).[7]

Syncope Syndromes

Neurocardiogenic Syncope

The mechanism for neurocardiogenic syncope (also termed vasovagal, neurally mediated, neurocardiogenic, vasodepressor) is not completely understood. It can be initiated by venous pooling leading to decreased central blood volume and stroke volume, causing a compensatory increase in sympathetic activity. In susceptible patients, this increase in sympathetic activity can trigger the Bezold-Jarisch reflex, leading to bradycardia and/or hypotension. This reflex occurs because cardiac sensory receptors in the posteroinferior left ventricle become stimulated and send signals to the vasomotor center in the medulla. This leads to increased parasympathetic activity, decreased sympathetic activity, and bradycardia (note that this pathway can be inhibited by atropine). Therefore, the overall response is one that one would expect to see related to elevated blood pressure, not reduced blood pressure. The paradoxical response results in hypotension, which is further exacerbated by decreased venous return from pooling of blood in the limbs. Alcohol also impairs vasoconstriction and may thus exacerbate the loss of compensatory adjustments. Catecholamine release itself (as with fear, panic, and other stimuli) may trigger the ventricular contraction and thus the Bezold-Jarisch reflex.

Clinically, patients with neurocardiogenic syncope will maintain normal blood pressure and cerebral perfusion immediately upon standing or upon another precipitating event, only to experience a sudden drop in blood pressure with bradycardia. They may feel lightheaded and may experience autonomic prodromal symptoms such as nausea, vomiting, pallor, diaphoresis, and epigastric discomfort.

Orthostatic Syncope

Orthostatic syncope occurs when the normal compensatory mechanisms that counter the effects of gravity are impaired. Clinically, patients with orthostatic syncope have a gradual decrease in blood pressure over time after standing from a lying or sitting position, rather than the abrupt decrease seen in neurocardiogenic syncope. They may lack the autonomic responses (nausea, vomiting, pallor, diaphoresis, and epigastric discomfort) often seen in neurocardiogenic syncope. Patients tend to be elderly, diabetic, and/or receiving cardiovascular medications. Orthostatic syncope can occur in the setting of volume depletion, such as blood or other fluid loss, or with vasodilation; it can be exacerbated by alcohol or by medical disorders affecting autonomic regulation (e.g., Shy–Drager syndrome or diabetes mellitus). Prolonged bed rest may result in cardiovascular deconditioning and orthostatic syncope because of diminished responses to upright posture. Of note, and complicating the diagnostic process, is that orthostatic hypotension is common in the elderly and reported in up to 40% of asymptomatic patients older than 70 years, and 23% of asymptomatic patients younger than 60 years.[8] Consequently, the finding of orthostatic hypotension must be carefully placed in the context of the patient's history and other physical findings.

Situational Syncope

Situational syncope, often referred to as "swooning" in the past, may be mediated by neuroautonomic mechanisms similar to those causing neurocardiogenic syncope, but is precipitated by a "triggering" event. Events such as injury, pain, hunger, fear, crowding, sight of blood, prolonged standing, or anxiety may result in a catecholamine surge that stimulates cardiac mechanoreceptors, resulting in the same feedback loop described for neurocardiogenic syncope. Other causes for situational syncope, such as urination, defecation, coughing, sneezing, and swallowing, may be found in the setting of decreased venous return (as from the Valsalva maneuver) and enhanced vagal tone.

Carotid Sinus Syndrome

This has been defined as syncope or presyncope when carotid sinus massage produces asystole (cardioinhibitory) for 3 or more seconds, or hypotension or mixed when both cardioinhibitory and vasodepressor responses occur.[9]

Seizure

Seizures are discussed in Chapter 12, but a few points are worth noting. The loss of consciousness in seizure is usually abrupt in onset, and an antecedent aura may not occur or be remembered. The postseizure ("postictal") return to consciousness is slow, however, confusion after an unexplained episode of unconsciousness points strongly toward seizure, as does an accompanying transient focal neurologic deficit (Todd's paralysis). Patients may appear confused after a syncopal episode, but usually for no more than 20 to 30 seconds. Transient cerebral anoxia may cause a brief (usually less than 6 to 8 seconds) episode of seizure activity (convulsive syncope) and may be difficult to distinguish from a true underlying epileptic event. Other discriminating factors are discussed later in the chapter.

Psychogenic Syncope

Up to 20% of patients with unexplained syncope may have psychogenic syncope.[10] Syncope may be one of the manifestations of anxiety, panic, somatization, and conversion disorder. However, this is a difficult diagnosis and should be considered a diagnosis of exclusion and one that is almost never made in the emergency department.

Syncope in Children and Adolescents

Syncope in children and adolescents is a common and generally benign event, and the tendency to faint in childhood may be familial.[11] It is common during acute illness, as a response to other noxious emotional or psychologic stimuli, or related to medications or alcohol. Orthostatic syncope is common.[12] Serious causes are rare yet important (e.g., hypertrophic cardiomyopathy, prolonged QT syndrome, myocarditis, anomalous origin of left coronary artery, Wolff–Parkinson–White syndrome). Exertional syncope, a positive family history suggestive of long QT syndrome, sudden death at a young age, or a cardiac murmur on physical examination can be "red flags" for possibly serious etiologies.

Breath-holding spells may cause syncope. The term *breath-holding*, implying a voluntary prolonged inspiration, is a misnomer. Breath-holding usually occurs during expiration and is involuntary.[13] There are two types of breath-holding–related syncope: cyanotic and pallid. In cyanotic breath-holding spells, the child holds the breath at the end of a bout of crying and becomes cyanotic and limp with loss of consciousness. There is rapid return of normal color, respirations, and consciousness. In the pallid variety, the child seems to be responding to a mild irritation and breath-holding may not be obvious. The child usually, but not always, becomes pale and has a sudden syncopal episode.

The pathophysiology of breath-holding spells is thought to involve carotid sinus hypersensitivity and brief cerebral anoxia on the basis of brief cardiac asystole. Some children may have these on a daily basis, and a breath-holding spell can occasionally precipitate an anoxic seizure. Breath-holding spells are usually benign, and most children outgrow them by the age of 5 years.[14]

Drug-Induced Syncope

A number of drugs, usually those with cardiovascular effects, may precipitate syncope. Some common examples are nitrates, β-blockers, vasodilators, calcium channel blockers, angiotensin-converting enzyme inhibitors, phenothiazines, and alcohol.[15] Medications (e.g., quinidine, procainamide, disopyramide, flecainide, amiodarone, sotalol) can precipitate syncope by causing hypotension and conduction delays, by prolonging the QTc, and by stimulating arrhythmias including torsades de pointes. Drug-related syncope is more common in elderly patients, especially when they are taking multiple medications.[16]

Diagnosis

History

A detailed history of the event, if available, can be the most helpful part of the evaluation. A reliable witness can often provide the key to making the correct diagnosis. A history of events leading up to and immediately following the suspected syncopal episode is particularly helpful. Aspects of the history that may be useful, if available, are listed in Table 13-3. The duration of a "warning" period of minutes, sometimes several minutes, suggests vasovagal syncope; a very short warning period (e.g., 10 seconds or less) suggests cardiac syncope.[7] The diagnosis of neurogenic syncope has been associated with historical features of palpitations, blurred vision, nausea, warmth, diaphoresis, or lightheadedness before the event; and nausea, warmth, diaphoresis, or fatigue after the event.[7] The duration of any postevent alteration of consciousness is particularly helpful, as it is usually brief with true syncope and prolonged with a seizure. Severe sudden onset headache accompanying a syncopal episode, if not owing to injury from a fall, suggests the possibility of an acute intracranial hemorrhage (e.g., intraparenchymal hemorrhage, subarachnoid hemorrhage).

TABLE 13-3
ELEMENTS OF SYNCOPE HISTORY

Body position at the time of event
Activity: physical, emotional
Prodromal feelings: warmth, nausea, diaphoresis, visual loss, odors, heart rate and
  rhythm, pain, lightheadedness
Physical result of event: fall, injury, pain
Current illness/medical history
Motor activity during event
Incontinence
Tongue biting
Duration of event
Rate of return to normal level of consciousness
Skin color
Pulse, respiratory activity, shortness of breath
Neurologic symptoms: headache, weakness, numbness, speech or visual
  problems
Alcohol use
Medication use
History of similar events
Family history

The most common neurogenic cause of syncope is a seizure. Brainstem ischemia may cause "drop attacks"; however, drop attacks, by definition, do not involve loss of consciousness, and the involvement of other brainstem structures usually results in additional neurologic signs and symptoms (vertigo, diplopia, dysarthria, ataxia, limb numbness or weakness, or facial paresthesias). Transient ischemic attacks (TIAs) that are related to carotid artery disease (anterior circulation) virtually never cause syncope. Factors favoring seizure include a history of similar events in the past that are stereotypic and not associated with body position, lateral tongue biting, disorientation, observed motor activity during the event, and a postictal period of prolonged confusion or sleepiness.[16] Factors that more strongly favor syncope are sweating, nausea before the event, and being oriented immediately after the event. It should be kept in mind that cardiac syncope may be associated with brief tonic or tonic–clonic muscular activity at onset, and some forms of partial epilepsy may have bradycardia associated with them.[17] In trying to distinguish syncope from seizure, incontinence and trauma from the event are not especially discriminating.

Physical Examination

Some elements of the physical and neurologic examination tend to be more helpful than others. Vital signs should be at the patient's baseline by the time they are evaluated in the emergency department (ED). Persistent hypotension, bradyarrhythmias, tachyarrhythmias, or hypoxia are concerning and must be investigated. Systolic blood pressure less than 90 mm Hg has been identified as a high-risk marker for morbidity and mortality in patients with syncope.[18] Orthostatic hypotension is a finding that requires further evaluation. It can be misleading, as patients with other causes of syncope may have blood pressure declines of 20 mm Hg or more upon changing from the supine to the upright posture; also, orthostatic hypotension is common in the elderly and in ED patients without syncope.[19] The recurrence of presyncope or even syncope upon standing is probably more significant than any particular numeric blood pressure change.

On cardiac examination, murmurs reflecting valvular heart disease, particularly aortic stenosis or idiopathic hypertrophic subaortic stenosis (IHSS) or arrhythmias, can suggest cardiac syncope. Clinical findings suggesting underlying congestive heart failure correlate with high risk of sudden death in the syncope patient.[18] Focal neurologic findings may be a result of seizure if they were not preexisting. The tip of the tongue may sustain a laceration when the patient with syncope falls for any reason and strikes their chin, but a laceration of the side of the tongue is suggestive of a seizure,[20] as is disorientation after the event. Although testing for carotid sinus sensitivity (CSS) is rarely done in the ED setting, it may be diagnostic, as CSS is a rare cause of syncope[21]; however, CSS may also be present in many normal people. Testing for CSS itself carries a small risk of adverse neurologic outcome (stroke or TIA). Contraindications to testing for CSS include carotid bruit, stroke, recent myocardial infarction, or history of serious cardiac dysrhythmia. The abdominal examination should assess for evidence of tenderness and/or distension, which might suggest predisposing medical conditions to syncope, e.g., aortic abdominal aneurysm. A stool guaiac test looking for gastrointestinal bleeding may be helpful in select patients.

The American College of Emergency Physicians (ACEP) has published a clinical policy on syncope and makes one level A recommendation (high certainty) and two level B recommendations (moderate certainty) regarding the history and physical examination; there are no level C recommendations (low certainty).[22]

Level A: "Use history or physical examination findings consistent with heart failure to help identify patients at higher risk of an adverse event."
Level B: "Consider older age, structural heart disease, or a history of coronary artery disease as risk factors for adverse outcome." "Consider younger patients with syncope that is nonexertional, without history or signs of cardiovascular disease, a family history of sudden death, and without comorbidities to be at low risk of adverse events."

Diagnostic Testing

The ACEP policy makes two recommendations related to diagnostic testing in their clinical policy on syncope[22]:

Level A: "Obtain a standard 12-lead ECG in patients with syncope."
Level C: "Laboratory testing and advance investigative testing such as echocardiography or cranial CT scanning need not be routinely performed unless guided by specific findings in the history or physical examination."

Laboratory Evaluation

Laboratory evaluations are rarely helpful in diagnosing the cause of a syncopal event.[22] Although a low hemoglobin may precipitate orthostatic syncope, the history is usually more suggestive, and orthostasis can occur without low hemoglobin. However, a hematocrit less than 30% has been found as a useful predictor of adverse outcomes.[22] Creatine phosphokinase has not been shown to be of diagnostic benefit in differentiating syncope from seizure.[23] A pregnancy test should be obtained in women of childbearing age. Electrolytes, although commonly obtained, rarely lead to determining the cause of syncopal event. Abnormal electrolyte levels may be consistent with etiologies discovered by other methods but are unlikely to be differentially diagnostic by themselves. Cardiac enzymes may also be useful in select patient populations; in one series of 791 patients, 11 myocardial infarctions were diagnosed though it is unclear if these cases could be identified by other findings.[22]

Electrocardiography/Rhythm Strip

An ECG or cardiac rhythm recording may reveal the substrate for a rhythm disturbance, or an actual rhythm disturbance, and is usually obtained when history and physical examination do not reveal a diagnosis. The diagnostic yield of an ECG is less than 5%; however it is a low-cost/high-return test.[22] The ECG should be carefully analyzed for evidence of preexcitation syndromes (delta wave) prolonged QTc, Brugada syndrome (incomplete RBBB with ST elevation in V2 and V3), complete heart block, supraventricular tachycardia, or ventricular tachycardia.

Prolonged ECG Monitoring

Holter or patient-activated loop recorders may be useful beyond the initial patient evaluation in excluding an arrhythmic cause for syncope when symptoms are found to occur in the absence of a recorded arrhythmia, or in the rare instance when arrhythmic syncope is frequent enough to occur during monitoring. Four factors have been found to identify patients who could benefit from prolonged monitoring: age >65 years, male gender, history of heart disease, and the presence of a nonsinus rhythm on the initial ECG.[23]

Brain Computed Tomography/Magnetic Resonance Imaging

There is no evidence to support the routine use of emergent neuroimaging in patients with syncope. The decision to obtain a CT scan or MRI scan is based on the history and physical examination. Such imaging may be obtained in some patients in order to further evaluate symptomatology suggestive of the possibility of TIA, stroke, or the sequelae of trauma.

Other Testing

There is no evidence to support the routine use of transthoracic echocardiography in the evaluation of syncope. Tilt table testing (sometimes performed with pharmacologic enhancement) may be useful for the further evaluation of patients without heart disease, when initial history and physical are nonrevealing, or in patients with heart disease without arrhythmias.[24] Neither electroencephalograms (EEG) nor carotid Doppler ultrasound has been shown to be of benefit in the acute evaluation of the patient with syncope.

Disposition: Risk Stratification

The majority of patients with syncope do not have life-threatening conditions and do not need to be hospitalized. The challenge for the emergency physician is to identify those patients at risk for an adverse outcome. Investigators have tried to design prediction models to distinguish those patients needing hospital admission from those who can be safely discharged home. Martin et al. studied 626 patients in order to identify predictors of arrhythmia and 1-year mortality. Four features were identified—abnormal ECG, history of ventricular arrhythmia, history of congestive heart failure, and age >45 years.[25] Colivicchi et al. studied 598 patients and identified four predictors of 1-year mortality: age >65 years, lack of a prodrome, abnormal ECG, and history of cardiovascular disease.[2] The most recent risk stratification model by Quinn et al. looked at 7-day adverse outcomes and reported five predictors (the San Francisco Syncope Rule): abnormal ECG, shortness of breath, systolic blood pressure less than 90 mm Hg upon arrival in the ED, hematocrit less than 30%, and congestive heart failure by history or by physical examination.[18] None of these three prediction models have been validated to have 100% sensitivity; however, they provide a framework for clinical decision making. The ACEP Clinical Policy on syncope makes two level B recommendations regarding who should be admitted after an episode of syncope of unclear cause[22]:

Level B recommendations:

"Admit patients with syncope and evidence of heart failure or structural heart diseases."
"Admit patients with syncope and other factors that lead to stratification as high risk: older age and associated comorbidities, abnormal ECG, hematocrit less than 30%, history or presence of heart failure, coronary artery disease, or structural heart disease."

REFERENCES

1. Quinn J, McDermott D, Stiell I, et al. Prospective validation of the San Francisco syncope rule to predict patients with serious outcomes. *Ann Emerg Med.* 2006;47:448-454.
2. Colivicchi F, Ammirati F, Melina D, et al.; OESIL Study Investigators. Development and prospective validation of a risk stratification system for patient with syncope in the emergency department: the OESIL risk score. *Eur Heart J.* 2003;24:811-819.
3. Blanc J, L'Her C, Touiza A, et al. Prospective evaluation and outcome of patients admitted for syncope over a 1 year period. *Eur Heart J.* 2002;23:815-820.
4. Kapoor W, Karfp M, Maher Y, et al. Syncope of unknown origin. *JAMA.* 1982;247:2687-2691.
5. Chen L, Shen W, Mahoney D, et al. Prevalence of syncope in a population aged more than 45 years. *Am J Med.* 2006;119:1088-1095.
6. Sun B, Emond J, Camargo C. Direct medical costs of syncope related hospitalizations in the United States. *Am J Cardiol.* 2005;95:668-671.
7. Soteriades E, Evans J, Larson M, et al. Incidence and prognosis of syncope. *N Engl J Med.* 2002;347:878-885.
8. Calkins H, Shyr Y, Frumin H, et al. The value of the clinical history in the differentiation of syncope due to ventricular tachycardia, atrioventricular block, and neurocardiogenic syncope. *Am J Med.* 1995;98:365-373.
9. Atkin D, Hanusa B, Sefcik T, et al. Syncope and orthostatic hypotension. *Am J Med.* 1990; 91:179-185.
10. Linzer M et al. Psychiatric syncope. *Psychosomatics.* 1990;31:181-188.
11. Driscoll DJ et al. Syncope in children and adolescents. *J Am Coll Cardiol.* 1997;29:1039.
12. Ross B et al. Abnormal responses to orthostatic testing in children and adolescents with recurrent unexplained syncope. *Am Heart J.* 1991;122:748-754.
13. DiMario F. Breath-holding spells in childhood. *Am J Dis Child.* 1992;146:125-131.

14. DiMario FJ Jr. Prospective study of children with cyanotic and pallid breath-holding spells. *Pediatrics*. 2001;107:265-269.

15. Hanion J, Linzer M, MacMillian J, et al. Syncope and presyncope associated with probable adverse drug reactions. *Arch Intern Med*. 1990;150:2309-2312.

16. Hoefnagels WA et al. Transient loss of consciousness: the value of the history for distinguishing seizure from syncope. *J Neurol*. 1991;238:39-43.

17. Demps C, Jagoda A. A case of bradycardia and asystole following a seizure. *Am J Emerg Med*. 1998;16:582-585.

18. Quinn J, Stiell I, McDermott D, et al. Derivation of the San Francisco syncope rule to predict patients with short-term serious outcomes. *Ann Emerg Med*. 2004;43:224-232.

19. Koxiol-Mclain J, Lowenstein S, Fuller B. Orthostatic vital signs in emergency department patients. *Ann Emerg Med*. 1999;20:606-610.

20. Benbadis SR et al. Value of tongue biting in the diagnosis of seizures. *Arch Intern Med*. 1995;155:2346.

21. Richardson DA et al. Prevalence of cardioinhibitory carotid sinus hypersensitivity in patients 50 years or over presenting to the accident and emergency department with "unexplained" or "recurrent" falls. *Pace*. 1997;20:820.

22. Huff JS, Decker W, Quinn J, et al. Clinical policy: critical issues in the evaluation and management of adult patients presenting to the emergency department with syncope. *Ann Emerg Med*. 2007;49:431-444.

23. Bass E, Curtiss E, Arena V, et al. The duration of Holter monitoring in patients with syncope: is 24 hours enough? *Arch Intern Med*. 1990;150:1073-1078.

24. Chen L, Benditt D, Win-Kuang S. Management of syncope in adults: an update. *Mayo Clin Proc*. 2008;83:1280-1293.

25. Martin T, Hanusa B, Kapoor W. Risk stratification of patients with syncope. *Ann Emerg Med*. 1997;29:459-466.

14
THE DIZZY PATIENT

The principal problem in any patient complaining of "dizziness" is defining the problem. Dizziness is not a medical term and must be clarified (through careful history taking) and categorized into one of four general groups: vertigo, disequilibrium, presyncope, and nonspecified lightheadedness. The key for the clinician is to identify potentially life-threatening conditions, specifically distinguishing a central nervous system process from a peripheral one.

CLASSIFICATION

Vertigo

Vertigo is the feeling or sensation of movement. This may be described by the patient as swaying, spinning, whirling, leaning, or tilting. In general, when there is a definite illusion of movement, the problem lies somewhere along the peripheral or central nervous system pathways related to the vestibular apparatus.

Presyncope

Presyncopal episodes are often described by patients as dizziness. Unlike the vertiginous patient, however, these patients will describe an impending loss of consciousness. They feel as if they are about to faint and may describe the sensation as lightheadedness or "graying out" (see Chapter 13).

Disequilibrium

Equilibrium depends on a constant stream of sensory information from the vestibular, proprioceptive, and visual systems. This information is integrated by cerebellar centers and influenced by the extrapyramidal pathways to produce confident and rhythmic motion by the patient. Patients with various problems in any of these systems, such as the decreased proprioception as seen in diabetic patients with peripheral neuropathy or decreased vision, may experience disequilibrium. Most such patients have comorbidities with minor defects in multiple systems, which in combination produce a sense of imbalance, without a sensation of motion, however.

Nonspecified Lightheadedness

The most difficult patients are those who do not fall into any of the three groups mentioned above. These patients generally have extremely vague histories and are unable to pin down any specific symptoms. This group includes patients with hyperventilation syndromes, anxiety neuroses, and other psychiatric disorders. Diagnosing this group represents a considerable challenge to both the patience and the skill of the physician.

The focus of this chapter is to provide a framework for approaching the patient with a chief complaint of dizziness, primarily in order to distinguish central from peripheral etiologies. Hypoperfusion states causing presyncope, neuropathies causing disequilibrium, and systemic processes causing generalized weakness are presented in other chapters, although they are important conditions that should be considered when approaching these patients.

EPIDEMIOLOGY

Dizziness is a common component of many acute medical conditions. The incidence increases with age and is one of the most common chief complaints in patients over 75 years of age.[1] Dizziness accounts for up to 5% of emergency department (ED) visits and contributes to the ED presenting complaint in up to 24% of patients.[2] True vertigo accounts for approximately half of patients complaining of dizziness, 17% to 42% of who ultimately receive a diagnosis of benign paroxysmal positional vertigo (BPPV).[3] Of those patients with vertigo, vertebrobasilar insufficiency and posterior circulation stroke are the most concerning diagnoses to be considered and pose the greatest risk management concern for the practicing emergency physician.[4] Even in the absence of posterior circulation disease, dizziness from all causes is associated with disability and injury, especially from falls in the elderly.

PATHOPHYSIOLOGY OF VERTIGO

Vertigo results from dysfunction in the vestibular system from either its peripheral or central components. The peripheral vestibular apparatus includes the labyrinth located in the petrous portion of the temporal bone and the vestibular portion of the eighth cranial nerve, which courses through the cerebellopontine angle connecting the labyrinth to the brainstem. The labyrinth is composed of three semicircular canals, which register head rotation, and the otoliths (utricle and saccule), which sense head position relative to gravity. The central vestibular apparatus consists of vestibular nuclei at the pontomedullary junction in the brainstem; these nuclei are intimately connected to the nuclei controlling eye movement and the cerebellum. Position is registered centrally based on balanced input from the paired labyrinths. Vertigo occurs when input from two labyrinths is unequal; the resulting unbalanced input creates the sensation of movement. In general, acute processes result in vertigo. Chronic processes, such as degenerative disease or expanding tumors, usually result in disequilibrium but not actual vertigo since the brain has time to accommodate to the deficit.

Differential Diagnosis

Central Vestibular Causes

Although less common than peripheral causes, central causes of vertigo are the most concerning (Table 14-1). Disorders include vertebrobasilar insufficiency, brainstem and cerebellum infarct, and hemorrhage; basilar artery migraine, cerebellopontine angle (CPA) tumors, and degenerative diseases are other considerations.

TABLE 14-1 —————————————————————————————
DIFFERENTIAL DIAGNOSIS OF DIZZINESS

Peripheral vestibular causes
Benign paroxysmal positional vertigo
Vestibular neuritis
Vestibular neuronitis
Labyrinthitis
Ménière's disease
Perilymphatic fistulas

Central neurologic causes
Transient ischemic attack/stroke
Vertebrobasilar ischemia
Cerebellopontine angle mass
Basilar artery migraine
Multiple sclerosis
Multisensory deficit syndrome/disequilibrium syndrome

Cardiopulmonary causes
Arrhythmias
Postural hypotension
Hypovolemia (anemia)
Myocardial ischemia
Structural cardiac or valvular disease
Hypoxia
Vasovagal episode (also neurologic)

Other
Drug effects
Thyroid disorder
Hyperventilation
Anxiety/panic disorder

TABLE 14-2

PERIPHERAL VERTIGO VERSUS CENTRAL VERTIGO

	Central	Peripheral
Intensity	Mild	Severe
Tinnitis	Rare	Common
CN findings	Frequent	None
Nystagmus		
Visual fixation	No inhibition	Inhibits
Horizontorotary	Rare	Common
Vertical	Common	Never
Latency	None	3–40 s
Fatigue	None	Yes

Table 14-2 summarizes findings that help to distinguish central from peripheral vertigo. In general, when compared with peripheral vertigo, the symptoms of central vertigo are less acute, more persistent, and associated with neurologic deficits. Symptoms associated with brainstem ischemia include diplopia, ataxia, dysarthria, or facial weakness. However, many exceptions exist, and clinicians must always have a high index of suspicion, especially in those patients with cardiovascular risk factors. Of note, even patients with no cardiovascular risk factors may develop central vertigo, e.g., from vertebral artery dissection or from cardiac emboli. Slowly growing lesions such as acoustic neuromas do not generally produce symptoms because compensatory mechanisms have time to evolve. Indeed, it is these compensatory mechanisms that facilitate recovery from acute insults. CPA tumors and posterior fossa masses may produce vertigo, or if their principal involvement is the cerebellum, they may produce only a feeling of unsteadiness. Such disequilibrium is usually unrelenting and progressive and may move to involve multiple cranial nerves and long tract signs.

Benign Paroxysmal Positional Vertigo

Benign paroxysmal positional vertigo is the most common cause of peripheral vertigo and most common cause of recurrent vertigo with a lifetime prevalence of 2.4%.[5] This syndrome is characterized by a rapid onset of vertigo, associated with a change of head position, which lasts less than 30 to 60 seconds (Table 14-3). Often, patients will

TABLE 14-3

CHARACTERISTIC FINDINGS IN BENIGN PAROXYSMAL POSITIONAL VERTIGO

Episodic periods of vertigo lasting less than 1 minute
Provoked by head movement
Nystagmus that has delayed onset and short duration
Fatigability of nystagmus on repeat testing
Reversal of nystagmus on returning to an upright position
Surpression of nystagmus with visual fixation

complain of the acute onset of symptoms after rolling over in bed, gazing upward, or bending forward. Findings include a horizontal/rotary nystagmus with associated nausea and/or vomiting. Characteristically, symptoms abate when the patient lies still with the eyes closed. The pathogenesis of this condition is thought to be due to the accumulation of free-floating calcium carbonate particulate debris that forms a plug in the posterior semicircular canal, which accounts for approximately 80% of cases of BPPV.[6] When the affected canal is down, as when the patient is in a recumbent position, the calcium carbonate plug acts as a plunger and stimulates the labyrinth. The latency reflects the time required for the plug to move in the canal and stimulate the system; fatigue reflects the process of the plug breaking apart. A history of prior head trauma has been linked to the onset of BPPV, presumably due to dislodged endolymphatic debris.

Ménière's Disease

Ménière's disease is a peripheral nervous system disorder resulting from an increase in endolymph volume (endolymphatic hydrops). Distention of the endolymphatic system results in vertigo, and the increased pressure on hair cells results in an associated hearing loss. The duration of the vertigo and nausea/vomiting in Ménière's disease tends to be hours rather than seconds, as in BPPV. Onset is most frequently in the fifth decade of life. It also differs from BPPV in that it is associated with a sensation of "fullness" in the affected ear with a fluctuating sensorineural hearing loss and tinnitus. Disequilibrium may also be present.

Vestibular Neuritis and Neuronitis

Vestibular neuritis results when the vestibular nerve becomes infected and results in an imbalance of input from the labyrinths causing vertigo. Vestibular neuronitis implies damage to the sensory neurons of vestibular ganglion; the two terms, neuritis and neuronitis, are often used for the same clinical syndrome reflecting difficulty localizing the site of the lesion since they often occur on a continuum. Neuronitis may evolve and involve damage to the brainstem vestibular nucleus and consequently result in hearing loss.

Vestibular neuritis and neuronitis cause a constellation of symptoms that includes acute-onset vertigo, nausea, vomiting, and disequilibrium. It is thought to be viral in etiology, generally occurring in otherwise healthy individuals. As mentioned above, hearing remains unimpaired when only the vestibular apparatus is involved, i.e., all audiologic testing is normal, versus impaired hearing that accompanies a neuronitis. No brainstem findings or other cranial nerve abnormalities are found. The time course of symptoms tends to be over a period of days, with symptoms usually peaking during the first day and then gradually improving over the next few days. As may be seen with all the peripheral causes of vertigo, the patients appear acutely and severely ill.

Labyrinthitis

Labyrinthitis may be differentiated from vestibular neuritis in that there is both nystagmus and vertigo along with hearing loss. Viral labyrinthitis has been reported in association with multiple-viral illness and is generally short-lived and of little consequence. Bacterial labyrinthitis, however, can occur in patients with middle ear disease with fistulas, or mastoid disease, or in association with meningitis. Viral labyrinthitis is generally pain-less; when pain is present, a bacterial etiology should be suspected. These patients rep-resent a medical emergency and require prompt diagnosis and treatment.

Posttraumatic Vestibular Syndromes

Perilymphatic fistulas between the middle and inner ear may result after trauma, after a forceful Valsalva maneuver, or after acute external pressure changes as in scuba diving. Replication of the patient's symptoms on Valsalva maneuver or pneumatic otoscopy, combined with a suggestive history, is diagnostic. Acute traumatic tympanic membrane rupture can also lead to immediate onset of vertigo, nausea, and/or vomiting associated with hearing loss. A similar constellation of symptoms can be seen in patients with frac-tures through the petrous portion of the temporal bone.

Disequilibrium Syndromes (Multisensory Deficits Syndromes)

A generalized feeling of unsteadiness in the nonvertiginous elderly patient usually rep-resents a multisensory deficits syndrome. These patients frequently relate that their problem is worse in the evening when they are fatigued and their visual inputs are dimin-ished. Such patients frequently do well in familiar surroundings where only minimal information is necessary for them to make decisions but do poorly in unfamiliar situa-tions. Multisensory deficits can be tremendously exaggerated by medications including those used to treat vertigo.

Other Causes

Other causes of dizziness include drug toxicity, hypoglycemia, anemia, hypothyroidism, and multiple sclerosis; psychiatric causes include anxiety and hyperventilation, although these diagnoses are ones of exclusion and rarely definitively made by emergency physi-cians. All tranquilizers, antiepileptic drugs, and antipsychotic drugs may, through multi-ple mechanisms, cause a combination of disequilibrium, near-syncope, and mild forms of vertigo that the patient may be unable to separate on a historical basis (Table 14-4). Ototoxic drugs that cause a sense of unsteadiness and hearing loss rarely actually cause vertigo since the deficits are bilateral.

Migraine-related vertigo accounts for up to 14% of vertigo cases in adults.[7] Making the diagnosis for migrainous vertigo involves first ruling out other causes of vertigo and criteria include episodes of vertigo, migraine according to International Headache Soci-ety criteria, and at least two of the following symptoms during the events: headache, pho-tophobia, phonophobia, visual, or other aura.

EVALUATION

Patients presenting with a complaint of dizziness require a complete set of vital signs and an assessment at triage for cardiovascular risk factors. Oxygenation and cardiovascular stability should be assessed; if fluid intake has been compromised, dehydration needs to be addressed. Patients with vertigo are at risk of vomiting, and thus appropriate precau-tions should be taken.

TABLE 14-4 —————————————————
DRUGS ASSOCIATED WITH DIZZINESS

Anticonvulsants
Alcohols
Aminoglycosides
Other antibiotics
Heavy metals
Cinchona alkaloids
Salicylates
Minor tranquilizers
Major tranquilizers
Diuretics
β-Blockers
α-Blockers
Centrally acting antihypertensives

Vertigo/dizziness may be a symptom of stroke; since many triage screens do not take posterior circulation deficits into consideration special care must be taken in select patients upon initial presentation to the emergency department.

History

The key to diagnosis of the dizzy patient lies in careful history taking, allowing the patient to describe the symptoms. The correct etiology of dizziness can be made by history alone in over half of patients seen[8] (Table 14-5). If patients report that they have a sense of motion or spinning, follow-up questions regarding relationship of symptoms to position and movement are important. The time course for various causes of vertigo may also be helpful: BPPV usually has an abrupt onset, vertebral basilar insufficiency may develop over minutes or have a stuttering course, Ménière's syndrome has vertigo that may last

TABLE 14-5 —————————————————
HISTORICAL FEATURES IMPORTANT TO CHARACTERIZE IN A PATIENT WITH A CHIEF COMPLAINT OF DIZZINESS/VERTIGO

- Sensation of motion, whirling, spinning, tilting, leaning
- Relation to change of position, sharp turns, specific positions
- Rate of onset and duration of symptoms
- Relation to autonomic nervous system stress
- Time of day
- Drugs and medications: prescription and nonprescription
- Associated symptoms: nausea, vomiting, blurred vision, loss of vision, motor weakness, hearing loss, tinnitus, headache, difficulty speaking or swallowing, incoordination
- Other medical problems (thyroid disease, diabetes, hypertension, stroke)

for hours, and vestibular neuronitis and labyrinthitis have persistent symptoms for days. Patients with near-syncope as the underlying mechanism of their dizziness will frequently have an increase of symptoms with autonomic stress. Information about the relationship to orthostatic change as well as swallowing, coughing, and urinating may be helpful. Patients with disequilibrium have particular difficulty when one of their sensory modalities is reduced. In particular, older patients with decreasing vision find that in the evening when rooms are inadequately lighted, they have considerably more difficulty in walking. Also, patients with multisensory deficits have greater difficulty as the day progresses and fatigue affects their system. A seemingly endless list of drugs may cause not only vertigo but also generalized weakness and/or autonomic changes that may be interpreted by the patient as dizziness. Many of the medications that affect blood pressure, electrolytes, or central or peripheral nervous system structures may be the cause of the patient's symptoms. A history of both prescription drugs and over-the-counter medications used should be elicited.

There are several caveats that need to be highlighted in the history of patients with dizziness/vertigo. Head motion or position that triggers the symptom suggests a peripheral etiology. However, this is true only if the events are brief and episodic; it is not true if the event is a single event that lasts hours to days and yet is exacerbated by position. Cardiac events and TIAs that cause vertigo are generally spontaneous and not position related; strokes may produce persistent dizziness or vertigo that is made worse with changes in position or turning of the head.[4]

Physical Examination

The physical and neurologic examination should be performed systematically with a focus on the vital signs, cardiovascular system, cranial nerves, posterior column, and sensory functions.

The head examination should assess for evidence of trauma. Examine the tympanic membranes and external auditory canals for the presence of infection or tympanic membrane rupture. Impacted cerumen or foreign body should not cause vertigo but may give a sense of disequilibrium. Clinical findings of otitis media raise concerns for a labyrinthitis. The eye examination includes checking for the presence of nystagmus.[3] Peripheral vestibular nystagmus is typically horizontal rotatory with a slow and fast component. The fast component points away from the affected side. It typically extinguishes with repeated testing or ocular fixation.[4] In peripheral disease the nystagmus is in a constant direction regardless of direction of gaze, although the intensity of the nystagmus may vary. The nystagmus increases in intensity with gaze in the direction of the fast phase. Visual fixation will reduce the intensity of nystagmus in peripheral disorders. Central disorders can produce nystagmus that changes direction with gaze (gaze-evoked nystagmus), although nystagmus can be present in only one direction of gaze. Vertical nystagmus that is spontaneous and nonfatigable represents a central pathology until proven otherwise. Visual fixation does not affect the degree of nystagmus produced by central disorders.

A cardiovascular examination should be done particularly in patients at risk for cardiovascular disease. The carotid arteries should be assessed for bruits. Bruits suggest carotid stenosis, which may suggest cerebrovascular insufficiency as a cause of the patient's symptoms. A systolic murmur suggests aortic stenosis, which may explain near-syncope or syncope also associated with exertion.

Neurologic Examination

The neurologic examination in the patient with dizziness/vertigo focuses on cranial nerves III, IV, VI, VII, VIII, and IX, and on cerebellar function. Failure to ambulate patients and to assess for ataxia has been identified as a common pitfall in the failure to diagnose stroke in patients presenting with dizziness/vertigo.[9] Patients presenting to the emergency department with a complaint of dizziness, vertigo, or imbalance who have a normal neurologic examination have less than 1% chance of having an underlying stroke as the etiology of their presentation.[9]

Cranial nerve VIII deficits may help elucidate the etiology of vertigo. The best general test of cranial nerve VIII is the use of soft whispered speech. The test is performed by having the examiner whisper letters and numbers in one ear while masking sound in the opposite ear. Masking can be accomplished by simply rubbing the fingers or hair in front of the opposite ear. Soft-whispered speech, whispered-speech, loud-whispered speech, spoken-speech, loud-spoken speech, and finally no response are the levels generally employed for the whispered-speech test.

The Weber test and Rinne test (see Chapter 3) are used to differentiate conduction from neurosensory disorders.

Cerebellar function is assessed using finger-to-nose, finger-to-finger, and rapid alternating movement tests. Ambulation is a key component of the evaluation, although care must be taken to ensure the patient does not fall. Patients with peripheral vertigo are typically able to walk without assistance, whereas patients with an acute cerebellar infarction or hemorrhage are generally unable to ambulate unassisted. Romberg testing is used to distinguish somatosensory deficits from cerebellar processes (see Chapter 3, on the neurologic examination).

Diagnostic Maneuvers

The Dix-Hallpike maneuver (Fig. 14-1) (sometimes referred to as the Nylen–Bárány maneuver) is a provocative test designed to precipitate BPPV originating from the posterior semicircular canal (the majority of cases of BPPV) and thus to help distinguish BPPV from central vertigo. It will not be helpful in diagnosing other types of peripheral vertigo. Before doing the test, the clinician should warn the patient that the maneuver may precipitate the vertigo and associated vomiting. The maneuver begins with the patient in the upright position with the head turned 45 degrees to the right; the patient is then quickly moved from the sitting position to a supine position with the head hanging off the edge of the stretcher with the neck extended and the chin pointing slightly upward. The maneuver is then repeated from the sitting position with the head turned 45 degrees to the left. When positive, the patient will, after a brief (up to 60 seconds) latency period, complain of a sensation of rotational vertigo, accompanied by nystagmus. The nystagmus tends to be horizontal or rotatory, with the superior aspect of the eye bearing toward the dependent ear. The sensitivity of the maneuver for BPPV is approximately 80% with a negative predictive value of 52%; therefore, a negative test does not rule out the diagnosis of BPPV.[3] Repetition of the maneuver leads to a reduction in the intensity of vestibular symptoms, and thus it is also used in therapeutic management. A video of the maneuver can be found at www.neurology.org/cgi/content/full/70/22/2067.

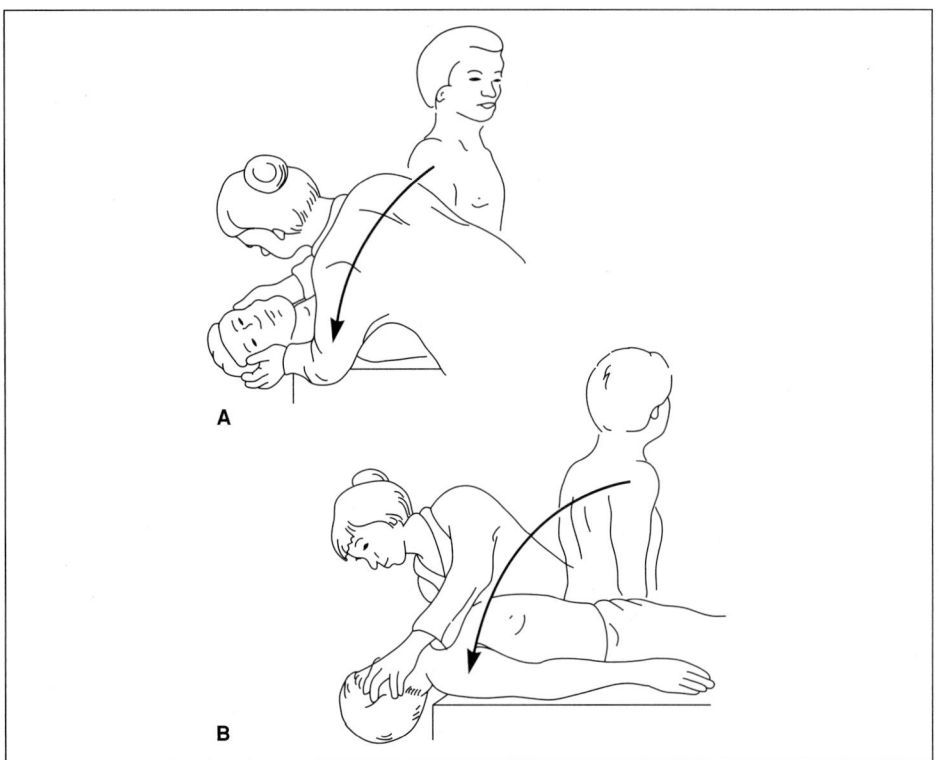

FIGURE 14-1 Dix-Hallpike test. (A) For testing the right posterior semicircular canal, the patient sits on the examination table and turns his or her head to the right 45 degrees. This places the posterior semicircular canal in the sagittal plane. The examiner stands facing the patient on the patient's right side or behind the patient. (B) The patient is then moved by the examiner from the seated to the supine position with the head slightly hanging over the edge of the table. The right ear is down and the chin is pointing slightly up. The eyes are observed for the characteristic nystagmus. (Reprinted with permission from Lalwani AK. *Current Diagnosis & Treatment in Otolaryngology—Head & Neck Surgery*. 2nd ed. New York: The McGraw-Hill Companies Inc; 2008.)

Diagnostic Testing

No one panel of tests is indicated for all patients with a complaint of dizziness; instead, testing is tailored to clinical suspicion with a low testing threshold for anemia, hypoglycemia, and pregnancy. Likewise, a single 12-lead ECG is rarely definitive but is indicated along with continuous rhythm monitoring when dysrhythmias are in the differential diagnosis.

Neuroimaging is not recommended in clear cases of BPPV.[3] It is indicated in patients with signs of a central process, focal neurologic deficits, headache, or risk factors for cerebrovascular disease for which no other explanation of the symptoms can be found. A noncontrast head computed tomography (CT) scan is a reasonable screening test for patients with suspected central lesions causing vertigo, but it has limitations that preclude it from being definitive. Magnetic resonance (MR) brain imaging and angiography are preferred except for detecting acute hemorrhage. MR imaging is more likely to detect subtle brainstem or inferior cerebellar infarction, whereas CT or MR angiography is indicated to assess for vertebrobasilar occlusive disease. Decision making for advanced neuroimaging must take into consideration the patient's presentation, risk factors, and availability for follow-up care.

Special mention needs to be made regarding the patient with sudden onset of headache, severe vertigo, vomiting, and cerebellar incoordination. Such patients should be considered as having an acute cerebellar hemorrhage and are best treated as if they have a life-threatening emergency. An emergent noncontrast head CT is indicated. Along with vertigo, patients with acute cerebellar hemorrhage often present with unilateral ataxia, small pupils, vomiting, and diaphoresis. Paralysis of conjugate lateral gaze or sixth nerve palsies may also be seen.

Specialized Neurologic Testing

Audiometry is used in evaluating dizzy patients with unilateral hearing loss. It is helpful in diagnosing Ménière's disease and acoustic neuromas. It is not recommended in the diagnostic evaluation of BPPV.[3] Vestibular function testing involves a battery of tests designed to record nystagmus in response to labyrinthine stimulation or voluntary eye movements. It may be helpful in cases of atypical nystagmus, and vestibular dysfunction of unclear etiology; it is not recommended in patients with BPPV.[3]

EMERGENCY DEPARTMENT MANAGEMENT

Management of vertigo depends on the underlying etiology. Rest, reassurance, antiemetics, and fluids provide the framework for supportive care of these patients. Treatment of acute posterior circulation stroke is time dependent and may include thrombolysis (see Chapter 5).

Therapeutic Maneuvers

The canalith repositioning maneuver (CRP), often called the Epley maneuver (Fig. 14-2), is a noninvasive bedside intervention designed to reposition particulate debris from the posterior semicircular canal to the utricle[3,6] (Table 14-6). Once the particulate matter is repositioned, abnormal vestibular input is eliminated. The CRP is reported to have a 40% to 95% success rate in patients with posterior canal BPPV, with a reported odds ratio of 5.1 in favor of conversion of a negative Dix-Hallpike test.[3] A video of the maneuver can be found at www.neurology.org/cgi/content/full/70/22/2067. Originally, patients were instructed to restrict postmaneuver activities, to wear a soft collar, and to remain in an upright position for up to 48 hours; these steps are not supported by the literature and no longer recommended.[6]

Vestibular rehabilitation exercises are used to promote habituation, adaptation to vertigo. These exercises can consist of repetitive side-to-side head movements performed while lying down, or may involve use of the CRP. Both have been shown to decrease the intensity of vertiginous episodes in BPPV and to facilitate recovery. These exercises can be provided as part of the discharge instructions.[3]

Vestibular Suppressants

Four categories of medications have been used in the management of vertigo: antihistamines, anticholinergics, phenothiazines, and benzodiazepines. The biggest advantage in

TABLE 14-6

CANALITH REPOSITIONING MANEUVER (EPLEY MANEUVER) FOR TREATING BENIGN PAROXYSMAL POSITIONAL VERTIGO

1. Begin with the patient in a sitting position with the head turned 45 degrees toward the side that was positive in the Dix-Hallpike test: calcium carbonate debris settles in the bottom of the posterior canal.
2. Rapidly lay patient down with the head hanging 30 degrees off the edge of the gurney for 30 s.
3. Rotate head clockwise to opposite side so that the other ear is toward the floor for 30 s.
4. Rotate the head so that the face is toward the floor (this will require the patient's body to move from the supine position to the left lateral decubitus position) for 30 s: in this position the debris should enter the common crus of the posterior and anterior semicircular canals.
5. Sit the patient up.

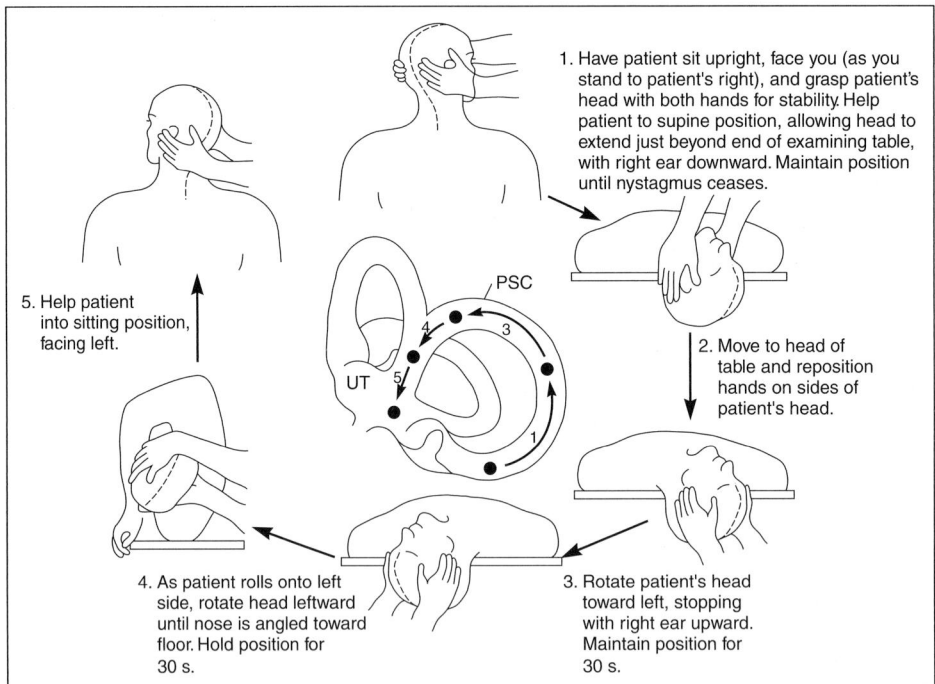

FIGURE 14-2 Epley maneuver. The patient is taken through four moves, starting in the sitting position with the head turned at a 45 degree angle toward the affected side. (1) The patient is placed into the Dix-Hallpike position (supine with the affected ear down) until the vertigo and nystagmus subside. (3) The patient's head is then turned to the opposite side, causing the affected ear to be up and the unaffected ear to be down. (4) The whole body and head are then turned away from the affected side to a lateral decubitus position, with the head in a face-down position. (5) The last step is to bring the patient back to a sitting position with the head turned toward the unaffected shoulder. (Reprinted with permission from Lalwani AK. *Current Diagnosis & Treatment in Otolaryngology—Head & Neck Surgery*. 2nd ed. New York: The McGraw-Hill Companies Inc; 2008.)

these agents is most likely their antiemetic effect. There is no evidence that any medication is effective in treating BPPV and the CRP is the intervention of choice.[6]

Antihistamines and anticholinergics may work through inhibiting muscarinic acetylcholine receptors. Meclizine is probably the most commonly used antihistamine although dimenhydrinate and diphenhydramine are alternatives. The benzodiazepines may work through inhibiting GABA receptors. In patients with prominent nausea or vomiting, the phenothiazine antiemetics such as promethazine or prochlorperazine may be effective. It is key to emphasize that all the medications mentioned may cause drowsiness and indeed may exacerbate symptoms in patients with disequilibrium syndromes, presyncope, or vertigo/dizziness of undefined etiology. Long-term use of these medications may also impair vestibular compensation.

DISPOSITION

Patients with suspected posterior circulation disease require hospitalization or consultation with a neurologist. Admission may be necessary for patients with severe symptoms accompanied by disequilibrium despite therapy (particularly the elderly at risk for falling). Patients discharged home should be advised not to drive and to minimize situations in which falling could cause harm. The canalith repositioning procedure is recommended in the literature as the treatment of choice for BPPV. Vestibular suppressant medications are of questionable value and potentially dangerous in patients with disequilibrium, presyncope, and undifferentiated dizziness. Patients with BPPV should be instructed on the importance of vestibular rehabilitation exercises and the possibility of recurrent symptoms.

SUMMARY

Successful ED management of a patient with an acute complaint of dizziness is built on a careful history and physical examination. The history focuses on symptom description and time course. The physical examination investigates abnormal vital signs, the presence of nystagmus (horizontal or vertical, fatiguing or nonfatigable), hearing loss, evidence of head trauma, or neurologic deficits. For patients with peripheral vestibular symptoms, the Dix-Hallpike maneuver may be confirmatory. Patients with peripheral vertigo do not need extensive diagnostic testing but instead require supportive care that includes hydration and the canolith repositioning procedure. Patients who have acute neurologic deficits should have emergent neuroimaging with appropriate neurology or neurosurgical consultation.

REFERENCES

1. Tinetti ME, Williams CS, Gill TM. Dizziness among older adults: a possible geriatric syndrome. *Ann Intern Med.* 2000;132:337-344.
2. Newman-Toker D, Cannon L, Stofferahn M, et al. Imprecision in patient reports of dizziness symptom quality: a cross-sectional study conducted in an acute care setting. *Mayo Clin Proc.* 2007;82:1329-1340.

3. Bhattacharyya N, Baugh R, Orvidas L, et al. Clinical practice guideline: benign paroxysmal positional vertigo. *Otolaryngol Head Neck Surg*. 2008;139:S47-S81.

4. Stanton V, Hsieh Y, Camargo C, et al. Overreliance on symptom quality in diagnosing dizziness: results of a multicenter survey of emergency physicians. *Mayo Clin Proc*. 2007;82:1319-1328.

5. van Brevern M, Radtke A, Lezius F, et al. Epidemiology of benign paroxysmal positional vertigo: a population based study. *J Neurol Neurosurg Psychiatry*. 2007;78:710-715.

6. Fife T, Iverson T, Lempert J, et al. Practice parameter: therapies for benign paroxysmal positional vertigo. *Neurology*. 2008;70:2067-2074.

7. Reploeg M, Goebel J. Migraine associated dizziness: patient characteristics and management options. *Otol Neurotol*. 2002;12:364-371.

8. Hoffman RM, Einstadter D, Kroenke K. Evaluating dizziness. *Am J Med*. 1999;107:468-478.

9. Kerber K, Brown D, Lisabeth L, et al. Stroke among patients with dizziness, vertigo, and imbalance in the emergency department: a population based study. *Stroke*. 2006;37:2482-2487.

NECK AND BACK PAIN

Acute and chronic neck and back pains are extremely common in the general population and as presenting complaints in the acute care setting.[1-3] This chapter focuses on evaluation of the patient who presents with neck or back pain with either no trauma or with minor trauma such as bending, lifting, or minor falls. Issues related to major trauma are covered in Chapter 10. A variety of disease entities from muscle spasm to metastatic cancer can be associated with such complaints. The majority of patients who present to an acute care setting have medically benign conditions that usually resolve with conservative management[4,5] but may recur and produce longer-term problems in a minority.[6] Because of the difficulty in correlating signs and symptoms with pathological changes on imaging studies, up to 85% of patients with low back pain cannot be given a specific diagnosis,[7,8] and most fall into the nonspecific category of "mechanical" neck or back pain. Therefore, an important component of the initial evaluation is to decide whether the patient has signs or symptoms that could represent more serious pathology and risk to the patient's neurologic well-being, "red flags." This can usually be accomplished with the history and physical examination. Only a few entities can threaten the integrity of the spinal cord/central nervous system (CNS) or nerve roots and thus represent the potential for acute decompensation. These are listed in Table 15-1. The signs and symptoms that comprise the red flags for these entities are discussed in their respective sections in this chapter. Some of the entities, such as epidural abscess, typically progress if untreated, and some, such as herniated nucleus pulposus, can have a variable course, many times with spontaneous symptomatic resolution. Thus, not all these entities represent equivalent risk to the patient. Although other life-threatening conditions such as acute myocardial infarction, aortic aneurysm, or dissection can present with a component of neck or back pain, they are not covered in this text. The focus of this chapter is the patient with pain caused by a disease process related to the spine.

TABLE 15-1

POTENTIAL IMMEDIATE THREATS TO SPINAL CORD/
CNS/NERVE ROOT INTEGRITY

1. Spinal abscess (epidural, subdural)
2. Bony compression: fractures (including pathologic), dislocations
3. Herniated nucleus pulposus
4. Hematoma (epidural, subdural)
5. Subarachnoid hemorrhage (spinal, intracranial)
6. Arterial dissection/infarction

HISTORICAL FEATURES

Among the most important diagnostic historical features are the age of the patient, the duration of pain, the location of the pain, the magnitude of forces in cases of trauma, the radiation in specific nerve root patterns, the relation to neck or back movement, the mode of onset, underlying medical conditions, systemic complaints, and atypical features (Tables 15-2 and 15-3). Referral of pain from other areas, such as the chest or abdomen, may suggest nonneurologic etiologies. Patients younger than 18 years or older than 50 years are at increased risk for more serious underlying pathology such as tumor or infection in both age groups, and abdominal aortic aneurysm and cancer in the older population. The prognosis for patients with recent onset of low back pain is generally good, with rapid diminution; though not always complete resolution of pain and prompt (within 2 weeks) return to work. The majority, but not all, have substantial improvement or no symptoms at 6 months to 1 year, though recurrences are common.[9–11] Most guidelines suggest that as most benign causes for acute back or neck pain, when treated with conservative management, resolve or are significantly improved within 6 to 8 weeks.[12,13] Pain lasting longer raises suspicion of more serious underlying pathology. Features significantly correlated with back pain as a result of malignancy include a past history of cancer, hematocrit <30%, a markedly elevated sedimentation rate, or the subjective judgment of the clinician that cancer is the cause. Traditional predictors such as age >50 years, pain unrelieved by bed rest, pain of greater than 1-month

TABLE 15-2

HISTORICAL FEATURES OF BACK AND NECK PAIN

1. Localization
2. Radiation of the pain
3. Mechanism of injury, rate of onset
4. Relation to movement
5. Associated neurologic symptoms (e.g., weakness)
6. Urinary control
7. Underlying disease entities
8. Weight loss
9. Fever

TABLE 15-3 ——————————————

HISTORICAL FEATURES OF LOW BACK PAIN

Disease to be Detected	Medical History	Sensitivity	Specificity
Cancer	Age ≥50 y	0.77	0.71
	History of cancer	0.31	0.98
	Unexplained weight loss	0.15	0.94
	Failure to improve with a month of therapy	0.31	0.90
	No relief with bed rest	>0.90	0.46
	Duration of pain >1 mo	0.50	0.81
Spinal osteomyelitis	IV drug abuse, UTI or skin infection	0.40	N/A
Compression fracture	Age ≥50 y	0.84	0.61
	Age ≥70 y	0.22	0.96
	Trauma	0.30	0.85
	Corticosteroid use	0.06	0.995
Herniated disk	Sciatica	0.95	0.88
Spinal stenosis	Pseudoclaudication	0.60	N/A
	Age ≥50 y	0.90	0.70
Ankylosing spondylitis	4 out of 5 responses[a]	0.23	0.82
	Age at onset ≤40 y	1.00	0.07
	Pain not relieved supine	0.80	0.49
	Morning back stiffness	0.64	0.59
	Pain duration ≥3 mo	0.71	0.54

[a] Five questions were asked before age 40: did problem begin slowly, persists for at least 3 months, morning stiffness, improvement with exercise.
Adapted from Deyo RA, Rainville J, Kent DL. What can the history and physical examination tell us about low back pain? *JAMA.* 1992;268(6):760-765.

duration, and leukocytosis have little predictive power, but may raise concern. Atypical features such as night pain raise concern for tumor or infection, as do systemic complaints such as fever, chills, night sweats, or unexplained weight loss. A history of immunocompromise or IV drug use also represents increased risk for spinal infection. Back pain radiating below the knee raises suspicion for nerve root irritation. Bilateral sciatic pain worsened by activity, prolonged standing, and back extension can suggest lumbar stenosis. Such pain is usually relieved by rest and forward flexion of the back.

Associated Neurologic Symptoms

Concomitant onset of problems with loss of bowel or bladder control and/or muscle weakness may indicate that an emergency exists. Acute loss of bladder innervation usually results in urinary retention, with possibly subsequent overflow incontinence. Loss of bowel control usually does not occur acutely. Most conditions that pose a potential threat to the patient's neurologic well-being have associated neurologic signs and/or symptoms. The presence of neurologic symptoms strongly influences the neurologic examination. The results of both the history and the physical examination form the basis for decisions about the need for additional testing.

Underlying Disease

Spinal column pain with or without associated physical findings may have different implications in patients with underlying disease such as severe collagen vascular disease, IV drug use, sickle cell anemia, metabolic bone disease, or (especially) a known history of cancer. A history of a febrile illness may suggest an infectious etiology. Many of these historical features associated with back pain have been studied, and their respective sensitivities and specificities are summarized in Table 15-3. While it is difficult to apply such numbers to individual patients, the figures do indicate the relative importance of various elements of the history. Comparable data for neck pain is not available.

Examination

General Physical Examination

Observation of patients performing common movements such as walking, sitting, and standing may reveal helpful information about their complaints and activity limitations; patient "guarding" to avoid pain exacerbation is also a useful observation (Table 15-4). Most patients with mechanical low back pain find certain positions and postures more comfortable.

Vital Signs

Checking temperature may be useful in the patient with a suspected spinal column disease and a history suggestive of a febrile illness. A patient with complaints of back pain

TABLE 15-4

EXAMINATION ELEMENTS FOR NECK AND BACK PAIN

General physical examination
Temperature
Spine: palpation, range of motion
Abdomen
Neurologic examination
Motor bulk, strength
Straight leg raising (back)
Sensation
Reflexes
Spurling's sign (see text)

and an elevated temperature (or a recent history of an elevated temperature) may have an acute infectious process that may or may not be revealed on the general physical and neurologic examination. It is uncommon but not rare that patients with an infectious process related to the spine do not have a fever at the time of presentation. A past history of a febrile illness may be the only clue to an infectious etiology.

Spine

Direct inspection and palpation of the spine can be helpful. Point tenderness will help to guide further evaluations and may reveal evidence of direct trauma or underlying infection. Areas of redness or warmth may also indicate underlying infection but are nonspecific. Palpation of the musculature in both the neck and lumbar regions may reveal spasm, which may be the result of, or contributing to, the patient's pain. Noting the range of motion of the spine in flexion, extension, rotation, and lateral bending may help with a determination of the extent of the painful conditions, but it is not differentially diagnostic.

Abdomen

While the focus of this chapter is the patient with spinal pain (i.e., without other somatic complaints such as abdominal pain), abdominal diseases may present with back pain, which predominates over the abdominal pain. Back pain with tenderness in the costovertebral angles may suggest renal involvement. Severe low back pain with a tender pulsatile abdominal mass indicates the possibility of an abdominal aortic aneurysm. While usually associated initially with chest pain, an aortic dissection may also result in back pain. A patient with a palpable bladder, or suspicion of such, may be in urinary retention as a result of cauda equina or spinal cord compression. Ultrasonic bladder scanning is a noninvasive test that may be used to estimate post-void residual urine.

Rectal Examination

If there is a significant question about spinal cord or cauda equina dysfunction such as with a complaint of urinary retention or perineal numbness, examination for rectal tone is important. Loss of the bulbocavernosus reflex or loss of rectal sphincter tone can reflect interruption of the S2 to S4 reflex arc, which is active in bladder contractions. This reflex is elicited by placing the examiner's gloved finger in the rectum and squeezing the head of the penis in men or tugging on a Foley catheter in women or men. A prompt contraction of the rectal sphincter is the normal response.

Neurologic Examination

The emphasis in the neurologic examination should be directed on the basis of findings that reflect possible spinal nerve root, spinal cord, cauda equina, and/or associated peripheral motor or sensory nerve involvement. The examination is tailored to the suspected area of involvement of the spine and any history of neurologic deficit, with emphasis on the upper extremities in patients with neck concerns and the lower extremities in patients with back pain.

Motor Examination

Motor examination includes looking at the specific muscles innervated by the appropriate cervical nerve roots and lumbar and sacral nerve roots (Table 15-5). Motor strength is usually compared side to side. In the legs, testing plantarflexion strength is best done by having the patient walk, if he or she is able, on his or her toes. Patient with mild plantar flexion weakness may be able to overcome the examiner's hand resistance in testing plantar flexion strength. In the patient with acute back pain, motor bulk is rarely affected, and abnormal motor movements are rarely seen. Patients who have such findings should be suspected of having more long-standing neurologic involvement.

Sensory Examination

As with the motor examination, attention should be paid to sensory involvement of the cervical and lumbosacral roots/spinal cord as indicated by the history. The sensory examination is important in patients who are thought to have thoracic spinal root involvement. Since the musculature is essentially impossible to evaluate in this region, sensory findings may be the only clue to thoracic spinal root problems. Sensation is of particular importance in assessing the lower lumbar nerve roots in cases of suspected lower lumbar/sacral root or conus medullaris involvement. Loss of sensation around the genitalia and rectal areas is a good indication of involvement of the lower spinal cord (conus medullaris) or cauda equina. Stroking the skin next to the rectum should cause a contraction of the sphincter ("anal wink") in patients with an intact S2 to S4 reflex arc.

Reflexes

Reflex analogues of the various indicated nerve roots are indicated in Table 15-5. Pathologic reflexes such as the Babinski sign in the foot or Trömner's sign (see Glossary) in the hand may be indicative of long-term upper motor neuron dysfunction and do not occur in cases of isolated nerve root dysfunction.

ANCILLARY TESTING

Laboratory Testing

In the acute evaluation of neck and back pain, laboratory tests are of little to no value in assessing the patient. In diagnosed cases of epidural abscess/vertebral osteomyelitis, nonspecific markers of inflammation (the sedimentation rate and C-reactive protein) are usually, but not always elevated[14–17]; however their prospective use in nonselected patients has not been studied. Likewise, a complete blood count with elevated white blood cells may be seen but is not very sensitive or specific. Metabolic bone disease and cancer generally require evaluation beyond the scope of the acute care setting.

Management

In patients in whom there is no definite cause for back pain, in whom there are no focal neurologic findings, and no red flags, symptomatic treatment is usually the appropriate initial management strategy.

TABLE 15-5 — NERVE ROOT INNERVATIONS

Nerve Root	Pain	Sensory Loss	Motor Loss	Reflex Loss
C5	Neck, shoulder, upper arm	Lateral shoulder	Deltoid, biceps	Biceps
C6	Neck, shoulder, extending down to lateral aspect of arm involving thumb and forefinger	C6 dermatome out to thumb and forefinger	Biceps	Biceps
C7	Neck and lateral aspect of the arm to third and fourth fingers	C7 dermatome third and fourth digits	Triceps and extensor carpal ulna radius	Triceps
C8	Ulnar aspect at forearm and fifth digit hand	C8 nerve root including fifth digit	Intrinsic muscles of the hand and wrist extensors	None
T1-T12	Isolated dermatome of specific nerve root	Dermatomes; specific nerve root	Essentially untestable	None
L4	Upper thigh Anterior surface of inner thigh	Anterior Medial surface of thigh L4 distribution down to medial aspect of the foot	Quadriceps	Knee jerk
L5	Lateral aspect of the thigh and outer side of calf across dorsum of the foot to great toe	L5 dermatome usually involving the great toe	Extensor hallucis longus	None
S1	Pain in back of the thigh and calf involving the toes	S1 distribution usually involving fourth and fifth toes, back of thigh	Gastrocnemius plantar flexion	Ankle jerk
S2-S4	Perineum	Perianal-saddle area	Bladder	Bulbocavernosus and anal wink

Imaging

With most acute presentations of nontraumatic neck and back pain, radiographic evaluation is not usually indicated or helpful.

Cervical Spine Evaluation

Cervical spine X-rays should be considered for the initial evaluation of patients who complain of posttraumatic neck pain. For consideration of significant neurotrauma, see Chapter 10.

Lumbosacral Spine Evaluation

Indications for plain film X-rays of the lumbosacral spine have been studied extensively. Direct trauma to the lumbar spine with tenderness on physical examination probably reflects the most compelling reason for emergency X-ray evaluation. In patients with lifting, straining, or bending injuries unassociated with direct trauma, there is little evidence to suggest that X-ray evaluation is helpful for initial management. Since this group represents the largest proportion of back pain patients seen in the acute care setting, careful selection of which patients even need X-ray evaluation is important. Plain lumbosacral spine radiographs have been used historically in those patients with pain unimproved for 1 month, those with a history of cancer, those who are older than 50 years, and those with suspected vertebral infection. Under these circumstances, one is looking to include or exclude signs of vertebral involvement from infection or malignancy, spinal stenosis, spondylolisthesis, and nonpathologic vertebral fractures. There are other imaging modalities that will better define each of these entities (see Chapter 2) but an initial plain film may be useful.

Computed Tomography

A plain (no intravenous or intrathecal contrast material administered) CT scan may help to define osseous abnormalities (fractures, extensive degenerative changes, etc.). It is not sensitive for spinal cord or cauda equina compression, most intrinsic spinal canal abnormalities, or for ligamentous instability. CT scanning with intrathecal contrast material ("CT myelography") is an excellent test to define spinal cord/cauda equina compression and can substitute for MRI if MRI is not available.

Magnetic Resonance Imaging

Magnetic resonance imaging (MRI) is a more sensitive test for assessing for intrinsic spinal canal abnormalities including spinal cord abnormalities, frank spinal cord compression, and extracanalicular processes extending into the spinal canal or neural foramina such as herniated disk material and/or spinal stenosis of any etiology. It is the diagnostic modality of choice, if available, in nontraumatic acute myelopathy to exclude mass lesions compressing the spinal cord. In asymptomatic patients, lumbar MRI will reveal incidental disk herniations in about one third, disk bulges in one-half to two-thirds, and disk degeneration in up to 90% of scans.[18,19] Twenty percent of asymptomatic patients older than 60 years may have findings consistent with lumbar spinal stenosis on imaging studies. These findings make correlation of symptoms and signs with radiographic imaging problematic. Imaging is probably useful in evaluating

TABLE 15-6 ————————————————————————————————
CAUSES OF BACK AND NECK PAIN

1. Myofascial syndromes
2. Disks, nerve root syndromes
3. Degenerative diseases of the spine: spondylosis, osteoporosis
4. Malignancy
5. Spondylolysis and spondylolisthesis
6. Neurologic complications of underlying disease
7. Acute myelitis
8. Spinal epidural abscess or hematoma
9. Referred pain: gynecologic, urologic, abdominal, vascular
10. Psychiatric

only for potential red flags and/or planning surgery in patients with indications for surgery.[20,21]

SPECIFIC DISEASE ENTITIES

The combination of history and the physical examination should allow the examiner to categorize neck and back pain into specific etiologies (Table 15-6).

Myofascial Conditions; Acute Soft-Tissue Conditions

All forms of trauma, but particularly high-speed automobile-type trauma associated with a rapid deceleration mechanism, may produce forces that may cause considerable strain on muscular and ligamentous elements supporting the spinal column. Neck muscle tenderness following rapid-deceleration injuries, with or without resultant spasm, represents a common problem. In patients who have normal neurologic examinations and in selected cases normal static cervical spine films, a conservative approach to management with symptomatic relief is advised. In rare instances, ligamentous instability may not be revealed on initial radiography, and follow-up imaging (e.g., lateral flexion/extension radiography, MRI) may be indicated for those patients not improving.

Muscular tenderness in the lower back without specific findings on neurologic examination usually entails a conservative approach. In patients with mild to moderate pain, simply avoiding painful activities and receiving analgesics generally suffice. Bed rest, although once popular, is probably not helpful. Pelvic traction appears to offer no advantage.[22]

Nerve Root Syndromes

Specific nerve roots along the spinal column may be compressed by either bulging/herniated disks or vertebral spondylosis or a combination. These disease processes may be indistinguishable from each other on a clinical basis and indeed may be distinguished only by spinal imaging. Initial management of both problems is the same, and rarely do patients require surgery. Table 15-5 delineates the common nerve root compression syndromes for both the cervical and lumbosacral regions.

In general, patients with nerve root compression syndromes will complain of dull, aching, often intermittent pain, which may become suddenly worse with straining, coughing, or sneezing. Numbness in the appropriate dermatome distribution commonly occurs. Such pain is usually relieved by lying down. It may radiate in specific nerve root distributions. Symptoms typical of cervical radiculopathy include neck pain usually worsened with rotation or flexion of the neck, with associated shooting pain in one arm with possibly a combination of sensory loss, motor loss, and/or reflex changes in the appropriate dermatome.[23] Cervical disk pain can be referred to the subscapular region. With cervical root compressions, symptomatology is often made worse by pushing down on the patient's head while turning the head to the side of the patient's symptoms, which puts compressive force on the cervical spine (Spurling's test).

In the lumbar region, aching pain in a buttock radiating into the lateral aspect of the ipsilateral thigh and leg, usually termed sciatica, is a common presenting complaint. These symptoms can generally be magnified by straight leg raising with the patient lying supine with the hip flexed (Lasègue's sign). For this test to be done properly, the patient must be relaxed and should not assist in lifting the leg. All lifting should be done by the examiner. The only sign considered reliable for disk herniation is radiating pain in the leg (sciatica) that occurs between 30 and 70 degrees of elevation. Back pain alone is nonspecific. Contralateral straight leg raising, with radiating pain in the leg opposite to the one being lifted, is considered very suspicious for herniated nucleus pulposus.[24] In patients with low back pain without sciatica, it is estimated that the likelihood of disk herniation is 1 in 1000.[8]

The piriformis syndrome occurs when the piriformis muscle compresses the sciatic nerve at the level of the sciatic notch creating symptoms similar to sciatica. These include buttock and leg pain with or without back pain and with or without neurologic symptoms and/or signs referable to the sciatic nerve. It can be found in patients with sciatica, but without findings for lumbar disk herniation on imaging studies. Patients have worsening pain when the hip is placed into flexion, adduction, and internal rotation (FADIR)[25,26] and with prolonged sitting. There may be a history of direct trauma to the buttocks, or prolonged sitting on hard surfaces.

When lumbosacral disks herniate laterally, they may cause irritation of the nerve root. In a small number of cases, the disk may herniate in the midline, causing compression of the cauda equina. A complete acute cauda equina compression syndrome is characterized by low back pain with perineal numbness, acute urinary retention (occurring in 90%),[8] diminished or lost rectal tone (60%–80%), and paralysis in the legs. As the compression may involve the distal spinal cord (conus medullaris), depending on the spinal level of involvement by the mass, in addition to the nerve roots of the cauda equina, a Babinski sign may be found. Such compression with definite neurologic deficits represents a medical emergency. Surgical decompression may be indicated emergently. Diagnostic imaging such as MRI or, if MRI is not readily available, a CT myelogram can define the lesion best prior to decompression. Midline herniation of a disk in the cervical region with cord compression may cause spasticity in both the arms (depending on the level) and the legs with loss of posterior column sensory function below the level of the involvement.

Midline spinal cord compression in the lower thoracic and upper lumbar regions will cause compression of the distal spinal cord or cauda equina. It should be noted that the spinal cord (conus medullaris) usually ends between the L1 and L2 vertebral body levels. Lesions below this level may affect multiple nerve roots of the cauda equina but will not involve the spinal cord. Lumbosacral lesions may present with loss of sphincter tone, exertional leg pain, and decreasing strength. The vast majority of nerve root compression syndromes can be handled conservatively.

Degenerative Disease of the Spine

Degenerative disease of the spine, or spondylosis, is a common problem with elderly patients. The degenerative process is a result of collapse of the nucleus pulposus with resultant bulging and/or frank tearing of the anulus fibrosus. Calcification of the anulus fibers causes hypertrophic changes, including spurs, or osteophytes. Thickening of the ligamentum flava may also occur and all or some of these processes may result in spinal stenosis. Patients with cervical spinal stenosis may develop spinal cord compression with spasticity in the legs or loss of proprioception in the legs with a wide-based gait.

Symptoms typical of lumbar spinal stenosis include neurogenic claudication, which is a discomfort radiating into, or predominantly present in the thigh and lower leg, which worsens with prolonged walking. It is typically worsened by lumbar extension and improves with lumbar flexion.[27] Patients with lumbar spinal stenosis may walk bent forward at the waist. While typical lumbar stenosis is more common in elderly patients as a result of the degenerative changes indicated above, it may appear in younger patients with congenital abnormalities of the spine such as shortened pedicles and/or spondylolysis/spondylolisthesis. Symptoms caused by spondylolysis/spondylolisthesis may include nerve root compression and/or spinal cord irritation and compression depending upon the level of involvement.

Spondylolysis and Spondylolisthesis

Spondylolysis is a condition in which the posterior portion of the vertebral arch is separated from the vertebral body at the level of the pars interarticularis (that portion of the anterior neural arch located between the superior and inferior articular processes) by vertically oriented clefts. The underlying etiology is related to "repetitive microfractures" of, or congenital defects of, the neural arch, which may not become symptomatic for many years. When spondylolysis is present, spondylolisthesis, which is forward displacement of one vertebral body over the immediate caudad-vertebral body, may also occur. Spondylolysis and spondylolisthesis generally cause low back pain, which may begin gradually or may be associated with an injury. Because spondylolisthesis usually occurs at the L5 to S1 level, the spinal cord is not involved. With severe displacement, however, compression of nerve roots may occur.

Neurologic Complications of Underlying Spinal Disease

A particular problem in the acute care setting is the patient with a known disease of the spine, who may have long-standing back pain, whose back pain has become worse. Patients with ankylosing spondylitis, rheumatoid arthritis, Paget's disease, metastatic cancer, metabolic bone disease, or osteoporotic compression fractures may have back or neck pain. The history and physical examination are used to determine whether there is involvement of the spinal cord or spinal roots. Patients with evidence suggesting spinal cord involvement may require immediate imaging evaluation (e.g., MRI). As in other forms of spinal cord or root compression, proper follow-up examinations may be necessary to determine the need for intervention. Patients with rheumatoid arthritis may have neurologic complications from subluxation of the vertebrae. Atlantoaxial subluxation may result in compression of the upper cervical spinal cord.

Transverse Myelitis

Myelitis is a nonspecific term designating inflammation of the spinal cord. Myelopathy is an even more nonspecific term indicating dysfunction of the spinal cord. Transverse myelitis may be partial or complete and refers to a process in which a lesion extends horizontally across the spinal cord, resulting in loss of neurologic function below the level of the lesion. Symptoms and signs such as urinary retention or overflow incontinence, saddle anesthesia, major motor weakness in the arms or legs (paraparesis, quadraparesis), long track signs, and sensory levels raise suspicion for either intrinsic cord abnormalities or extrinsic cord compression. Extrinsic cord compression can be due to tumors (benign or malignant, primary or metastatic), abscess, or hematomas.[28] Inflammatory myelopathies can be extremely variable with respect to the degree of back pain. Symptoms may come on in a matter of hours, days, or weeks and may be impossible to differentiate from structurally compressive lesions of the spinal cord without imaging, optimally MRI.

Differential diagnosis of acute spinal cord lesions requires careful attention to the progression of symptoms. Acute myelitis and acute polyneuritis (Guillain–Barré syndrome) may present as ascending polyneuropathies. The spinal cord symptomatology caused by epidural abscesses, epidural hematomas, and spinal cord tumors tends to be focal in nature and does not have an ascending quality. Table 15-7 emphasizes the differential diagnosis in acute myelopathy.

Spinal Epidural Abscess and Epidural Hematomas

A rare but potentially dangerous cause of symptomatic back pain is spinal epidural abscess. The spinal epidural abscess is usually the direct result of vertebral osteomyelitis

TABLE 15-7

CAUSES OF MYELOPATHY

Primary infectious viral syndromes or bacterial, spirochetal, rickettsial, fungal, or parasitic conditions
Postinfectious or parainfectious myelitis
Toxic, metabolic
Radiation myelitis
Idiopathic
Myelopathy: compression from tumor, abscess, hematoma
Other: vascular occlusion

or diskitis,[29] so patients generally have exquisite point tenderness on back examination; however, this finding is nonspecific.[8] Rarely, remote infections seed the epidural space directly without involvement of overlying bone. Spinal epidural abscess may proceed to compress and/or infarct the spinal cord or nerve roots, giving a cord dysfunction syndrome indistinguishable from that of the midline disk herniation or spondylosis. Patients may have an acute presentation with rapid progression of symptoms or a chronic course over months. The pain may be particularly severe, unrelieved by rest, and worse at night. Patients with IV drug abuse, immunocompromised status, sickle cell anemia, osteomyelitis, recent spinal surgery,[30] spinal injections, or infection elsewhere in the body are more prone to this condition. The patient usually has a history of a febrile illness but may not be febrile on presentation, making consideration of an infectious etiology difficult. Early diagnosis can be very difficult.[31] Rarely does the patient appear septic. Management of suspected epidural abscess requires imaging evaluation, optimally MRI, and immediate consideration of surgery combined with long-term antibiotic therapy. The most common organism isolated is *Staphylococcus*, and includes MRSA,[15] but a wide variety of infectious organisms can be found. An elevated sedimentation rate, although nonspecific, is typically found. The white blood cell count may or may not be elevated, and a normal white blood cell count does not exclude the diagnosis. Blood cultures may be positive.[32] Plain radiographic findings lag behind clinical symptoms by several weeks and may take up to 2 months to become positive for associated vertebral osteomyelitis and still will not demonstrate the extent of spinal canal or paraspinal involvement. Positive plain radiographic findings include osseous destruction and less specific vertebral end-plate irregularities and disk space narrowing.

Another rare, but important cause of pain is spontaneous epidural hematomas with resultant spinal cord compression. This may occur during anticoagulation[33] or thrombolytic therapy[34] or from spontaneous hemorrhage from the posterior internal vertebral venous plexus.[35] They cannot be distinguished from other causes of cord compression without imaging evaluation.

Other Spinal Hemorrhage

Another very rare cause for sudden, severe back or neck pain and possible sciatica with neurologic symptomatology is spinal subarachnoid hemorrhage. A vascular malformation of the spinal cord can bleed, with associated sudden severe pain, neurologic symptoms and signs related to the spinal cord segments involved. Aortic dissection may mimic this presentation. Intracranial subarachnoid hemorrhage may rapidly migrate to the cervical and lumbar subarachnoid space, with resultant severe neck or back pain. This entity is covered in Chapter 7. Migration of blood to the intracranial subarachnoid space from spinal subarachnoid hemorrhage may produce a headache. Spontaneous bleeding from intraspinal tumors may present with similar symptoms.

BACK PAIN IN CHILDREN AND ADOLESCENTS

Back pain is an uncommon complaint in children and adolescents. It may, however, indicate significant illness or injury. Whereas in adults where the vast majority of cases of back pain do not represent significant or serious medical illness, and usually resolve with

TABLE 15-8

BACK AND NECK PAIN IN CHILDREN AND ADOLESCENTS

Benign bony tumors
Osteoid osteoma
Benign osteoblastoma

Malignancy
Ewing's tumor
Osteogenic sarcoma
Neuroblastoma
Wilms' tumor
Lymphoma
Leukemia
Bone cyst

Developmental
Spondylolisthesis/spondylolysis
Scheuermann's disease

Inflammatory
Diskitis
Vertebral osteomyelitis/epidural abscess
Collagen vascular disease
Ankylosing spondylitis

Mechanical
Fracture
Hip joint disease
Muscle spasm/strain
Herniated nucleus pulposus

conservative measures, this is not necessarily the case in the child or adolescent. Minimal back pain may be the result of a significant illness. Herniation of an intervertebral disk, although possible, is very uncommon in this age group. Other significant causes for consideration include vertebral fracture (if there has been significant injury), overuse injuries, spondylolysis/spondylolisthesis, intervertebral diskitis, vertebral osteomyelitis, ankylosis spondylitis, neoplasms, Scheuermann's disease, and juvenile rheumatoid arthritis (Table 15-8). It should be noted that the usual childhood idiopathic scoliosis is uncommonly painful.

PATIENTS WITH RECURRENT BACK OR NECK PAIN IN THE EMERGENCY DEPARTMENT

The primary issue with most patients who present to an acute care setting with an exacerbation of an ongoing back or neck problem is symptomatic relief. However, some patients will have progression of an underlying benign process (such as disk disease), whereas others may have a new etiology mimicking prior symptoms. These patients are the most problematic. One should consider red flags that might indicate the entities covered in Table 15-1. Depending on the findings, and the date and type of prior imaging, repeat imaging such as MRI may be necessary. The findings that tend to push one to more rapid consideration of definitive diagnostic imaging are objective weakness and difficulty with urinary control, or signs of myelopathy. The extent of any neurologic deficit and the degree of pain relief obtained in the acute care setting will dictate the location (inpatient versus outpatient) and timing (urgent versus more routinely scheduled) for such studies. Contact with prior treating physicians and review of prior imaging studies may be helpful in determining whether imaging studies may be indicated. There is a paucity of good-quality studies to guide the management of many benign disorders of the spine, and the decisions to recommend surgical treatment are largely experience based and subjective.

Referred Pain

The scope of this book does not permit a full discussion of each entity that may present with back pain. Note that renal stones, acute pyelonephritis, abdominal aortic aneurysms, and other retroperitoneal conditions may all present as back pain. Lower lumbar and sacral back pain may be related to lesions of the genitalia in both men and women. Prostatitis and diverticulitis may also present as back pain. The elderly patient with sudden onset of nontraumatic low back pain with abdominal pain should be considered at risk for having an expanding or rupturing abdominal aortic aneurysm.

References

1. Walker B. The prevalence of low back pain: a systematic review of the literature from 1966 to 1998. *J Spinal Disord*. 2000;13:205-217.
2. Walker B, Muller R, Grant WD. Low back pain in Australian adults. Prevalence and associated disability. *J Manipulative Physiol Ther*. 2004;27(4):238-244.
3. Deyo RA, Mirza SK, Martin BI. Back pain prevalence and visit rates estimates from U.S. national surveys, 2002. *Spine (Phila Pa 1976)*. 2006;31(23):2724-2727.
4. Cherkin DC. A comparison of physical therapy, chiropractic manipulation, and provision of an educational booklet for the treatment of patients with low back pain. *N Engl J Med*. 1998;339:1021-1029.
5. Grotle M, Brox JI, Glomsrod B, et al. Prognostic factors in first-time care seekers due to acute low back pain. *Eur J Pain*. 2007;11:290-298.
6. Van den Hoogen, Hans JM, Koes BW, et al. The prognosis of low back pain in general practice. *Spine*. 1997;22(13):1515-1521.
7. Hestbaek L, Leboeuf-Yde C, Manniche C. Low back pain: what is the long-term course. A review of studies of general populations. *Eur Spine J*. 2003;12:149-165.
8. Deyo RA, Rainville J, Kent DL. What can the history and physical examination tell us about low back pain? *JAMA*. 1992;268(6):760-765.
9. Atlas SJ, Deyo RA. Evaluating and managing acute low back pain in the primary care setting. *J Gen Intern Med*. 2001;16:120-131.

10. Schiottz-Christensen B, Nielsen GL, Hansen VK, et al. Long-term prognosis of acute low back pain in patients seen in general practice: a 1 year prospective follow-up study. *Fam Pract*. 1999;16:223-232.

11. Henschke N, Maher GC, Refshauge KM, et al. Prognosis in patients with recent onset low back pain in Australian primary care: inception cohort study. *BMJ*. 2008;337:a171.

12. Pengel LHM, Herbert RD, Maher CG, et al. Acute low back pain: systematic review of its prognosis. *BMJ*. 2003;327:323.

13. Henschke N, Maher CG, Refshauge KM, et al. Prognosis of acute low back pain: design of a prospective inception cohort study. *BMC Musculoskelet Disord*. 2006;7:54.

14. Koes BW, van Tuler MW, Ostelo R, et al. Clinical guidelines for management of low back pain in primary care: an international comparison. *Spine*. 2001;26:2504-2513.

15. Auletta JJ, John CC. Spinal epidural Abscesses in children: a 15-year experience and review of the literature. *Clin Infect Dis*. 2001;32:9-16.

16. Fernandez M, Carrol CL, Baker CJ. Discitis and vertebral osteomyelitis in children: an 18-year review. *Pediatrics*. 2000;105:1299-1304.

17. An HS, Seldomridge A. Spinal infections: diagnostic tests and imaging studies. *Clin Orthop Relat Res*. 2006;444:27-33.

18. Jarvik JG, Hollongsworth W, Brook M. Rapid magnetic resonance imaging vs radiographs for patients with low back pain: a randomized controlled trial. *JAMA*. 2003;289:2810-2818.

19. Jensen MC, Brant-Zawadzki MN, Obuchowski N, et al. Magnetic resonance imaging of the lumbar spine in people without back pain. *N Engl J Med*. 1994;331:2:69-73.

20. Chou R, Rongwei F, Carrino JA, et al. Imaging strategies for low-back pain: systematic review and meta-analysis. *Lancet*. 2009;373:463-472.

21. Jarvik JG, Deyo RA. Diagnostic evaluation of low back pain with emphasis on imaging. *Ann Intern Med*. 2002;137:586-597.

22. Beurskens AJ et al. Efficiency of traction for nonspecific low back pain. 12-week and 6-month results of a randomized clinical trial. *Spine*. 1997;22:2756-2762.

23. Carettr S, Fehlings MG. Cervical radiculopathy. *N Engl J Med*. 2005;353:392-399.

24. Deyo RA, Loeser JD, Bigos SJ. Herniated lumbar intervertebral disk. *Ann Intern Med*. 1990; 112:598-603.

25. Boyajian-O'Neill LA, McClain RL, Coleman MK, et al. Diagnosis and management of piriformis syndrome: an osteopathic approach. *J Am Osteopath Assoc*. 2008;108:657-664.

26. Papadopoulos EC, Khan SN. Piriformis syndrome and low back pain: a new classification and review of the literature. *Orthop Clin North Am*. 2004;35:65-71.

27. Katz JN, Harris MB. Lumbar spinal stenosis. *N Engl J Med*. 2008;358:818-825.

28. Schmidt RD, Markovchick V. Nontraumatic spinal cord compression. *J Emerg Med*. 1992;10: 189-199.

29. Mackenzie AR et al. Spinal epidural abscess: the importance of early diagnosis and treatment. *J Neurol Neurosurg Psychiatry*. 1998;65:209-212.

30. Calderone RR, Larsen JM. Overview and classification of spinal infections. *Orthop Clin North Am*. 1996;27:1-8.

31. Sampath P, Rigamonti D. Spinal epidural abscess: a review of epidemiology, diagnosis, and treatment. *J Spinal Disord*. 1999;12:89-93.

32. Chao D, Nand A. Spinal epidural abscess: a diagnostic challenge. *Am Fam Physician*. 2002;65: 1341-1346.

33. Rodriguez Y, Baena R, et al. Spinal epidural hematoma during anticoagulant therapy. A case report and review of the literature. *J Neurosurg Sci*. 1995;39:87-94.

34. Sawin PD, Traynelis VC, Follett KA. Spinal epidural hematoma following coronary thrombolysis with tissue plasminogen activator. Report of two cases. *J Neurosurg*. 1995;83:350-353.

35. Groen RJ, Ponssen H. The spontaneous spinal epidural hematoma. A study of the etiology. *J Neurol Sci*. 1990;98:121-138.

GLOSSARY

abdominal epilepsy   Attacks of severe abdominal pain, either as an aura to a seizure or by themselves without a seizure.

abducens nerve   Sixth cranial nerve; provides innervation to lateral rectus muscle of eye, the action of which abducts the eye.

absence attacks   Petit mal epilepsy; consists of sudden fixed vacuous stare without response to environment of short duration (10–30 seconds). There may be minor eyelid fluttering.

abulia   Lack of spontaneity or effervescence of personality.

acalculia   Inability to perform mathematical calculations (not simple memory tasks such as 2 + 2 = 4).

acoustic neuroma (neurinoma)   A benign tumor originating from the eighth cranial nerve.

Adie's pupil   A pupil that responds poorly and slowly to light (and slowly dilates in the dark); responds better in convergence. Usually unilateral, the pupil is dilated in average light and is usually found in women with absent tendon reflexes. The pupil is unusually sensitive to 2.5% methacholine (mecholyl).

AED   An abbreviation frequently used for antiepileptic drug.

agnosia   The loss of ability to recognize the import of sensory stimuli agraphia. The loss of ability to write in the absence of paralysis.

akinetic mutism   Severe deficiency or loss of movement and lack of speech. Patient appears asleep but can be aroused, and eyes will follow. Causative lesions involve reticular activating system in upper pons and midbrain such as basilar artery thrombosis. Also called coma vigil.

alexia   Inability to read.

Alzheimer's disease   A dementing illness with characteristic brain atrophy, senile plaques, and neurofibrillary tangles. Peak onset at age 50 to 60 years but reported in widely varying age groups.

amaurosis fugax   "Fleeting blindness" with temporary monocular visual loss due to ocular vascular insufficiency, commonly embolic in etiology. Amaurosis implies blindness without apparent eye lesion.

amblyopia   Defect in vision resulting from imperfect sensation of the retina without organic eye lesion.

amnestic–confabulatory syndrome (Wernicke–Korsakoff syndrome)   A confusional state characterized by retrograde amnesia and anterograde amnesia. Confabulation need not continually be present, but the patient must be alert and other cognitive functions that do not depend on memory may be impaired only to a minor degree.

analgesia   Loss of ability to perceive painful stimuli.

anesthesia   Loss of ability to perceive all sensory stimuli.

anesthesia dolorosa   An extremely intense, deep-seated pain located cortically and usually caused by severe involvement of thalamic structures.

anisocoria   Unequal pupils.

anomic aphasia   Difficulty naming objects, conditions, or qualities without serious limitations in speaking or writing.

anosognosia   Loss of ability to recognize hemiplegia; more broadly used, lack of ability to recognize any neurologic deficit or other disease or disability.

anterior circulation Refers to circulation supplied by internal carotid artery. Anterior spinal artery (cord) syndrome. See pages 20 and 21.

Anton's syndrome Cortical blindness with denial of blindness (anosognosia) caused by bilateral lesions in occipital lobes.

aphasia Loss of powers of speech without paralysis of muscles required for word production.

aphasia, anomic A variety of conduction aphasia in which conversational speech is fluent but with lack of substantive words and great difficulty in finding words, at times causing total inability to name objects.

aphasia, Broca's An expressive aphasia in which the patients know what they wish to say but are unable to say it. Unable to talk, repeat, or read aloud.

aphasia, conduction A variety of fluent aphasia, similar to Wernicke's aphasia except that the speech is more broken and there are more hesitations for word finding. Many clichés and four- to five-word phrases are interjected. Comprehension is normal; repetition is poor.

aphasia, global Total loss of language ability with inability to speak or comprehend written or spoken words, read, write, repeat, or name.

aphasia, Wernicke's A type of fluent aphasia with high volume of word output but no meaningful or substantive words, so that no meaning is conveyed. Frequently one word is substituted for another.

apneustic breathing A respiratory pattern with a pause at full inspiration. Reflects abnormality at middle or caudal pontine level.

apoplexy Refers to sudden hemorrhage from any organ or, as in apoplectic stroke, to a sudden vascular lesion of brain marked by coma and paralysis.

apraxia A disturbance in the performance of skilled acts.

aqueduct of Sylvius A channel for circulation of spinal fluid through the midbrain and upper pons connecting the third and fourth ventricles.

arachnoiditis An inflammatory reaction in the arachnoid membrane, which forms the external limit of the cerebrospinal fluid-containing space.

Argyll Robertson pupil A pupil that does not react to light (directly or consensually) but does constrict on accommodation.

Arnold–Chiari malformation A congenital malformation of the lower brainstem characterized by displacement of midline cerebellar structures into the spinal canal and a distorted elongated pons and medulla.

aseptic meningeal reaction Increased white cells in spinal fluid due to a nonbacterial cause, e.g., viral, chemical.

asterixis See page 188.

ataxia Failure of coordination of movements.

automatisms A condition in which an individual is consciously or unconsciously, but involuntarily, compelled to the performance of certain (often purposeless) motor or verbal acts, for example, yawning.

Babinski sign An extensor toe sign consisting of dorsiflexion of the great toe, fanning of the toes in response to scraping the plantar aspect of the foot from the heel to metatarsophalangeal joints. Indicative of pyramidal (motor) tract dysfunction above age 18 months to 2 years.

basal ganglion Gray matter located with the thalamus deep in the cerebral hemisphere.

Beevor's sign Upward movement of the umbilicus on contracting the abdominal muscles due to paralysis of lower abdominal muscles.

Bell's palsy See pages 157–158.

Bell's phenomenon Upward rotation of the eyeball; an attempted eye closure in patients with Bell's palsy.

bitemporal hemianopsia Visual field loss in both lateral (temporal) areas, usually as a result of disease at the optic chiasm.

Broca's aphasia   See *aphasia.*

Broca's area   An area in the posterior portion of the inferior frontal gyrus of the dominant hemisphere.

Brown–Sequard syndrome   See pages 274–275.

Brudzinski's sign (neck)   Passive flexion of the head on the chest followed by flexion of both thighs and legs so that both lower extremities may be flexed on the pelvis. A sign of meningeal irritation; also found in partial decerebration.

bulbar palsy   Weakness accompanied by atrophy and fasciculations of muscles supplied by motor nuclei of tongue, pharyngeal muscles, palate, and sometimes lips. Characteristically there is dysphagia, dysarthria, and regurgitation of foods with difficulty protruding the tongue.

Bulbocavernosus reflex   A sharp contraction of the bulbocavernous and ischiocavernosus muscles when the glands penis is suddenly compressed or tapped.

caloric testing   See page 106t.

carotid sinus syndrome   Syncope and bradycardia produced by mechanical stimulation of the carotid sinus. An exaggerated normal response.

carpal tunnel syndrome   Compression of the median nerve at the wrist as it passes through the carpal tunnel. Features include numbness and paresthesias in the first three digits of the hand with weakness and possibly atrophy of the median nerve-supplied muscles. Paresthesias typically worse at night, precipitating shaking of hands.

carpopedal spasm   Also referred to as carpopedal contractions, this is a spasm of the feet and hands associated with hyperventilation, calcium deprivatoin, and tetany.

catalepsy   Sudden loss of voluntary motion of the entire body with diffuse muscular rigidity; similar to catatonia.

cataplexy   Attacks of limb weakness with loss of tone precipitated by emotional stimuli; usually associated with narcolepsy.

cauda equina   Latin for a horse's tail: the bundle of spinal nerve routes arising from the lumbar enlargement and conus medullaris and running through the lower part of the subarachnoid space within the vertebral column.

causalgia   A distressing type of burning pain accompanied by vasomotor and trophic changes; usually secondary to nerve injury.

central cord syndrome   See page 275.

cerebellopontine angle syndrome   Tinnitus with progressive deafness, numbness, and/or pain in the ipsilateral face, ipsilateral facial palsy, vertigo, ipsilateral dysmetria, and ipsilateral sixth nerve palsy; commonly due to acoustic neurinomas.

cerebral palsy   A nonspecific term used to describe a disorder of motor function that begins in infancy; characterized by spasticity and/or involuntary movements; caused by brain dysfunction.

Chaddock's sign   An extensor toe sign with response and significance similar to Babinski's sign; produced by blunt stimulation of the lateral aspect of the foot.

Charcot-Marie-tooth disease   A familial peripheral neuropathy characterized pathologically by hypertrophic peripheral nerves; commonly affects distal limb musculature, resulting in weakness at ankles, atrophic calf muscles, high arches; occasionally involves hand involvement. The hypertrophied peripheral nerves may be palpable. The expression of this disease is very variable.

chorea   188, 193t.

Chvostek's sign   Tapping over the facial nerve in front of the ear causing spasm or titanic contraction of some or all of the facial muscles. Chvostek's sign represents hyperexcitability of motor nerves to mechanical stimulation.

clonus   A series of rhythmic muscle contractions caused by sudden passive stretching of the muscle.

cluster headache   See page 211t.

coma   See Chapter 4.

coma vigil Also know as akinetic mutism. Imprecise term applied to a number of situations. Most commonly used when the lesion disconnects the cerebral hemispheres from all areas below the oculomotor nucleus in the brain stem.

complicated migraine A term used when the neurologic deficit, e.g., hemiplegia, persists after the classic or hemiplegic migraine, thus simulating a cerebral infarction.

concussion See Chapter 10.

conjugate gaze A condition in which the visual axes of the two eyes are parallel in all positions of gaze.

constructional apraxia Inability to draw geometric figures or to write with eyes open; figures drawn may have major parts missing or misplaced; usually due to a lesion in the angular gyrus.

conus medullaris Medullary cone; a tapering lower extremity of the spinal cord.

corneal reflex Reflex eyelid closure on stimulation of the cornea as by a wisp of cotton; mediated by fifth or seventh cranial nerves.

cortical blindness A condition in which blindness is due to dysfunction in the occipital cortex and pupillary reflexes are preserved. See *Anton's syndrome*.

cortical denial syndrome Inability to perceive sensory stimuli contralaterally when the stimuli are applied bilaterally simultaneously with preservation of ability to perceive that stimulus when it alone is applied; referred to as sensory extinction or inattention.

cortical sensation Functions usually considered to be mediated by the cerebral cortex (parietal lobe), which include stereognosis (perceiving and recognizing form by touch), barognosis (perception of weight), topesthesia (ability to localize a tactile sensation), graphesthesia (recognition of letters or numbers written on the skin), and two-point discrimination.

cremasteric reflex Contraction of cremaster muscle with elevation of the testicle on stroking the inner upper thigh with a blunt object; innervated by ilioinguinal and genitofemoral nerves via Ll and L2 cord segments.

Creutzfeldt-Jakob disease A degenerative disease producing rapidly progressive mental deterioration in midlife with pyramidal and extrapyramidal signs including hyperkinesias, abnormal tone, dysphagia, and dysarthria.

CT: helical (spiral) scanning The latest generation of CT scanners where a patient is slowly, but constantly, moved through the scanner gantry as the X-ray beam continuously passes around the patient. This results in data collection in a "spiral" pattern (similar to a collapsed or stretched "slinky" toy depending on the speed that the patient moves through the scanner with respect to the speed of the X-ray tube moving around the patient). Collected data can be interpolated or extrapolated by the CT computer to generate images of varying thickness as required for evaluation of certain structures (e.g., submillimeter sections are often obtained to evaluate inner ear structures or sometimes for the evaluation of nondisplaced spinal fractures while 5- to 8-mm sections are usually adequate to evaluate for acute intracranial hemorrhage). Such scanners are now standard and are used to scan large portions of a patient in a short period of time and also to perform CT angiography and perfusion CT.

CT: reconstruction algorithms Once a CT scan has been performed, images can be reconstructed by the CT computer using a variety of different algorithms. Images can then be viewed using different windows (see page 31). Most CT studies are automatically reconstructed (i.e., the collected data is turned into a viewable image) using a "bone" (also called "edge" or "detail") algorithm to increase the sharpness of osseous structures with respect to nearby nonosseous structures on the final images. All CT studies are also reconstructed with a "soft tissue" algorithm to better resolve structures with similar, but not identical, X-ray absorption (e.g., muscles, fluid, cerebral tissues, etc.). Generating images with different algorithms must be performed at the time scans are obtained or shortly thereafter; such images are routinely generated by Radiology Departments and almost never have to be specifically requested.

Dandy-Walker syndrome A congenital form of obstructive hydrocephalus with enlargement of the fourth ventricle out of proportion to the other ventricles, caused by atresia of the foramen of Luschka and Magendie. This cystic enlargement of the fourth ventricle is associated with multiple other congenital anomalies. The clinical presentation is extremely variable and is basically similar to other forms of hydrocephalus.

decerebrate rigidity (posturing) See page 305.

decorticate rigidity Abnormal posturing with upper extremity flexion and lower extremity extension indicating lesions involving the upper brain stem and cortex.

déjà vu A sensation of unreality characterized by feeling familiar with what ought to be an unfamiliar situation.

delirium Acute encephalopathy.

delirium tremens An alcohol-withdrawal syndrome characterized by confusion, delusions, hallucinations, tremor, agitation, sleeplessness, and autonomic hyperactivity (fever, tachycardia, sweating).

dementia Deterioration or loss of previously acquired intellectual functions.

demyelinating diseases Diseases associated with destruction of the myelin sheath surrounding nerve axons, resulting in defective functioning of that neuron. Multiple sclerosis is the most common of the more than two dozen entities considered.

Devic's disease One of the demyelinating diseases, also termed neuromyelitis optica. The clinical features consist of the acute simultaneous occurrence of transverse myelitis and optic neuritis. Most consider it simply a variant of multiple sclerosis.

diplopia Double vision.

dissociated sensory loss Impairment of some sensory modalities with preservation of others.

drop attack Sudden collapse of the legs without loss of consciousness.

dysautonomia Dysfunction of the autonomic nervous system manifested by orthostatic hypotension, impotence, loss of sweating, and urinary and fecal incontinence.

dysdiadochokinesia Inability to perform rapid alternating movements such as pronating and supinating the hand.

dysgraphia Difficulty writing in the absence of paralysis.

dyslexia Difficulty reading.

dysmetria Loss of ability to gauge distance, speed, or power of a movement.

dysphagia Difficulty swallowing.

dysphasia Difficulty with language functions.

Eaton-Lambert syndrome A general term to describe generalized weakness associated with various cancer syndromes.

EEG The record obtained by means of an electroencephalogram—an apparatus consisting of amplifiers and write-out systems for recording the electrical potential of the brain that arrive from electrodes attached to the scalp.

EMG (electromyogram) A graphic representation of the electrical currents associated with muscular action.

encephalitis See pages 103, 208.

encephalopathy Acute alteration of higher intellectual function.

end-point nystagmus (end-position nystagmus) A few rapid nystagmoid movements seen on extreme deviation of the eyes; usually seen on lateral deviation.

endovascular angiography (rotational angiography) Rotational angiography (sometimes called "spin" angiography) refers to endovascular cerebral angiography performed while the X-ray tube and detectors literally move around the patient during the injection of the contrast material. This results in a three-dimensional (3D) image set, which can be "post-processed" with special software. Such image processing has been shown to be able to identify otherwise occult (on standard endovascular angiography) findings such as small aneurysms or aneurysm neck pathology that might determine whether endovascular coiling or surgical clipping of an aneurysm should be performed. While the equipment (including computers and software) to perform rotational angiography have been available for 10 years, it remains expensive and not yet widely disseminated. However, at many institutions, it is already considered a crucial adjunct to standard multiplanar endovascular angiography and may well be considered the gold standard for aneurysm detection, particularly smaller aneurysms, in the near future.

ENG (electronystagmography)   A method of nystagmography based on electrooculography; skin electrodes are placed at outer canthi to register horizontal nystagmus or above and below each eye for vertical nystagmus.

enophthalmos   Inward protrusion of the eye.

essential tremor   See page 187.

extinction phenomena   See *cortical denial syndrome*.

extrapyramidal signs   Motor signs referable to disturbance in tone (usually rigid), movement (hyperkinesia or bradykinesia), and associated movements.

febrile seizures   Convulsions associated with fever in children between the ages of 6 months and 3 years without focal neurologic findings and normal spinal fluid examination.

fibrinolysis   A hydrolysis of fibrin either as a naturally occurring mechanism of the body or induced by administered fibrinolytic-thrombolytic agents such as streptokinase, urokinase, t-PA.

finger agnosia   Inability to recognize, name, or select individual fingers of either the patient or examiner. Usually points to involvement of the angular gyrus.

foot drop   Inability to dorsiflex the foot, due to either weakness of the tibialis anterior muscle (peroneus tertius, extensor digitorum longus, and extensor hallucis longus assist) or its nerve supply, or the deep peroneal nerve or its segmental innervation, L4, L5.

Foster Kennedy syndrome   Anosmia and optic atrophy on the side of a subfrontal mass with contralateral papilledema.

Friedreich's ataxia   A hereditary spinal ataxia, usually manifesting at puberty. Manifestations include ataxia, hyporeflexia, paresthesias, loss of vibration and position sense, dysarthria, skeletal deformities, and other variable nonneurologic findings.

Froment's sign   A sign of weakness of the adductor pollicis, usually caused by ulnar nerve dysfunction. The patient tries to hold a piece of paper, which the examiner tries to pull out between the ulnar side of the extended thumb and the radial side of the second metacarpophalangeal joint by contracting the adductor pollicis. The sign is positive if the patient flexes the thumb at the interphalangeal joint.

gegenhalten   Resistance to changes in posture or position of a limb, resulting in a rigid hypertonicity; seen in extrapyramidal disorders.

Gerstmann's syndrome   Finger agnosia, left-right disorientation, acalculia, and agraphia; usually due to lesion in dominant parietal lobe.

Gilles de la Tourette's syndrome (Tourette's syndrome)   See page 192.

global aphasia   See *aphasia*.

globus hystericus   A feeling of constriction or foreign body in the throat; of psychogenic origin.

Gowers' sign   Sciatic pain produced by passive dorsiflexion of the foot with patient supine, legs extended.

grand mal seizure   Major motor seizure; tonic–clonic seizure; generalized convulsions associated with loss of consciousness and jerking movements of all extremities. Also associated with increased tone, defecation, urination; often preceded by an aura.

graphesthesia   See *cortical sensation*.

Guillain-Barré syndrome   See pages 168–170, 244, 357.

Habit spasms (tics)   A form of tic. A sudden, violent, involuntary muscular contraction.

Hallpike maneuver   Nylen–Bárány test. See Chapter 14.

hemianopia   Loss of one-half of a visual field.

hemiballismus   Violent flinging of the extremities contralateral to a lesion in the Subthalamic Nucleus.

hemiplegic migraine   See pages 208–211, 212t

hepatic coma   See pages 110t, 117

histamine (cluster) headache   See page 211t.

Hoffmann's reflex   Flexion of the terminal phalanx of the thumb and the second and third phalanges of the other fingers when any of the middle fingers is flicked upward.

Hoffmann's sign   Sudden brief flexion of the distal phalanx of the patient's long finger, with the wrist and hand supported, produces sudden flexion of the other fingers and flexion and adduction of the thumb. A pyramidal tract sign.

Hoover's sign   See page 290

Horner's syndrome   See pages 98, 107, 217

Horton's headache   Cluster headache; see page 211t

Hutchinson's pupil   A unilaterally dilated, fixed pupil.

hypalgesia   Diminished pain sensation.

hyperacusis   Abnormally acute or painful hearing.

hyperpathia   Increased sensitivity to pain and a deep aching painful sensation generally related to thalamic lesions.

hypesthesia   Diminished tactile sensation.

hypnagogic hallucinations   Hallucinations that occur as one begins to fall asleep.

idiopathic intracranial hypertension   By definition the ideology of idiopathic intracranial hypertension is not known. At this time it should be regarded as any gradual elevation of cerebrospinal fluid pressure without an anatomically or biochemically explainable ideology.

intention tremor   A tremor that occurs or worsens on volitional movement.

interictal   Periods between seizures.

internuclear ophthalmoplegia   A paresis of eye adduction in horizontal gaze by not convergent. A lesion in the medial longitudinal fasciculus may be unilateral or bilateral.

Jacksonian seizure   Involuntary tonic–clonic movements usually starting in one extremity or side of the face; may go on to altered consciousness. When the seizures remain limited to one side of the body, consciousness is usually retained. Localization of the seizure focus is usually to the contralateral motor context.

jake palsy   Acute peripheral neuritis producing weakness.

jamais vu   A feeling of unreality characterized by lack of familiarity with what ought to be a familiar sensation. The opposite of déjà vu.

Kernig's sign   With the patient supine and the thigh flexed at a right angle to the trunk, complete extension of the leg is impossible. This sign indicates meningeal irritation and is seen in many forms of meningitis.

Kernohan's notch   Also called *crus phenomenon*. A syndrome in which supratentorial pressure causes herniation and compression of the third nerve with the various pressure forces pushing the brainstem to the opposite side, causing compression of the contralateral cerebral peduncle and corticospinal tracts against the sharp edge of the tentorium. This results in hemiplegia ipsilateral to the side of the compressed third nerve.

Korsakoff's psychosis   A psychotic state characterized by failure of memory, imaginary reminiscences, and sometimes marked hallucinations with agitation. It is usually seen in association with acute polyneuritis.

lacunar infarction   Infarction of small penetrating arteries of the brain; usually related to severe hypertension. These infarcts may be asymptomatic but can result in such syndromes as (1) pure motor strokes, (2) pure sensory strokes, (3) clumsy hand-dysarthria syndrome, and (4) various other isolated neurologic lesions.

Lasegue's sign   With the patient supine and the hip flexed when the knee is extended, pain or muscular spasm is present, indicating irritation of the sciatic nerve.

lateral medullary syndrome   See *Wallenberg's syndrome*.

lethargy   A morbid drowsiness from which the patient can be aroused and can appear to be awake and cognizant of surroundings but falls back into inattention or sleep as soon as the stimulus is removed.

Lhermitte's sign   Sudden tingling or electric shock–type sensations up and down the spinal cord when the patient's head is flexed or extended. This has been reported to be positive with meningeal irritation, multiple sclerosis, and cervical cord compressions.

locked-in syndrome   Also called *Count of Monte Cristo syndrome*. Vascular lesion involving the motor pathways of the pons, which are destroyed, sparing the reticular system. This results in paralysis of all lower cranial nerves and extremities but with consciousness present. The patient retains vertical eye movements and will be able to look up on command.

low-pressure (normal-pressure) hydrocephalus   A pathologic increase of cerebrospinal fluid within the skull in which there is dilation of cerebral ventricles and neurologic disturbances but spinal fluid pressure is normal.

macula (macula lutea)   A small yellow-orange area on the inner surface of the retina at a point corresponding to the posterior pull of the eyeball, which serves as the central point of focus for the visual axis.

Magendie's foramen   The anatomic opening on the dorsal aspect of the fourth ventricle, which allows cerebrospinal fluid to enter the subarachnoid space. Obstruction of this structure and the accompanying foramen of Luschka results in noncommunicating hydrocephalus.

marche à petit pas   A short-stepped shuffling gait with a lack of associated hip and arm movements; frequently seen in diffuse cerebral and Parkinson's disease.

Marcus Gunn phenomenon (jaw winking)   A partial ptosis of congenital origin in which opening the mouth and chewing in lateral movements of the jaw cause exaggerated reflex elevation of the ptotic lids. This pathologic movement is presumed to be on the basis of abnormal proprioceptive impulses from the pterygoid muscles, which are relayed to the oculomotor nucleus.

Marcus Gunn pupillary sign   A pathologic light reflex indicating decreased stimuli being transmitted from one eye. On testing the involved eye, the central light reflex causes the pupil to dilate. When the light is moved to the affected eye because of the lack of total light reaching the midbrain, the pupil fails to hold and may actually dilate. These changes can be accentuated by rapid alternate stimulation of the eye with a bright light, the swinging flashlight test.

Ménière's disease   A disease of the inner ear characterized clinically by vertigo, tinnitus, nausea and vomiting, and progressive deafness related to increased pressure in the endolymphatic fluid of the inner ear.

meningitis   Any inflammation of the covering membranes of the brain and spinal cord; may be due to various types of infections, chemical irritation, or underlying disease.

meningocele   A protrusion of the protective membranes (meninges) of the brain or spinal cord through a defect in the skull or spinal column.

meralgia paraesthetica   Tingling and burning that progress to numbness in the lateral lower thigh due to compression or irritation of the lateral femoral cutaneous nerve.

micturition syncope   Sudden loss of consciousness due to an acute decrease in cerebral blood flow precipitated by active urination. The mechanism is thought to be increased parasympathetic activity causing bradycardia and hypotension.

migraine with aura   Classic migraine—those migraine headaches accompanied by visual, auditory, or some other sensory episode prior to the onset of the actual head pain.

migraine without aura   Throbbing, pulsatile headaches that meet the criteria for a migraine headache but are not preceded by any auditory, visual, or other sensory experiences prior to the onset of the head pain.

miosis   Decrease in size of the pupillary aperture; contraction of the pupil.

miotic   Relates to contraction of the pupil or an agent that causes the pupil to contract.

Mobius' syndrome   A congenital facial diplegia. The clinical picture includes paralysis or paresis of the ocular muscles together with paralysis or paresis of the facial muscles. The pathologic basis appears to be hypoplasia of the nuclear centers in the brainstem.

mononeuritis multiplex Inflammation of several nerves simultaneously in anatomically unrelated portions of the body, generally on an inflammatory vasculitis basis. Diabetes mellitus and collagen vascular diseases are the most common causes.

mononeuropathy Involvement of a single nerve by a disease process.

monoplegia An isolated paralysis of only one limb.

Moro reflex A postural and righting reflex seen in infants. A body startle reflex in which a sudden noise or movement directed toward the body of the infant or a blow on the bed next to the infant causes extension on all limbs and the spine. The reflex is normal during the first 4 to 5 months of life.

MRI: echo planar imaging (EPI) A type of MR scanning sequence that allows very rapid acquisition of spatial localization data so that scan times can be dramatically reduced, albeit with an associated loss of image quality and the creation of new artifacts. EPI scanning sequences are used for diffusion MR, perfusion MR and some functional MR scans where data needs to be more rapidly acquired than with more standard MR scanning protocols or, the use of standard MR scanning protocols would result in unacceptably long scan times. In addition, relatively uncooperative patients (both adult and pediatric) and in utero (i.e., fetal) MR scanning sometimes employ EPI scanning techniques to shorten overall scan times.

MRI: functional MRI (fMRI) Functional MRI (fMRI) is a somewhat vague term that usually refers to using various MRI techniques to assess cerebral cortical activation of different regions of the brain. It currently does not have a role in evaluating acute neurologic changes. (It should be noted that some researchers include MR spectroscopy and diffusion MRI as subtypes of fMRI.)

MRI: T1, T2, and FLAIR T1 and T2 refer to intrinsic characteristics of a water molecule being imaged. Before a set of scans is obtained, the MR machine is programmed by the technologist to "bring out" either the T1 or T2 characteristics of the tissue being scanned, hence the delineation "T1-weighted scan" or "T2-weighted scan." The term *FLAIR* is an abbreviation for "fluid-attenuated inversion recovery" and is a type of T2-weighted scan where the signal from pure water is nulled so that it is black instead of white (pure water normally appears white on standard T2-weighted scanning). FLAIR scans are useful as most pathologic processes are white on T2-weighted scans and by using a FLAIR scanning sequence, normal fluids, which can be distracting to the interpreter of an MR image, are rendered black so they do not obscure underlying pathology either within the brain or in the subarachnoid space.

MRI: windows Unlike CT, there is no correlation between any given "window" settings and the appearance of an image. The reason for this is beyond the scope of this text, but reflects the fact that CT attenuation values essentially reflect the electron density of an image pixel while an MR "intensity" (i.e., proton signal strength) value would have to be calibrated for each patient for all of the different MR imaging sequences performed and also for each of the myriad selected background MR machine imaging parameters (e.g., homogeneity of the magnetic field, receiver coil position, and dozens more). Such calibration would have to be performed for all patients before each of their respective scans and would take a prohibitively long time to perform. Therefore, for any series of MR images on a given patient, the "windows," which optimally demonstrate structures, need to be individually selected by the technologist performing the scan or at a workstation by whoever is reviewing the study.

mydriasis Dilation of the pupil.

mydriatic Any agent that dilates the pupil; a cycloplegic.

Myelitis A general term for inflammation of white matter. Originally referring to both bone and nervous tissue is now reserved for inflammations of the spinal cord.

myelomeningocele Protrusion of both the spinal cord and its covering membranes through a defect of the bony spinal column.

Myelopathy A general term for disturbances or diseases of the spinal cord.

myoclonus   Sudden spasm or twitching of a muscle group frequently seen at the moment of sleep.

myokymia   Quivering or fibrillary tremor; twitching of isolated muscle groups usually around the head and neck region; may occur as a benign and transient condition or may be associated with multiple sclerosis or brainstem disease.

myopia   Nearsightedness; trouble viewing distant objects; may be the result of increased refractive error or elongation of the eyeball.

narcolepsy   Uncontrollable and paroxysmal attacks of sleep. Has been associated with lesions of the posterior hypothalamus, but the actual pathologic process is unknown.

neurogenic claudication   Paresthesia in the back, buttocks, and lower limbs caused by mechanical disturbances resulting from posture or by ischemia of the cauda equina.

nonconvulsive status epilepticus   A continuing state of seizure activity in which the patient does not present with outward manifestations such as tonic–clonic motor activity.

normal-pressure hydrocephalus   A hydrocephalic syndrome with anatomic changes in the brain but cerebrospinal fluid pressure within the normal range when measured with standard lumbar puncture technique.

Nylen–Bárány maneuver   A test for positional nystagmus in vertigo. Usually referred to as the Hallpike test. See Chapter 14.

nystagmus   Rhythmic oscillation of the eyeballs. Multiple types associated with various structural and metabolic abnormalities. The unifying factor in all types is brainstem-initiated eye deviation with rapid cortical correction phase.

oculogyric crisis   Uncontrollable rotation movements of the eyeballs.

ophthalmoplegia   Paralysis of one or both eyes in one or more directions of gaze.

opisthotonus   A tetanic contraction with hyperextension of the spine and extremities.

opsoclonus   Erratic, rapid, nonrhythmic movements of the eyes in both horizontal and vertical directions.

palinopsia   The retention of a visual image or its recurrence after the stimulus has been withdrawn. Most often associated with disease of the parietal occipital region.

palmar grasp reflex   A pathological frontal lobe release sign in which stroking of the palm results in an involuntary grasping motion by the patient.

palmomental reflex   Contraction of the ipsilateral mentalis and orbicularis oris muscles in response to stimulation of the thenar area of the hand. A frontal-lobe release sign.

papilledema   Swelling of the optic nerve head, which may be due to increased intracranial pressure, orbital disease, intraocular disease, or systemic disease.

papillitis   Inflammation of the optic nerve head with edema. Appearance may be confused with papilledema.

paracusia   A paradoxic increase in hearing in deaf people in an environment of increased noise.

paralysis   Loss of strength of voluntary movement in a limb or muscle.

paraplegia   Paralysis of both lower extremities involving the lower portion of the trunk.

paresis   Partial or incomplete paralysis.

Parinaud's syndrome   Loss of upward gaze usually due to a lesion in the pineal gland causing pressure on the superior colliculus.

Parkinson's disease (paralysis agitans)   A diffuse degenerative disease of the brain with both early and severe involvement of the basal ganglions. Associated with rigidity and tremor and progressing to include organic brain syndrome.

Patrick's sign   Pain in the hip when the heel of the painful extremity is placed upon the opposite knee and the thigh is depressed downward. Positive Patrick's sign generally indicates hip joint disease, but it is usually absent in disease entities involving the sciatic nerve.

peripheral neuropathy   A general term for any damage to the nervous system that lies outside the brain and spinal cord. *Neuritis* may also be used to denote any type of damage to the peripheral nerves regardless of etiology, although many physicians reserve the term for conditions of infectious origins.

petit mal seizure   Absence spells; attacks occurring mostly in children characterized by short duration (10–30 seconds) of altered consciousness. Motor tone is usually preserved.

Phalen's sign   In patients with median nerve compression in the carpal tunnel, painful paresthesias reproduced by holding the wrists in extreme flexion for 2 minutes.

phantom limb   A sensation of the continued presence of an absent portion of the body, which may manifest as pain, paresthesias, or sensation of movement.

phantom sensation   Spontaneous sensations referred to previously denervated and insensitive areas; frequently associated with lesions of the spinal cord or cauda equina.

phrenic neuralgia   Dysfunction of the phrenic nerve from any cause. Most common etiologies include infection, surgery, developmental anomalies, tumors, and idiopathic causes. Diaphragmatic spasms and paresthesias in the distribution of the phrenic nerve may come out in advance of the paralysis. Although it is usually unilateral, bilateral cases do exist and are life-threatening.

piriformis syndrome   Pain in the distribution of the sciatic nerve when the nerve is irritated in the area of the piriformis muscle or is otherwise compressed.

plantar reflex   The normal plantar response, i.e., plantar movement or flexion of the toes upon stroking the sole of the foot.

posterior circulation   The arterial supply of the brain derived from the two vertebral arteries and their union, the basilar artery. The areas supplied include sections of the occipital lobe, midbrain, pons, and medulla, as well as portions of the spinal cord.

posterior column signs   Physical examination findings indicative of pathology in the posterior columns of the spinal cord. The posterior columns include the fasciculus gracilis and fasciculus cuneatus. Clinically the syndrome is characterized by alteration of vibration and position sense.

postherpetic neuralgia   Persistent motor and sensory dysfunction in peripheral nerves affected by herpes zoster after the skin manifestations have resolved. Most common manifestations are dysesthesias and paresthesias.

presbycusis   Loss of ability to perceive or discriminate sounds, which is a part of the natural aging process.

presenile dementia   A term that may be used interchangeably with Alzheimer's disease. The pathology includes gross atrophy of the brain with widening of the cortical sulci and enlargement of the ventricles. The clinical picture includes onset of dementia in the fifth and sixth decades.

primary lateral sclerosis   A general term for idiopathic involvement of the corticospinal tracts.

prion diseases   Any of a number of slow viral diseases of the brain including Creutzfeldt–Jakob disease, Gerstmann–Straussler–Scheinker syndrome, and kuru.

proprioception   Sensory information derived from the peripheral end organs of the nerves in muscles, tendons, and joints that supply the central nervous system with information regarding position and movement of body parts.

pseudobulbar palsy   Diminution of musculature associated with the brainstem (bulb) due to pathology located in supranuclear areas of the brain. In contrast to actual bulbar palsy due to involvement of the cranial nerve nuclei and peripheral nerves, this is an upper motor neuron process with little to no muscular atrophy. Frequently associated with personality changes that include spasmotic laughing or crying or both simultaneously.

pseudotumor cerebri   Benign intracranial hypertension. Increased intracranial pressure in the setting of an otherwise normal patient. Diffuse edema of the brain with no identifiable masked lesion or ventricular system abnormality. Along with idiopathic forms, it has been seen in conjunction with infectious disease, toxins, trauma, and generalized diffuse neuritis.

psychogenic seizures   Also known as pseudoseizures or hysterical seizures, these are seizures produced by physiologic episodes that can be mistaken for seizures or that lead to seizures that are not truly epileptic in nature. Malingering disorders such as Munchausen syndrome and malingering are conscious events and are differentiated from psychogenic seizures by the fact that the patient knows full well what is going on. The patient is not deliberately feigning the attacks and may have no conscious awareness of what is going on. These can be extremely difficult diagnoses and are sometimes made with the combination of simultaneous time-link video recordings and EEG recordings.

psychomotor seizure   A partial seizure with complex symptomatology and impairment of consciousness. Attacks are characterized by repetitive motor acts or activity inappropriate for the patient's situation.

quadrantanopia   Loss of a quarter of a visual field as bounded by a vertical and horizontal radius. May be unilateral or bilateral, superior or inferior. Usually homonymous but may occasionally be bitemporal or binasal.

radiculopathy   Any disease process affecting the intradural portion of a spinal nerve route prior to its entrance into the intravertebral foramen or a portion of the foramen and the nerve plexus.

Raeder's (paratrigeminal) syndrome   An inflammation of the anatomic space containing the components of the fifth cranial nerve, the carotid artery and its sympathetic fibers, and the third, fourth, and sixth cranial nerves. The syndrome is characterized by paralysis of occulosympathetic pathways, which may involve sweating along with facial pain and involvement of the third, fourth, and sixth cranial nerves singly or in combination. Etiologies of the syndrome include carotid artery aneurysms, tumors, ophthalmic herpes, and spreading infections from chronic maxillary sinusitis. In rare cases, trauma may be the etiology.

Ramsay Hunt syndrome   Herpes zoster auricularis with vesicles on the tympanic membrane and on the face between the ear and mastoid regions, often associated with facial paralysis, loss of taste over the anterior two-thirds of the tongue, and deep protracted facial pain.

retrobulbar neuritis   Inflammation of the optic nerve accompanied by defects in vision and no observable change in the funduscopic examination. The term *papillitis* is used to refer to inflammatory optic neuritis with observable changes in the optic nerve head.

Reye's syndrome   Encephalopathy associated with fatty degeneration of the liver; seen almost exclusively in children. The disease process is characterized by persistent vomiting usually following a viral illness such as influenza or varicella. Generalized seizures and progressive lethargy and coma rapidly follow.

Rinne's test   A tuning-fork test used to delineate the predominance of either bone or air conduction in patients with hearing loss. (See Chapter 14.)

risus sardonicus   A tight or drawn facial appearance seen with facial muscular spasm; often associated with tetanus.

Romberg's sign   A test of both equilibrium and dorsal column sensation. (See Chapter 3.)

saccades   The general term for rapid eye movements such as the fast phase of nystagmus or the rapid eye movements seen in REM sleep.

Saturday night palsy   A colloquial term for compression neuropathy of the radial nerve in the upper arm; usually reserved for patients whose radial neuropathy is the result of their own malpositioning and lack of activity for prolonged periods.

Schilder's disease   A generalized term for diffuse sclerosis characterized by degeneration of white matter in the central nervous system. Has more recently been divided into multiple hereditary and nonhereditary specific disease patterns.

scotoma   A spot of varying size and shape within a visual field in which there is no vision.

seizure   The sudden onset of a disease with alteration in neurologic discharge. A convulsion. See also *febrile seizure, grand mal seizure, Jacksonian seizure, petit mal seizure,* and *psychomotor seizure.*

sleep paralysis   Associated with narcolepsy. Periods of paralysis developing during relaxation or just before going to sleep.

snout reflex   A contraction of both the upper and lower portions of the orbicularis oris and muscles about the nose, causing protrusion of the lips induced by tapping or touching the lower lips. This is a sign of the loss of frontal lobe functions seen in dementia.

spatial agnosia   Disorganization of spatial judgment in which patients cannot find their way in familiar surroundings. Also characterized by inability to perform constructional tasks such as copying and drawing.

spinal ataxia   A group of diseases characterized by gait disturbance and incoordination. Spinal ataxias differ from generalized cerebellar ataxia in that there is also diminished vibration and position sense and altered deep tendon reflexes, pyramidal track signs, or other evidence of involvement of spinal cord or peripheral nerves.

spinal shock   Weakness, decreased reflexes, decreased sensation; seen immediately following injury to the spinal cord.

Spurling's Test   With the head inclined to the painful side of the neck–axial pressure causes increased pain in the involved ridicular distribution.

stereognosis   The ability to understand the form of an object by means of the sense of touch. A parietal lobe function.

stupor   A state of loss of response to the environment in which consciousness may be impaired in varying degrees. The patient is difficult to rouse but can be brought to purposeful response with noxious verbal or physical stimulation. The patient promptly falls back into a nonresponsive mode when not being stimulated.

subarachnoid space   The area between the arachnoid and pia mater layers of the meninges; contains the cerebrospinal fluid.

subdural space   The potential space between the dura mater and arachnoid layers of the meninges.

subhyaloid hemorrhage   Bleeding into the space between the retina and the vitreous; almost exclusively found in association with subarachnoid hemorrhage from aneurysmal rupture.

supranuclear palsy   Decreased movement of the musculature supplied by the cranial nerves secondary to upper motor neuron disease involving the cortex, subcortical structures, or cortiospinal tracts.

supratentorial   The space above the tentorium cerebelli including the anterior and middle fossa of the skull; containing the cerebral cortex, deep cortical structures, and thalamic structures.

swallow syncope   Transient loss of consciousness secondary to bradycardia with resultant inadequate cerebral profusion initiated by the act of swallowing; a response mediated through the vagus nerve.

syringobulbia   A condition of dysfunction of the lower brainstem (bulb) secondary to cavitation and expansion of the primitive central cord of the nervous system. The brainstem analog of syringomyelia.

syringomyelia   A disease of the spinal cord principally in the cervical region; marked by the presence of expansion of fluid-filled cavities in the region of the primitive central cord. Clinically there is pain and temperature loss as well as decreased motor strength in the upper limbs with relative preservation of motor and sensory findings in the lower extremities. As the disease progresses, upper motor neuron findings in the lower extremities, such as hyperreflexia and spasticities, begin to appear.

tabes dorsalis   A sequela of syphilis with a chronic progressive sclerosis of the posterior spinal roots and posterior columns of the spinal cord and peripheral nerves. The clinical picture includes ataxia with lancinating pains in the extremities and markedly decreased position and vibration sense. Optic nerve atrophy and trophic disorders of the joints are not uncommon.

tarsal tunnel syndrome   Entrapment of the posterior tibial nerve in the region of the medial malleolus of the tibia; symptoms consist of pain, tingling, and numbness in the sole of the foot aggravated by standing and walking.

tectum   Any covering or roofing structure in the nervous system referring to the dorsalmost portion of the brainstem.

tegmentum   The portion of the brainstem dorsal to the cerebral peduncles and the pons.

tensilon test   Edrophonium chloride test; the use of a coinhibiting drug given to diagnose myasthenia gravis. (See Chapter 6.)

thalamic pain   Associated with cerebral hemorrhage or thrombosis involving thalamic structures; symptoms include alteration of sensory stimuli from the contralateral side of the involved portion of the thalamus. All sensory stimuli from the affected areas take on unpleasant sensations and may be accompanied by a brain or deep aching pain (hyperpathia). This may progress to intractable, deep-seated pain (anesthesia dolorosa).

thrombolytics See *fibrinolysis*.

Tinel's sign A tingling sensation felt in the nerve when percussion is made over the site of the nerve.

tinnitus Subjective noises (i.e., ringing, whistling) in the ears as the result of involvement of the cochlear mechanisms.

Todd's paralysis Postictal motor dysfunction with usually rapid return to normal function. The area of paralysis may correlate with that area of the brain most involved in the seizure focus.

torticollis Twisting of the neck secondary to either neck muscle irritation from injury or from involuntary contraction of the neck muscles due to drugs or underlying neurologic disease.

Tourette's syndrome See page 192.

transient global amnesia An amnestic state involving recent memory but not instantaneous memory or passed memory. Thought to be due to decreased blood flow through the hippocampus. A form may come as intermittent episodes causing loss of memory covering days to weeks.

transient ischemic attack (TIA) Short-term neurologic dysfunction clearing within 14 hours secondary to inadequate central nervous system profusion secondary to multiple causes. To be labeled a TIA, all neurologic symptomatology must be resolved within 14 hours.

Transverse Myelitis Inflammation or disturbance of function at a specific level of the spinal cord.

Trömner's sign A reflex in which, with the fingers partially flexed, the volar aspect of the tip of the middle or index finger causes flexion of all four fingers and thumb.

Trousseau's sign Muscular spasm elicited by pressure over the nerves and arteries supplying the area of spasm.

ultrasound: color Doppler Similar to duplex Doppler US except that directional and flow information is superimposed (in color) over the standard grayscale US image. In combination with standard grayscale US, it is typically used to evaluate extracranial vasculature.

ultrasound: duplex Doppler Also called Doppler US, this technique utilizes a special ultrasound "probe" and software (which permit both time and frequency analysis of reflected US waves) for the evaluation of blood flow—both direction and velocity—in real time. Arterial and venous structures can both be evaluated. An image of the vessel being evaluated (in grayscale US) and a "tracing" reflecting flow velocities are created. From this data, significant restrictions to flow can be inferred and in some cases directly visualized.

ultrasound: intravascular (IVUS) Utilizes an intravascular probe (placed within a blood vessel utilizing a percutaneous technique similar to that used for endovascular angiography) which can exquisitely evaluate vascular walls and immediate perivascular tissues.

ultrasound: power Doppler Color Doppler ultrasound technique which can visualize vessels with a greater sensitivity than color Doppler US; however, it is more prone to image degradations due by patient or tissue motion than standard color Doppler techniques. It also does not display the relative direction of blood flow.

ultrasound: standard (Grayscale) Used to evaluate internal organs (both superficial and deep), muscles and many pathologic processes by generating "real-time" images using electromagnetic waves above the level of human hearing. Images can be obtained in nearly any plane and for any amount of time as the technique has no known risks. Three-dimensional imaging is now possible ("4D" when one considers the "real-time" nature of US).

uncinate fit A type of focal seizure preceded by an aura of disagreeable smells.

vasovagal syncope Sudden loss of consciousness due to inadequate cerebral profusion secondary to bradycardia on the basis of increased vagus nerve stimulation. (See Chapter 13.)

Wallenberg's syndrome Vascular occlusion of the posterior inferior cerebellar artery, which supplies the dorsal lateral portion of the medulla. Signs and symptoms include loss of cerebellar function ipsilateral to the lesion with a loss of pain and temperature sensation from the ipsilateral side of the face. This is accompanied by loss of pain and temperature sensation in the limbs and the trunk on the opposite side of the body. Deviation of the eyes or nystagmus may be present from irritation of the vestibular nuclei.

Weber's syndrome A lesion secondary to dysfunction in the basilar portion of the midbrain. Signs and symptoms include spastic paralysis of the contralateral arm and leg combined with external strabismus of the ipsilateral eye and ptosis. Concomitant involvement of the third cranial nerve results in the dilation of the ipsilateral pupil.

Weber's test A tuning-fork test used to determine whether a hearing loss is primarily on a conductive or neurosensory basis. (See Chapter 14.)

Wernicke's aphasia A fluent aphasia secondary to lesions involving the auditory cortex of the temporal lobe. It is a fluent aphasia characterized by active, well-articulated speech that makes little to no sense because patients cannot monitor their own speech processes.

Note: Page numbers followed by the letter "*t*" indicate tables and those followed by the letter "*f*" indicate figures.